Reversing Chronic Lyme Disease:
The New Paradigm Beyond Conventional Medicine

Reversing Chronic Lyme Disease:
The New Paradigm Beyond Conventional Medicine

A thorough examination of the Lyme chronicle, and a closer look at Borrelia Burgdorferi, veers from the path of the conventional model to a radically deeper level of healing.

Craig Bruner

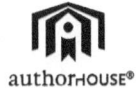

authorHOUSE®

AuthorHouse™ LLC
1663 Liberty Drive
Bloomington, IN 47403
www.authorhouse.com
Phone: 1-800-839-8640

Published by AuthorHouse   07/08/2013

ISBN: 978-1-4817-4147-7 (sc)
ISBN: 978-1-4817-4146-0 (e)

Library of Congress Control Number: 2013906930

CONTENTS

Disclaimer... vii

Preface... ix

Introduction...xv

Chapter 1:   The Hijacking of Conventional Medicine 1

Chapter 2:   The Origins of Lyme Disease (or Don't you Lyme
             to me!) 30

Chapter 3:   A Few of My Own Efforts...................................... 51

Chapter 4:   Borrelia Biochemistry... 64

Chapter 5:   Biofilms 80

Chapter 6:   The Infectious Process.. 96

Chapter 7:   The Limitations of Testing 102

Chapter 8:   Strains and How They Can Affect Test Results.............. 132

Chapter 9:   Therapies 137

Chapter 10: The Best Medicine 151

Chapter 11: Healing Substances 156

Chapter 12: Essential Oils 223

Chapter 13: Mixed Oxidants 244

Chapter 14: Anti-Biofilm Substances 278

Chapter 15: Antibiotics 292

Chapter 16: Putting it All Together....................................... 299

Bonus Chapter 17: The Fasting Factor: Achieving Level 6
             Healing 333

DISCLAIMER

This book is not intended to replace medical advice. Rather it is providing information to warn of the dangers of the conventional medical model, still being used by many traditional medical doctors with regards to Lyme disease treatments. By understanding the true nature of this disease and providing an in-depth discussion, the Lyme sufferer will become educated to an advanced level of understanding that will allow him/her to make more independent decisions with regard to treatment choices. This knowledge is your power to never again become a pawn in the political-medical battles wherein the patient is at the complete mercy of the medical system.

There are many good books on Lyme disease today. In the year 2000 when I first developed Lyme disease, much of this illness was still a mystery. Except for drug-based antibiotics, few other options were available to the Lyme victim. Due to the political battles now raging, the Lyme patient finds himself not only battling the disease, but the medical establishment itself. This has left many sufferers with no other option but to venture out on their own to find viable natural and non-drug treatments to do battle with. Today an explosion of new information and the sharing of that information have brought today's Lyme patient a ray of hope that didn't exist years ago. Back then only a few books were around whose information was sketchy and very limited on truly effective therapeutic options that the average person could employ.

I chose to write this book not necessarily as a comprehensive guide, but one which builds on past information, and also questions long-held ideas many of which are just plain false. In it you will find many new and old therapies that are based upon a realistic understanding of Borrelia Burgdorferi, the etiological or causative bacterial agent of Lyme disease. Understanding the biology and biochemistry of this bacterium are the keys to the proper development of effective treatments. For too many years Borrelia has been misunderstood, and as a result, the wrong approach to treatment has bred a generation of chronically ill victims that have little hope of ever being completely cured.

With this information, a new chapter is being written which illuminates a path to treatment seldom explored. Not only will you gain new insights into Lyme disease, but also more treatment options than one person could ever employ that can be uniquely tailored to his/her own needs. This book includes most of the major therapies that others have found success using, including several doctors versed in understanding the complexities of chronic Lyme disease.

Although I have had a deep interest in scientific research, biology, and health the greater part of my life, I am not a doctor, nor have I been formally trained in medicine. What I learned I had to learn on my own since I, like many reading this book, was left on my own out in the cold by conventional medicine. So, I chose to write this book as I wished someone had written for me when I first learned I had Lyme disease. The knowledge you will gain is what I wished someone had explained to me from the beginning. The therapies I will write about are not necessarily recommended for you, but written how I would recommend to myself if I were to start over again. So although you will find many options, they are your choice, as I give no recommendations. But I hope you will discover something that will help you make more informed decisions along your journey.

PREFACE

As is so often the case in this internet age, what is news today is ancient history tomorrow. What you are about to learn as a whole has taken years of cumulative research sifting through hundreds of articles, scientific journals, and interviews to gain a comprehensive understanding of the subject you are about to read. Understanding the chronic aspect of Lyme disease requires a much more thorough examination of the subject than is offered by the vast majority of the conventional medical community. When even many of the newer Lyme treatments don't bring the Lyme sufferer the degree of healing they had hoped; when resistance seems to be the rule rather than the exception; we seek to go deeper and farther than conventional medicine can take us.

In this book we deliberately confront the difficult questions and are not afraid to go deep into the evidence to gain a clear picture that reveals what the scientific evidence is telling us as to what makes Lyme disease resistant to most conventional treatments. We will learn what the biology of Borrelia Burgdorferi (Bb) is telling us about itself, and take this information to turn the tables against this pathogen. But more importantly, we will delve deeply into the subject of finding solutions to the very problems that seem almost insurmountable to conventional medicine.

As the title says, this book deals with chronic Lyme disease. All references herein, unless otherwise stated address the chronic aspect of the disease or what some call stages 2 and/or 3. Stage 1 or early disseminated Lyme, is a description of a small window of time immediately following exposure wherein spirochetes are vulnerable to antibiotics or anti-microbials, and have not yet migrated to remote locations in the body out of their reach, or have not yet morphed into a resistant form. This needs to be made clear from the beginning since stage 1 is a potentially curable form of the disease, and the addressing of that form is entirely different than chronic Lyme. Therefore, *Lyme disease* in this book refers to that stage beyond which a short course or two of antibiotics can completely cure the infection.

If you are reading this, then you likely don't have all the answers you are looking for when it comes to Lyme disease. What a confusing illness this is, not just because of how the illness manifests itself in different people, but also because there are so many opinions and inconsistencies given to us about how the disease is diagnosed, what constitutes a diagnosis, co-infection questions, which tests to use, false positives or negatives, etc. And the treatments that people have tried could fill volumes. Why do some treatments work for some people, yet others seem to find no benefit whatsoever? Why do some doctors think that Lyme disease is rare, while others seem to think it is in fact a very common and growing pandemic? Even worse, some think it is easy to cure, while others have learned the extreme stubbornness that Lyme can express given even the most intense therapies. In spite of all this, some don't even believe chronic Lyme exists since they are of the school that believes most all bacterial infections can easily be cured with a course or two of antibiotics; while others falsely rely on testing, and in the absence of positive tests, discount the illness altogether.

This is happening because most doctors view Borrelia Burgdorferi as they would any other bacterial infection. They begin from that premise, and design their course of diagnoses and therapies around an incorrect assumption. When their patients therefore do not respond to these therapies or their symptoms are not resolved, rather than reexamine their premise, they conclude it must be something else. With all the available research today on Borrelia Burgdorferi biochemistry and our understanding of its pleomorphic capabilities, and with all we have learned of its capacity to evade the immune system and antimicrobial medications, and especially with the recent explosion of information about biofilms and their connection to chronic disease, it is difficult to believe that many doctors are still holding on to an old paradigm. Why is an antiquated scientific model still being accepted when the answers seem so obvious even to the untrained lay man? Scientific literature is filled with research demonstrating that even long term antibiotics usually do not resolve this bacterial infection. Yet even tests prove the infection is still there.

How did doctors jump to the conclusion that their patients do not or no longer have the disease after a few treatments? Whatever happened to physicians being men of science that explored the unexplained, who didn't treat their patients based upon antiquated assumptions, or who followed blindly the dogma some medical society holds that flies in the face of reality? Whatever happened to doctors asking the question, "How do I resolve these apparent inconsistencies, and stop ignoring the obvious?" In the 1985 song *No One is to Blame* by English pop-artist Howard Jones the relevance to Lyme disease could not have been better sung when he wrote, "Doctor says I'm cured, but I still feel the pain."

This book was written in response to a very real need to give practical help, hope, and potential treatment therapies to sufferers of chronic Lyme disease, many of which are not currently known to most people. Due to the strict reins placed upon medical doctors by the FDA, medical boards, as well as insurance companies, even they are looking outside the box into the alternative health field to find treatment options that may offer hope to their patients. But since chronic Lyme disease has been the target of denial by some doctors holding on to an old paradigm that is not consistent with patient symptoms, many patients have been left on their own with nowhere to turn for help.

Due to the unique nature of the Lyme bacterium Borrelia Burgdorferi, Lyme disease is more like being cured of scurvy, than say polio. Scurvy can come back if you develop a vitamin C deficiency again. Lyme disease can return since (in this author's opinion) it may be impossible to completely eradicate the bacteria in all of its forms from the body, as even many healthy people probably have some form of the bacteria living in them. This goes against conventional medical dogma which says you can only get Lyme disease from a tick bite, which will be seen, flies in the face of scientific evidence.

As anyone knows who has suffered from this disease, they often get little consistent help from their doctors who truly don't know how to help them without driving them to the poor house with endless tests that are often times inconclusive, and antibiotic therapy that has shown to be almost completely ineffective at curing the illness for those with chronic Lyme. Patients end up drifting from doctor to doctor searching for an answer.

I decided it was time to take matters into my own hands by researching all I could to understand what makes this such a difficult illness to treat. What you will read is my own personal story how I struggled with health issues long before contracting Lyme disease that almost ended my life, and the almost miraculous recovery due to a new therapy, only to later contract Lyme disease and start me on a whole new journey. By spending years researching Lyme disease and the biochemistry of the Borrelia Burgdorferi, I discovered that its greatest strength could be turned against it, by using a different method than that employed by conventional medicine and without the use of antibiotics to restore my health. These I will share with you. They are unique and some will not be found in any other book currently available.

Should you decide to explore this yourself, I believe you will find a world of options that took me literally years to research. Perhaps no other book you will read will offer you more options for your arsenal, and the unique treatments that hold the potential for healing that the average person can learn him/herself.

Although the primary focus of this book is to identify therapies that can successfully address chronic Lyme disease, and all of which are non-prescription drug in nature, it needs to be understood that we are not advocating the complete replacement of antibiotics. They have their own capacity to deal with infections. However since most Lyme sufferers begin with antibiotics, when they fail, learning of alternatives to aid them is vital from those that have already used them and found them to be highly effective.

A word of advice: Lyme patients often out of necessity become an educated lot. They research to the core, and learn many valuable things along the way. Also along the way they find many different viewpoints and even contradictory opinions. So much of what we learn is theoretical, based upon some evidence, but has not yet been "proven". That's ok too. It's all part of the learning process that allows ideas to act like stepping stones. As we read and learn though, we will invariably become confronted with information that is sometimes conflicting. And there are some who have a very strong tendency to read and study everything with a hyper critical attitude. They want to tear apart some theory or idea someone else espouses. This has its place, as even many of the things you will read in this book are very confrontational at times. But remember why you are reading this: To see if you can glean something that will be useful to you in your journey to wellness. Do not become bogged down on those areas that seem to you to be controversial, or that you may even utterly disagree with. If you do this, you will be hindering your ability to remain open to those things that may be helpful to you. Learn to let go of what is not important, and soak up what is. I don't even agree with some things I wrote 5 years ago in my first book! I may rewrite a book later that contradicts things I have written now. Remain open as you read. The important thing is to learn what you can, and let go of what you disagree with.

INTRODUCTION

Several years ago I took a trip to Mexico to see a certain doctor about a Lyme treatment that was not generally available here in the US, and wanted to see if it would have an affect on my Lyme disease. When I arrived and began my consultation with him sharing my symptom history and story, he immediately thought that based upon some of my symptoms that I had candidiasis (a systemic fungal infection). I did have candidiasis some 10 years earlier and had been cured completely and without any further symptoms due to treatments of energy medicine after all other alternative and allopathic treatments failed. I had explained this to him, but in far greater detail. I could tell by his disbelieving smile while I was sharing that he wasn't "buying my story". He shared with me that he was absolutely convinced that most people who come to see him with Lyme disease don't actually have the disease, but have something else, and that Lyme was actually very rare. Not only that, but he said "many people who come to see us have actually convinced themselves that they have Lyme disease so they won't be open to be treated for what they really have, and won't go thru the treatments necessary to get better." Although that makes absolutely no sense whatsoever, it was the same kind of lecture that we as Lyme patients have heard before. We are told that we "jump from doctor to doctor to get attention or sympathy." It is a "psychological problem that is in your head."

At this point as you can imagine I was having to hold back my heating-up emotions because as I later learned, his specialty as a physician was the treatment of Candida infections, and many people came to see him for Lyme only to have him convince them otherwise. However since I had already flown all the way to see him from Dallas, I was going to play along with him and give him his due for the time being. He told me he had a product that he has used on his patients that most people don't know about, many of whom had tried everything you could imagine, even powerful prescription antifungals, and ended up finding success using the product. In fact he said "I had used it myself when I didn't think anything else would work, and experienced a very significant herxheimer reaction" (die-off symptoms indicating the treatment was working). He said that if I would try it I would know within a day or two if it was working due to the herx reaction I would experience. Again, in his mind, he was sure I had Candida, and this product would prove it.

Since I didn't want to come across as an uncooperative patient I told him I would be open and try it. But I wasn't going to waste my time and money coming to another country for the expressed purpose of convincing a doctor I don't have a fungal infection.

So I took the product and went back to my hotel. For the next two days I took the natural herbal product at the maximum dosage. I knew from experience that Candida die-off would generally be experienced relatively quickly (although depending on the severity, sometimes you have a delayed reaction.) By the end of the second day when no herx was experienced whatsoever, and with no reaction to the product at all, I decided to increase the dosage even more, and prepare to return to see the doctor the next day. I never had any positive or negative response from the medicine.

The next day I met with the doctor. "Doctor, I tried the product as you requested, and have had no reaction or benefit whatsoever. I am not trying to come across as a know it all. In fact, I think there is far more we don't know about Lyme disease than we realize. I noticed that your card says you are a specialist in treating Candidiasis. I find it interesting that 15-20 years ago or so when Candidiasis was still virtually unknown to the medical community, doctors at that time were not only skeptical of the illness, some even down-played its very existence. They said the exact same thing to their patients about Candidiasis as you are saying to me about my Lyme disease. They said it's actually very rare, or that we have convinced ourselves that we have the illness so we won't have to take responsibility for our lives, or that it's all psychological. Frankly, I am tired of it! Not too many years from now you are going to be convinced the same way all those doctors that denied the existence of Candidiasis have had to swallow their words and recognize this is real, not something in our heads."

I went on, "I have had Lyme disease for over 10 years, have been studying Lyme disease for nearly 7 years, have read hundreds of medical studies on Borrelia Burgdorferi and related species. I understand the symptoms, and how confusing they can be, the misdiagnoses, various theories and opinions that are out there, and the lack of agreement even by the most prestigious researchers and doctors. I spent 2 ½ years writing a research manual called **Lyme Disease, Energy Medicine, and the Biochemistry of Borrelia** and sent it out to some doctors to help give to them the most up-to-date information on the bacteria and possible protocols that might help them based upon research from medical doctors and PhD's alike doing all kinds of research from all sorts of angles. I am not one of your average patients who doesn't know what he is talking about!"

As we continued our conversation and having demonstrated that not only did his surefire treatment for Candida yield no results in me, he could see that I wasn't going to back down from what I knew just because someone had MD behind his name. I will also tell you that after spending a week at the clinic and several consultations for some different treatments we worked on, I was told by another patient I met at the clinic who also came to see him with Lyme disease that that doctor told him "Craig probably knows more about Lyme disease than any patient I know, and I am sure he probably has the disease."

The treatment I went to Mexico to try was intravenous activated sodium chlorite (aka MMS). Although oral treatments with MMS were inducing very significant herx (herxheimer) reactions, it was only able to go so deep unless I could take it intravenously. The doctor who owned and was the head of the clinic at the time wouldn't give permission to let my doctor try MMS IV's on me, not because he knew anything particular about whether it may or may not work, but he was not familiar with it and frankly wasn't willing to give it a try because they wanted me to try their treatments, IV silver and vitamin C. I did in fact try those treatments. But they yielded no noticeable results, probably because I had been so far along in my own treatments that most of the morphological forms that would have been vulnerable to IV silver were already killed off. And any benefit I would have received from IV Vitamin C was not even noticeable. (I had previously used high dose oral silver and C already in my therapies.)

Still having some symptoms, and not completely well, I was seeking something that would go even deeper to further rid me of my Lyme disease. So upon arriving home in Dallas, I learned of a MD who was offering many of the same alternative treatments as they did in Mexico. And of all places he was only about 25 miles from me! So I called his clinic to see about setting up an appointment to see him. "Sorry, but the doctor is not able to see new patients for several months. He is that far out in his schedule. Besides, he really doesn't treat Lyme patients. He usually refers them to another doctor who specializes in treating Lyme disease. (That doctor is apparently a LLMD, or Lyme literate medical doctor.) I can give you his number if you like?"

"Great" I thought. "I can see a LLMD in my area, and ask him about some of these treatments I am interested in." So I took down the number and called his office. The nurse answered the phone. I explained "My name is Craig Bruner. I have Lyme disease and was referred by another doctor." "Yes, that is what Dr . . . . specializes in" she said.

I then asked, "Can you tell me how many or what percentage of patients who have come to see the doctor end up being cured of the disease." She said, "He doesn't really cure them. We usually give to them antibiotics to help them feel better and to control the disease." Wow! That pretty much answered my question.

These are the kinds of stories Lyme patients live in, and they are all too common ones. It's hard enough to find a doctor who understands Lyme disease. But why would you want to spend your life without hope of being cured? It has almost come to a point where there are two religions called Lyme disease. One says it is very rare, can only happen in very strict circumstances, can only be diagnosed if you have a specific set of positive test results, and can be easily cured with a course or two of antibiotics. The other says it is in fact not an uncommon disease at all, has multiple vectors of infection so common, that a husband can even give it to his wife, or mother to child; is diagnosed based upon your symptoms, even if your test results were negative; and that unless you receive treatment very early, you will almost certainly develop long-term chronic Lyme disease and the hell that will follow unless you do something "out of the box" to stop it.

My friend, I will admit that with all I have learned, I feel inadequate to share with you what you will learn in this book because I am humbled by what we still as yet do not know, and how even what we do know seems to change almost daily as people all over the world, doctors, researchers, and patients alike gather pieces of the puzzle bit by bit to form a bigger picture of what is yet unknown. In recent years new information on Lyme therapies has spawned a number of authors writing on the subject of Lyme disease. This has been a much lacking area as so much research is being done that further illuminates our understanding of the genetics of Borrelia Burgdorferi, its microbiology, biochemistry, the relationship between immune factors and specific lipoproteins, etc, to the negligence of the most important topic of all—non-drug treatment options that sufferers can employ on their own.

Today there is such an over-dependance on the failing medical community that has by and large failed or even abandoned Lyme victims. Medical boards in many cases are setting diagnostic guidelines that literally prevent MD's from treating their patients with Lyme disease. It has even gone so far that some have actually ordered doctors in some states not to diagnose their patients with Lyme. This happened to me and angered me to the point that I decided to take matters into my own hands. I would no longer be a puppet in a corrupt system that manipulates doctors, protects insurance companies, and leaves victims to suffer and sometimes die or end their own lives due to the suffering they are forced to endure. Today the Hippocratic Oath should be called the Hypocrite oath, as the medical establishment has abandoned those once cherished values. This clearly does not represent the attitudes of all doctors.

My own search for non-drug treatments for Lyme was done almost exclusively without the help of medical doctors, not only because many seemed to have their own agenda by withholding help from Lyme patients, but also because it was clear that the therapies they had to offer were anemically ineffective at treating this long-term illness. Along the way I also researched and read books written by other authors, and many of the therapies they had used. In most cases I was disappointed to find a convenient absence of any mention either as to how these treatments had benefited them, or whether they were ultimately successful in eliminating their own Lyme disease. After all, what greater credibility could be given than to hear that what you are writing about actually worked? Although admittedly one common denominator with Lyme disease is that there is no one therapy that seems to work for everyone. And so of necessity it is not uncommon to see patients experiment for years using different forms of treatment until they find something that works. The sad thing is that even in those cases where something works, often it is short-lived as the nature of Bb is to possess many different forms, all of which are not susceptible to any one treatment, and morphing leads to adaptation.

I on the other hand will tell you up front how the therapies I have tried have benefited me and where I am in my current condition. But before I do this, I would like to explain something it took me years to learn, having known or heard testimonials of countless Lyme patients. Don't be fooled by many who claim to have "beaten the disease". That is not the same as being cured. There are many subtle variables in Lyme disease. The shorter term you have been infected, the greater chance you have of a complete recovery. However as time goes by with the infection unresolved, the more entrenched it becomes, and the more resistant to therapies. To those that persist however, many find that compared to their acute symptoms, significant reduction to the point where they have their life back seems almost cured. However depending on how long they've had the disease and/or how entrenched the infection has become, usually this is as far as is possible. The last 5-10% is the most difficult of all to resolve, and most Lyme disease victims are happy to have reached this point in their own healing process.

I however am not one to be satisfied with 95%, as often it is the 5% that is left unresolved that can be a source of persistent symptoms and infection that can be like a seed that spawns a relapse unless ongoing treatments keep the infection suppressed. It is this 5% that can be the most difficult to heal. Although I joined the "95% Club" some time ago, my final preoccupation has been with applying strategies that seek to ultimately eliminate the deeply entrenched and persistent biofilms which are believed to be the primary source of unresolved infection. We'll get to that later.

I have not yet shared with you my health journey that began many years before I ever developed Lyme disease. My story reads like a novel, and very few people have gone thru or experienced what I have, and emerged victorious. This too you will hear, later.

I am sure that those reading this will have come from different levels of learning of Lyme disease. To some this will all be new to you, and you will have to "catch up" since I have written this book from the standpoint that the reader has done at least enough homework to have a functional understanding of Lyme and the problems facing the elimination of this illness. Others will have been researching Lyme for a long time and are looking for a morsel of something new. There will probably be information that is new even to the most learned researcher. However, this book was written to fulfill two purposes. First, to help you have a deeper understanding of the organism that causes Lyme disease, and why it is so difficult to kill (hint: it is not primarily because it is pleomorphic, nor because it is a "stealth pathogen"), and as a result, why single or stand-alone treatments seldom work. Secondly and most importantly, to share with you what I have done personally that has brought me incredible success in my battle to reverse chronic Lyme.

My Story

There are some of you who would like to flip ahead and get right to the meat of the therapies. However learning what others have done can be very beneficial and insightful. Learning the mistakes others have made can save you years of suffering and pain. I think you will see that mine is a bit different story. Most people, particularly those who have had the illness for some time and have already spent perhaps even years taking medications without success, know the horror stories that take place with anyone taking antibiotics and/or who have had a chronic illness for any length of time. And if you have not yet experienced what I am about to share, it is good to warn you ahead of time to be alert of the condition mentioned in my preface called candidiasis. Taking antibiotics long-term, even certain natural antibacterials can have a devastating effect on your intestinal flora and gut which in turn can lead to "leaky gut syndrome". The gut is the residence of some 80% of the immune cells. When you take long-term antibiotics, you are not augmenting the immune system, you are actually suppressing it! That is the reason why very few people taking antibiotics (other than stage one Lyme) ever become cured of the disease. But I am getting ahead of myself.

THE EARLY YEARS

As a child I grew up constantly being sick from both sore throats and ear infections. Several times a year I would be put on antibiotics for an ear infection or sore throat, only to have to go again sometimes a few months later. That occurred for nearly my entire adolescence. I was also a hyper active child always getting into trouble from agitating my mother or brothers and sister. I recall one time when my mother said she was going to call the men in the white coats to come and take me away. That may sound amusing when you are an adult, but when you are 6 years old and she actually picks up the phone pretending to call them, you are terrified of being sent away by your own mother!

Several years after graduating from college, around the age of 25, I experienced a devastating emotional trauma that sent me into a deep depression that would consume my life for the next 18 years. I felt a deep sense of rejection and self-hatred because of some beliefs I held. Every waking thought for nearly 16 of those years was only one thing, I wanted to end my life. The only time I didn't wish myself dead was when I was sleeping. Not a moment went by did I ever have a happy thought. I was probably one of the most miserable human beings that had ever walked on this earth, quite literally. Although I tried to keep myself busy with activities and work, people I worked with knew something was bothering me, but none dared to ask. I can recall many times during work going to the back of the building, opening the back door, and weeping like a baby. It wasn't an isolated incident. I lived that way for 15 years. During that time I had seen several psychiatrists, and was only able to survive thanks to antidepressant medication. If I wasn't on my medication, it was as if voices were screaming in my ear. This was about the mid 1980's. And during the next 15 years I was on medication for depression. I had been on as many as 16 different drugs, in various combinations. So I became familiar with and interested in medicine for that reason.

However I had grown up always being health conscious. I had been actively involved in sports in high school and college, worked out regularly, never smoked, drank, or did any kind of recreational drug use, always took vitamins and health supplements. Yet due to my weakened immune system both from childhood, and now from the chronic depression, my body was aging quickly although still a young man. My job was as a cabinet maker in a large carpenter's shop. There I was constantly being exposed to all sorts of wood composites and plywoods filled with formaldehyde and other chemicals, adhesives, lacquers, solvents, glues, paints, stains and cleaners. And to make matters worse, I lived in Dallas, Texas which is notoriously one of the worst places in the country for allergies.

With all this toxicity weighing on my immune system, as well as the build-up of toxins from the medications I was taking, my body's immune system slowly began to collapse. I had developed a bursitis on my elbow that became infected beyond the ability for antibiotics to work, and had to have surgery to remove it. However upon having a culture done of the infection, it was learned that I had a bacterial infection called mycobacterium avium, which would require 1-2 years of being on two antibiotics.

So for the next year I faithfully took my medicine. However during that time some strange things began to happen. I began experiencing all kinds of symptoms, the pattern of which didn't follow anything in my life I had previously known. This went on for about a year. At the end of that time I knew I would need to be retested to see if I needed to continue on antibiotics, or if I had beaten the infection. Since the medicines were about $400 per month with no insurance, I was anxious to get off them as soon as possible. At the time I had been studying natural medicine and knew there were some natural alternatives to antibiotics, and decided to employ their use rather than continue taking the drugs.

As I had said, I had been experiencing all sorts of symptoms, but had been assuming that they must be the side effects from the antidepressants I had been taking for many years. Until one day, I finally decided to stop the antibiotics and begin taking two natural antibiotics, oral hydrogen peroxide therapy, and garlic capsules. The problem was that I started taking them both at the same time. And what I didn't know at the time was that I had been developing a severe systemic candida yeast infection over the past year due to taking the antibiotics. By destroying the good bacteria as well as the bad, my body didn't have any way of defending itself against the natural fungus and parasites that also naturally inhabit the intestines, which the good bacteria normally keep in check. My doctor never told at the time about the need to take probiotics. I was about to be in for a shock, as I began taking large doses of the two antimicrobials hoping to avert continuance on the two abx's (antibiotics) I had been on. Not only did I not know that I had been developing severe candida overgrowth, but what was worse, I wasn't aware that candidiasis was extremely vulnerable to oral hydrogen peroxide and garlic. I naturally had never heard of a herxheimer reaction either. But I was about to get a crash course in its meaning.

I was still working as a carpenter this time in my own shop, and suddenly found myself terribly ill. The brain fog well known in candida had intensified ten-fold over the already depressed state I was in, along with head-aches, itching, fatigue, intestinal problems, etc. But when I began stumbling around like a drunken man falling all over the place, I knew this was something extraordinary. When in time it only intensified, I knew it was time to see a doctor, but this time I needed a good one.

Over the years I had been suffering from agonizing suicidal depression, and yet I continued to persevere, not giving up. And if I had reason to find a gun and pull the trigger, it was nothing compared to adding on top of that what I was now experiencing. The sense of hopelessness, fear and uncertainty if I was going to even survive, let alone how I was going to pay for whatever was wrong with me, this was pushing me to the limits of my ability to remain rational. I truly no longer felt like a human being. The only feelings in my life were loneliness, pain, and like I was walking at the edge of my own sanity. Adding to that all the physical symptoms of my new illness, I truly entered into a world that was no longer real. I couldn't think straight, and felt like a walking zombie. But still for unknown reasons I never gave up.

My condition led me to search the yellow pages and fell upon a name that seemed to resonate with me, the Environmental Health Center of Dallas. Not being sure what was wrong with me, I suspected it may have something to do with my constant occupational exposure to environmental toxins. Little did I know that the magnitude of my health problems would soon be revealed.

I spent time telling my history and symptoms to my new physician there, as well as had several blood and stool tests done. I tested positive for gluten antigen. I also had rather extensive serial dilution endpoint titration done for quite a number of foods, candida, and environmental toxins. I was of course showing reactions to quite a large number of them, and was put on antigen injections. Having tested positive for candida, and having full-blown symptoms of candidiasis, I now began treatments which involved an elimination diet of all allergic foods, anti-sugar, anti-candida, and anti-gluten diets. I also began a full detox program, anti-fungal meds, nutritional supplements, probiotics, coffee enemas, daily antigen injections, and other therapies too involved to discuss.

For the first time in years I finally had hope and at least a partial explanation as to why I had been so sick for so long. I also began to become educated to another world of natural medicine that I had known nothing about. I learned about how the body was not just a machine, but an organism that must live in balance with my environment. I read everything I could on the subject of toxins and the body, nutrition, how the teeth affect your health, and quantum healing. Although emotionally I was a deeply broken man, I chose to not allow myself to focus on the way I felt, but to believe that one day something good would come of what was happening to me. Funny how when you don't have a friend in the world, and you lose even the capacity for friends, sometimes your ability to find love for yourself is all that is necessary to help you find some light to guide you thru the darkest of tunnels.

As time went on in my therapies, I slowly began experiencing relief, primarily due to my toxic and candida loads being reduced. However I was still not experiencing the healing I had hoped would come sooner rather than later. So I began seeing other types of practitioners. For the next several years I received so many different kinds of treatments I scarcely am able to remember them all. With all the desensitization injections, cleansing protocols and colonics, anti-gluten, anti-candida, anti-sugar diets, hormone therapy, homeopathic neutralization, IV H2O2 therapy, thyroid therapy, vitamin C I.V's, ultra-violet blood irradiation, ozone and infra-red saunas, herbal and supplement therapies, holograghic repatterning, meditation, acupuncture, chiropractic, osteopathic manipulation, amalgam and root canal removal, cavitation surgeries, and nearly 18 doctors later, part of me was much better, but another part still was not resolved.

In spite of attempting to balance and strengthen my immune system, remove my toxic environment, cleansing the body, lowering my candida load and eliminating allergic foods, my food allergies only intensified. In fact now, after several years of rather extensive and expensive therapies which involved some of the best therapies from some of the best doctors, I was now actually worsening. As time had gone by, I had to add more foods to my antigen injections. With all that I had done so far, still my body's hyper allergic reactions were not resolving. Week after week it seemed I was losing another food from the already dwindling supply of available non-allergic foods. In spite of my rotation and elimination diets, and antigen injections, it only worsened. Eventually in time, my list was so short, I could no longer even rotate them. I was losing weight fast. Due to the rate at which I was deteriorating, and having already exhausted virtually every possible therapy one could imagine, I was once again hearing hopelessness knocking at my door.

It is difficult to comprehend such a condition if you've never experienced it. Your body doesn't assimilate what you are eating, and what you do eat, your cramps are so severe you feel like fainting. You would rather simply not eat at all than eat food and react so severely. You slowly waste away because you simply cannot eat, very similar to Crohn's disease. It is a slow and grueling condition. It never stops, but only worsens. And you finally reach a point when it finally sinks in that this is not fixing itself. Due to the severe and weakened condition I was now in, I knew deep inside that it would only be a matter of time until I was so weak I would no longer have the energy to live anymore. I would become like those malnourished children you see in Africa. I was slowly turning into a skeleton. Deep inside, due to the decline of my condition, I knew that unless a miracle happened, I wouldn't have much longer to live. This had gone on too long. I was now so sick I couldn't even get out of bed at times. This was how far along my condition had declined.

Finally I saw my physician at the Environmental Health Center one last time. "Doctor, I have been receiving treatments from you for all this time, and had many other therapies for my condition as well. Not only am I not getting better, but I have been getting worse. I no longer have any non-allergic foods that I can eat." I was literally wasting away.

Then with my doctor's response, I felt like I received a death sentence. "Craig, sometimes all we can do is all we can do. We have done the best we can to help. I don't really know of anything else to help." At this point and in a brief second several years of efforts and therapies with all the hope and improvements flashed before my eyes. To think of all the ways your life would end, who would have thought it would be like this? But then with those words, a flicker of hope: "We have a nurse that works here that has been having good results with a new therapy. You should contact her."

What I learned about was a new therapy (at the time) that addressed the underlying causes of allergies. Medical doctors want to deal with what they can control thru chemistry. But controlling the body's own immune system going awry is not in the doctor's handbook. They manipulate the chemistry of the body thru their medicines, but do not deal with what gives rise to the problems to begin with.

A new field of medicine had been emerging that is actually based on old ancient wisdom, but that western medicine with all their pseudo-intellectualism would never accept. There is an invisible part of man that gives rise to our physical. Without that part of us, the body dies. It is the "real" us. Not the external, but the underlying internal. And it is this new field of quantum or energy medicine that addresses the underlying problems by correcting miscommunication and removing blocks that prevent the free flow energy from flowing to the physical part of us. The new therapy I was told about is called the Nambudripad Allergy Ellimination Technique or NAET for short. Although it was new and being practiced by only a few doctors at the time, the principle behind how it worked was so successful that in time several off-shoots and variations would be developed by different practitioners around the country and eventually around the world.

I met with a local practitioner who was a chiropractor, and found healing beyond anything I had ever experienced. After going thru some removal of energetic blockages that were initially preventing NAET from working, it began working like gang-busters. One food after another was slowly added back to my diet. I began to gain weight! The candidiasis which I had battled for 5 years was gone in 2-3 treatments. My anti-depressants were no longer needed as my depression began to lift with each subsequent treatment. I eventually learned to self-treat. In time, between my practitioners and my own treatments I have cleared hundreds of substances that I had previously been allergic to. Electromagnetic field stress, computer screen radiation, low pressure weather systems, hypersensitivity to chemical and environmental substances became a thing of the past, and now no one would ever believe that I even went thru what I did. My food allergies are completely gone. The affects of these treatments truly seemed in the realm of the miraculous. Perhaps it wasn't an actual miracle, but for me it was close enough.

There are some that hear of such therapies, but they simply do not make sense to them, and conclude that they must be attributed to the placebo affect. It is curious how that the placebo affect had every opportunity to work from the countless therapies that did in fact fail. But the "placebo affect" actually worked on the one therapy that made no sense at the time and in which I had the greatest doubt would work. Hmm?

Having had a strong inclination towards science from my childhood, I had always had a fascination with the how and why of the way things worked. And I especially was curious about NAET since it had a literal life-saving impact on my life. I had studied and understood the "esoteric" explanations of vibrational or energy medicine. But it wasn't until I studied the work of Dr. William F. Koch MD, PhD in Biochemistry that I understood how the effects of therapies such as NAET worked on a physical level. Much like a radio that can only receive signals that match the sending frequency, so cells have receptors that only receive what they recognize. And much like the newer radios that have the built in ability to automatically tune to a station's frequency, so our body's cells are suppose to recognize what is threatening and what is not. But if something blocks that signal and it becomes unrecognizable, then cells can react with "distortion" much like static that is heard by a radio that is not properly tuned to the right station. When that happens, whatever is distorting the frequency needs to be neutralized so that proper communication can be reestablished. (This is why it is called "energy medicine".)

This is what happens in allergies. Overly stressed or infected cells lose their normal capacity to receive signals, and what they end up hearing is "static". They begin to process energy signals outside of their normal range of action. What follows is the forcing of distorted frequencies by affecting other cells and their activities beyond the normal functions. Much like listening to a radio while driving in a car near power lines can cause static or even one radio station to be heard on another, so allergic reactions by cells force them to operate outside their normal function. Dr. Koch explained the allergy process on an energy level:

We have given a thorough description of the allergy mechanism in various writings and lectures in the past. Briefly we may say that in this condition the cell functional elements are made to work "under forced draft" beyond physiological control. They have adsorbed into their colloidal surfaces a fluorescent toxin which transfers the exothermic energy which is constantly evolved in the living cells, into the functional element affected. The specificity is determined by the similarity in spectral absorption range of the functional unit and the emission range of the fluorescent substance. So the energy transferred passes right into the chemical processes of the functional unit and forces its activity to proceed without the usual control. Thus are produced the hypersecretion of hay fever, the contraction of the bronchial musculature in asthma, the conduction of a constant series of impulses through the neurones associated in some thought complex resulting in the fixed ideas and delusions of insanity . . . Energy is transferred from the cell substance to a functional unit where it does not belong and forces function.[1]

Just as osteopathic realignment and manipulation is believed to improve circulation and immune response by removing obstructions which impede nerve communication, so the realigning of the normal flow of energy in the body can have powerful and lasting results. This became the basis of understanding how these new "energy medicines" function, by resetting the communication within cells, allergic reactions resolved on their own.

Having thoroughly gone off-topic, it was important to explain a very real scenario that happens in people that are put on antibiotics for long periods of time. As conventional medicine almost without exception confronts Lyme disease using often long-term antibiotics, the development of candida and related conditions becomes a very real and all too common result. The subsequent deterioration of health that cascades downhill can be cumulative and leaves Lyme sufferers with more diseases than they started with. Although this part of my story ended with a happy ending, the terrible nightmarish journey could have been avoided altogether by understanding the dangers that long-term anti-biotic therapy can have, no matter what the illness that mandated it to begin with. Iatrogenesis is a term meaning "doctor-induced illness." That is truly what I had.

However this was not the end of my story. In fact, it was only the beginning. Well into my treatments of which I was having tremendous success, I had severely injured a ligament in my lower back. Being forced to continue to work since I had no savings or insurance to pay for treatments, the healing process was slow. In time the intense pain turned chronic, and the unhealed injury seemed to trigger a cascade of symptoms. My depression intensified again, only this time it was different. It was much more severe and of a different nature than my previous depression. I was experiencing a different kind of brain fog, this time with forgetfulness, inability to concentrate, writing words in the wrong order, bouts of rage, hyper anxiety, feeling like something was in my brain, almost like electrical shocks. My ligament tear was radiating with intense pain throughout my lower hip joints and lower back. The pain went up my spine and developed a stiff neck. It intensified when eating carbohydrates, and would subside upon fasting. But allergy testing revealed that I was not reacting to any of the foods I was eating. I began to develop joint pain, which became chronic. I developed extreme fatigue, cardiac pain, heart palpitations, and fluttering, swollen lymph glands, sleeplessness, headaches, numbness in my hands and feet, profuse sweating at night, blood in the urine and intestines, strange feelings almost like crawling and electrical shocks under the skin, sores in the mouth and nasal foul odors, sore throat, knee inflammation, facial twitching. These were all the beginnings of what I would later come to know as Lyme disease. It seemed that the onion affect had finally reached the core. We have heard that Lyme disease has sometimes been known to develop from a trauma or an injury. I will explain this more in detail later. But that is how mine began. Not from a tick bite. Now my life would begin a whole new journey, one which you the reader may also know all too well.

If there is one thing a Lyme sufferer doesn't want to hear, that is another Lyme story. Every one of us is so burdened down with our own suffering and struggles, the last thing we want is to get further burdened with someone else's. Hope, not hopelessness.

On the other hand, they say misery loves company. However I think that it is important and helpful to share important insights and observations which we all can learn from.

Lyme sufferers who come from strong alternative therapy backgrounds like I did begin by taking a very naïve approach to the disease. Like many of you I figured it was like any other bacteria and that all I had to do was to take antibiotics or the right herbal supplement or group of substances for awhile, and I would eventually cure myself. But in time you realize it doesn't work that way with this disease. Joining several Lyme forums on the internet early on in my disease, other Lyme victims would share their stories about how they had the disease for 15, 20, 25 years or more. This baffled me how a bacterial infection could still be had after that many years, and especially with so many of them actively receiving treatment from medical doctors for as long. As I heard the stories and listened to what treatments were being received, I realized that all were coming from different approaches. Some had been taking antibiotics of all sorts and combinations, but only experiencing enough benefit to keep them going back to their doctors with some relieved symptoms, only to have their symptoms return upon stopping, then starting the entire process all over again with a new antibiotic or combination. In some of these patients, they eventually caught on that their doctors didn't really have the answers. So they turned to alternative therapies. And of course this opened up a whole new world of options which gave to them renewed hope.

That is about the time and place where I entered the scene. Before I ever sought a diagnosis thru Lyme tests, I had already seen several doctors and practitioners telling me that based upon my symptom history I probably had Lyme disease. I began taking colloidal silver and several herbal products I already knew were natural antibiotics. By listening to the stories of other Lyme sufferers, I instinctively felt that going to a medical doctor to be treated with antibiotics didn't seem to be the answer. Of course an argument can be made that many people that had experienced healing from taking antibiotics would probably no longer be attending many of these internet forums since they were no longer being bothered by the disease anyways. Still, one would think that you would hear of at least a few. But this wasn't happening. Even the people I personally knew that had the disease, several whom were doctors themselves and had access to every kind of medicine and treatment available were still suffering even after many years. I just wasn't hearing the "C" (cure) word from anybody. All I was hearing about were some medicines that were being tried with hopeful results. And with many users, "I'll get back with you later on my experience." This was often some new silver or herbal product. Someone always had something new they were told would cure the disease that some doctor or research group was promoting. Since this was all new to me at the time, in my naivety I simply went along and tried many of these products, only to find limited or temporary benefit. Those taking antibiotics faired no better. In fact their poor track record had already been established.

Later I graduated to another group of forums that addressed Lyme disease using Rife Machines and other electronic devices. I began hearing the stories of a few people who were having some success using them. Many would share that they were experiencing herxes from using these electronic devices. Certainly they were showing real promise as legitimate therapies, and had genuine relevance in the battle against Lyme. The problem was I rarely heard of anyone actually having been cured by using Rife machines. Certainly there were testimonials of users having benefited.

Although the majority of people on these forums, like me, were trying to learn more about these Rife and other electromagnetic-based devices based upon the hope that they might be able to duplicate the same results, there always seemed to be confusion as to which type of machine was best for any particular application; what are the best frequencies to use; how often; what other conjunctive therapies could and couldn't be used while "rifing", etc. Most people don't understand enough about electronics to build these devices themselves, and so are left with having to purchase them from others or have them custom built. And these are not cheap devices either. Some run as high as several thousand dollars or more depending on several factors. And with little assurance as to whether these would work for any particular person, let alone cure them, that's an awful big expense to put out. I know for a fact that rifing, even with the best machines simply does not work for everyone. I dare say perhaps even most people. By "work" I mean received benefit from killing off of spirochetes in the body and subsequently experiencing a reduction of symptoms. A very good book on the subject was written by Bryan Rosner called *Lyme Disease and Rife Machines*. He also mentions some other protocols in the book that some have found helpful in healing Lyme. I do not personally know Bryan. I have read his book. However I was a bit dismayed to find that no place in his book does he claim to have eliminated his own Lyme disease using Rife machines. Although he sites a few that claim to have done so. It is simply another potential therapy that has been researched that offers hope to some.

I personally had the opportunity to own and try Rife machines, several EMP (electromagnetic pulse) devices, and the violet ray bulb/multi-wave oscillator. As for the Rife, I spent quite bit of time and expense trying to receive benefit by being treated at a practitioner's office. However after several attempts I didn't notice any effects from use. So I purchased my own, trying a number of frequencies. Again, no luck.

Still hopeful that some form of electromagnetic device would benefit me, I learned of someone local that owned a device called the PAP-IMI, which was the world's most powerful therapeutic electromagnetic pulsing device. They agreed to let me try it for a series of sessions. Again, not a herx in site. Although the PAP-IMI is not a rife machine, electromagnetic pulsers had been used successfully by a number of Lyme patients. They were recieving a good response, particularly in those with Babesia coinfections (since Babesia utilizes iron in its metabolic processes, which is obviously vulnerable to EMP exposure.) Most of these types of devices seemed to take some users only so far, but seldom all the way to complete healing.

In hindsight I believe the reason I may not have benefited from these electromagnetic devices is in part due to the fact that I had been taking several herbal products at maximum dosage for quite a long time, and partly during my experiments with rifing. These of course would have affected Borrelia by driving it into pleomorphic forms which are not readily vulnerable to these machines. Since my antimicrobials were in fact working, I felt no need to stop them completely to experiment with Rife since most of the Rife users (at least the ones sharing their stories) didn't appear to be having any more success using their machines than I was with my therapies. I also knew that there were some that testified they were not benefiting from Rife at all even though they were not taking medicines. It is of course just like any other therapy in which there are a number of variables that allow certain things to work for some people, but not work for others.

There are several reasons for this. First, a person may not have true Lyme disease; hence they will not receive benefit from Borrelia Burgdorferi (hereafter known as Bb) Rife frequencies. They may have some other pathogen mimicking Bb such as Bartonella, Babesia, Ehrlichia, mycoplasma, etc. Or since the form of the bacteria which responds best to Rife is the spirochete form, the cyst or L-forms will have shown very little if any reaction to rifing. For the most part, Rife machines generally work against only a few forms of the bacteria. There is a great deal of experimentation necessary since not only must the frequencies match the microbe, but sometimes more than one type of machine is necessary. For some this type of therapy is a viable and effective option, but it can be a bit technical, expensive, and almost never leads to complete healing. So I moved on.

Two very popular herbal products that were being touted at the time were Samento (aka TOA-free cat's claw), and Carnivora. I recalled reading one article by an MD at the time stating in particular that Samento was a cure for Lyme disease. So I, like many others purchased and began using the product. I did indeed find a significant herxing taking place, which offered me hope. I felt that perhaps I had found the answer I had been looking for. So for several months I not only continued taking the product, but gradually increased my dosage.

Now here is something you need to pay close attention to. Because I am going to describe the process that one would logically expect to observe when taking a medicine to reduce an infection, and that one would especially expect to see with an infection such as Lyme disease. It is customary to begin by taking low dosages, gradually increase it over time thereby giving the body time to not only adjust to the product itself, but to process the toxins that result from the herx reaction. Then as the herxing subsides over time, once again the dosage would be increased. This would once again be followed by more herxing as the deeper and more resistant bacteria are reached. It would not be inaccurate to say that in many types of bacteria-based illnesses, theoretically you would expect to reach a saturation point where no more bacteria are present to be killed, and the medicine has done its job. This would normally be followed by a reduction and eventual elimination of symptoms.

Except what I found in my Lyme disease was that in time and with increased dosages, this wasn't happening. It's as if the Samento just stopped working. I didn't understand why this was happening at the time. But I eventually stopped taking it altogether since it was demonstrating no further benefit, yet clearly my symptoms remained. I later tried it again several months later, but this time had no results at all. As time went by, I later read of several other Lyme patients that had the same experience.

This is often the pattern that is seen when you continue to take one substance for Lyme infection, and that includes most antibiotics. Borrelia Burgdorferi morphs to avoid being killed. Although I had heard of this happening in Lyme disease, it was a bit of a reality check when I personally actually experienced it because at the time I didn't fully grasped *why* this was happening.

I then moved on to a product called Carnivora that I had also heard good things about. The same exact thing happened as the Samento. I experienced massive die-off symptoms, fatique, brain fog, etc. Yet this too eventually stopped working. It seemed that each new group of treatments I was trying was doing the same thing. They would work for awhile and I would experience die-off symptoms, only to eventually stop working altogether.

As time went by and I had continued to study the many different medicines that people were taking for Lyme disease, I seemed to find this common thread.

However I also made another observation. There always seemed to be someone somewhere who claimed that a certain therapy was showing real promise or benefit, or a particular antibiotic or group of antibiotics was helping them. Often you were being lead to believe they felt like they were on their way to being cured. At least so they said. But this was either almost never repeatable by others, or few people experienced the same benefit using the same treatment protocols. We as humans tend to have similar tendencies as some animal species in that we generally have a "herd mentality". That is, we mostly tend to be followers. When one claim is made, we run over to see if all the noise is real and buy that product. Then when that doesn't work we run over to try the next claim, only to be disappointed again. Although that is human nature and behavior springing from noble efforts to find healing which we all want, the problem is that in time we simply don't know who or what to believe anymore. We play follow the leader, only to find out that in most cases the leader was like the proverbial blind pig that found the acorn. Yet time revealed that any progress was short-lived. And the whole process started all over again.

Now let me say at this point that my illness seemed to be going thru a progression. I couldn't say that I was continually improving and always heading in the direction of feeling better. Sometimes, and for reasons unknown to me at the time, I would go through periods of regression where I would feel so terrible that I wondered if all of my efforts were having any overall benefit at all. It's just that I knew that I couldn't stop or go backwards. That simply wasn't an option. And yes, I was like many of you who felt so terrible, fatigued, horrible feelings in the brain of being detached from reality, depression, agony, like someone took the top of your skull off and stirred it with a stick. That was besides the joint pain, night sweats, sinus and urinary tract infections, sore throat, etc. However in the midst of this, I was mindful of a deep sense of wondering how and why this was not only such an illusive illness, but what was it about this particular bacterium that made it so unique? Why was it so hard to kill? So began my journey.

ENDNOTES

Koch, W.F. (1941). *An efficient single dose treatment for Diabetes on a full carbohydrate diet without insulin.* Pg3 Retrieved July 26, 2005, from William F. Koch Website, http://www.williamfkoch.com/kochframe2.htm

CHAPTER 1

The Hijacking of Conventional Medicine

"I don't care how I do it; I only want to get well."

Lyme patient

Before proceeding, I felt it important to take a look at how conventional medicine approaches healing, and why we have reached the point in this country where not only Lyme disease sufferers, but victims of many other illnesses are no longer seen as individuals in need of healing, but as commodities with potential for profit or loss. The conventional medicine model differs in its approach to healing from natural medicine, and can have serious consequences unless the patient is vigilantly educating him/herself from the dangers this approach can lead to. Obviously the fact that you are reading this book tells me that you are either open to alternative therapies, or have gone the conventional route and haven't received the help you are looking for. For many who are victims of Lyme, conventional medicine is often the first place they start because they would like an official diagnosis. But then as time passes on in their journey back to wellness, as they take their prescribed antibiotics and begin to feel better, they realize that they never really reach that place where they were before their infection. Their doctor may feel that they need an additional month or two of meds to knock it completely out, but then after that it seems to return again. Then again!

It has actually become commonplace to hear of other Lymies who have been on antibiotics for Lyme disease sometimes for many years, with little hope of a cure. Stories like these lead many of us to begin to wonder if this is all there is or if there is any realistic hope of getting well by taking the allopathic approach. After all, if antibiotics are the primary treatment of choice of conventional medicine, but they do not appear to be resolving a person's illness, what's the use wasting your time, energy and money on false hopes if all doctors are doing is giving you the same ride on a merry-go-round, except on a different horse each time?

Trouble is, if you have not been exposed to alternative medicine and understand how the entire underlying philosophy of natural medicine takes a completely different approach than conventional medicine, you may be on the fence as to how effective non-drug therapies can be. After all, isn't alternative medicine a "second-class" form of medicine that people use when all else has failed?

Even with the tremendous experience and success I have personally had using alternative medicine over the years, I had occasions of taking antibiotics for my Lyme disease. This was because the speed of my recovery wasn't as fast as I thought it should have been, (especially in those early years before I discovered much more potent substances). However upon switching to antibiotics, and I have been on quite a few different ones, I found that I was actually making less progress than I was on non-drug therapies I had been using.

Of course in the early days before doing thorough research on Borrelia Borgdorferi, I didn't understand that this bacterial infection did not fit the same mold as other kinds of infections, and that my expectations of a quick and complete recovery were completely unfounded. When I was not seeing the fast and complete resolution to my illness I had expected using the herbal approach, I immediately assumed that the problem was the medicine I was taking. In time however I learned that the lack of progress I was having using natural medicine was because I was simply replacing a drug with a natural substance, but was employing the same conventional medicine model. Therein lay my problem. It would take me years of wasted effort and therapies before I understood what was happening to me. Until I replaced the conventional model with a completely different one, I would continue to run from therapy to therapy looking for the pot at the end of the rainbow; or perhaps more accurately, the pill at the end of the tongue.

This will be the beginning of what you also will learn, since you too may find yourself having fallen into the same trap as those that have come before you, wasting your money going from doctor to doctor, and trying one antibiotic after another. Because Lyme disease usually is not just one problem, but a multi-layered one that needs to be addressed on many different levels, this approach will not be successful. You have multiple variations of the microbe, biofilm resistance, coinfections, impaired immune cells, toxic disturbance, severe emotional swings, energy depletion, etc. But even when it comes to using natural medicine, I will give you a hint: It is not necessarily the therapy you are using, but *how* you are using it that makes the world of difference. That is a trap that we all fall into.

So I decided to include a chapter that discusses conventional medicine in general, why that approach is often at odds with natural healing, and to clear up some misconceptions and outright lies that are held to help the reader understand how to form their own opinions, and open their minds to possibilities they would otherwise be closed to. But please keep in mind that this is a general discussion about the philosophy itself, and is not a reflection on any particular physician that practices allopathic or conventional medicine, as there are many fine doctors obviously, as well as varying degrees as to how that model is practiced. Alternative, or complimentary, or Integrative medicine as it is sometimes called, is gaining more popularity with people, and more and more MD's are incorporating nutraceuticals and non-drug therapies into their practices to the degree that they are allowed to by the FDA and AMA. And therein lies another problem. However if you are already well versed in the conventional vs alternative debate, you may want to skip this chapter.

FDA APPROVED

Doctors are only allowed to use "approved" therapies. The FDA, working together with the American Medical Association, has certain standards of practice. Those standards establish acceptable guidelines. Except often those guidelines have little to do with safety or whether or not they promote health. The entire allopathic medical system is set up in order to benefit either pharmaceutical companies, or industries that provide supplies or develop devices that work to further expand the medical system. If you want proof of this, ask yourself why the FDA has made it a legal definition that only drugs can cure an illness. Drugs are defined by the FDA: "Articles intended for use in the diagnosis, cure, mitigation, treatment, or prevention of disease" and "articles (other than food) intended to affect the structure or any function of the body of man or other animals" FD&C Act, sec. 201(g)(1). [1]

Thus, technically speaking and according to the FDA, any natural food product that can for example be used to mitigate (alleviate) your headache is a drug, if that is your intention for using it, and can be legally regulated as a drug. One can readily see the problems and far reaching consequences holding such an idea could ultimately have with regards to the taking of any natural product, if in fact your purpose for taking the products is to give to you some health benefit. With one sweeping statement the FDA has just told you that anything you take to stay healthy (prevention of disease) is considered a drug which is subject to legal regulation. This truly is beyond belief when one considers that the FDA therefore has set the legal guidelines to control everything you put in your body, with no defense-able recourse.

Practically speaking, as well as scientifically, this definition of a drug is a lie, and in fact is beyond absurd. It is important to understand the implications of this definition, since it has nothing to do with what is true or even what is scientifically correct. It has been, and is still being used for purposes of control. Some may say that this was not the FDA's intent. Oh contrair! They have used this absurd legal description abusively by making it illegal for any food seller to make any kind of health claim (without their permission). We know most illnesses in part involve a deficiency of some sort that can very often be resolved or at least alleviated by diet or by administration of therapeutic levels of certain nutritional supplements in order to bring the body back into balance.

However if a doctor claims to either cure or mitigate a disease using a natural product, then he is technically in violation of the law because he is claiming to have used an unapproved drug (i.e. food or nutritional supplement). This is the reason for the legal disclaimer being put on supplements. They must "legally declare" that the supplement (for which people are taking for health benefit) is not intended to be used in a way that would define it as a drug—in other words, has no health benefits! It is the proverbial elephant in the room no one wants to mention.

Of course most people are taking supplements in order to alleviate or prevent disease! But manufacturers cannot *tell you* the benefits (unless they legally deny, or disclaim them in the same breath) or risk violating the law.

How do they get away with this? By convincing Americans that they are looking out for their safety by preventing false claims from being made about a product's intended use.

That is why doctors and healthcare practitioners are in so much fear of the FDA. It does not matter how many Americans die in this system. What is important is that the public be convinced and ***thinks*** that the government is looking out for them. They often do this by bringing up charges against doctors that imply the physicians are deliberately and falsely attempting to defraud the public by using "snake oils", and "false promises" or "unapproved treatments" to financially take advantage of their patients. (Ironically, drugs defraud and kill people at frightening rates. But that is of course not objectionable to the FDA.)

Therefore anything that is not approved by the FDA for a specific intended use in the healing of disease technically can be outlawed. It would be one thing if in fact the spirit of the law was to protect consumers from fraudulent claims by charlatans who may seek to take advantage of the public. But in fact, the FDA makes it no secret that their intention is in fact to withhold from the public actual healing and curative modalities from legitimate, ethical, and compassionate doctors and individuals whose only motive is healing people from disease.

IS THE **FDA** TRULY PROTECTING THE PUBLIC?

*A health reporter named Edward J. McCabe reported how successful oxygen therapies were. In 1999 he was sentenced to 3 years in prison on the pre-text of tax evasion.

*Dr. Basil Earle Wainright was a physicist who invented a special device used to aid in carrying oxygen, ozone, and other polyatomic forms of oxygen to blood to kill viruses, and known to inactivate HIV. It was called Polyatomic Oxygen Therapy. He was put in prison for over 3 years. Six assassination attempts were made on his life while in prison.

*Dr George A. Freibott, IV Many assassination attempts were made on this doctor. He was the President of the American Naturopathic Association and consultant for International Association for Oxygen Therapy. The American Government approved him as an accepted expert witness on oxygen/oxidation therapies. He practiced Naturopathy. He also received anonymous phone calls to threaten his life.

*James Boyce, M.D. had his medical license revoked and was sentenced to 5 years in prison for using ozone therapy to turn 254 HIV+ to HIV-. The charge: using "unproven methods" in the practice of medicine.

*Dr William F. Koch: Was a medical doctor with an additional PhD in Biochemistry. He taught chemistry, histology and physiology. He invented a medicine called Glyoxylide as a cure for cancers, allergies, and viral infections. He proved its effectiveness against the FDA in court. He was sued and jailed by the FDA, and finally acquitted after 600 doctors testified on his behalf. He was poisoned in 1967.

*Dr. F.M. Eugene Blass: Invented "Homozon" (a supplement that uses magnesium oxide to deliver oxygen into the body as an oxygen therapy, and is mentioned later in this book). He was also murdered at his home nearly the same time as Dr. Koch.

*Dr Burzynski of Houston, Texas, Developed "antineoplastons" to treat "untreatable" brain tumors. He has been persecuted by the FDA for over 10 years. Dr. Richard Crout of the FDA explained the FDA's motive for targeting doctors who develop drugs to cure diseases. "I never have and never will approve a new drug to an individual, but only to a large pharmaceutical firm with unlimited finances." Dr. Burzynski has held his ground and even used his own financial resources to finance drug trials. See Antineoplastons: How the FDA Stops Medical Progress. http://cancermed.com/fdamore.htm>.

*Wilhelm Reich, M.D. One of the worst cases of FDA abuse of power in US history. Dr. Reich held unpopular views on medicine that didn't set well with the FDA. His research was confiscated and burned by the authorities. He was sent to prison for years where he eventually died a broken man. One of Dr. Reich's coworkers, Dr. Michael Silvert was also sent to prison and supposedly committed suicide after his release. Many of Dr. Reich's associates had their homes raided illegally without a warrant.

*Dr. Max Gerson developed a diet and dietary supplements for degenerative diseases and cancer. He was asked to testify before the US Senate of some of the cures that had occurred. However later the FDA forced him out of the country due to litigation against him.

*In 1987 the FDA attacked The Life Extension Foundation by raiding their business with armed agents, and seizing supplements and personal property. This lead to a multi-year legal battle where the FDA eventually was defeated in one of the worst legal blows against this agency in their history.

*The FDA spurred the Texas Dept. of Health and Texas Dept of Food and Drugs in 1992 to raid many large well-known health food stores seizing products such as vitamin C and other herbal products. Although no official charges against the stores or their owners were made, their property was never returned. They told the store owners, "Don't talk to the press, or we'll come down on you twice as hard."

*During 1993 some 40 different FDA-backed raids which included the DEA, IRS, Customs, and the US Postal service were made against natural food stores and natural product manufactures throughout the country. Entire stocks of products as well as bank accounts and property were confiscated. Even the US Postal Service illegally participated by preventing mail from being delivered so they could not carry out legal defense on their own behalf.

*Dr. Gary Davis, was a family practice physician from Tulsa, OK who developed a cure for AIDS by using goat serum. This has been verified by testimonies of actual users. He approached the FDA for approval. Later however, he had his laboratory burned down. He was finally poisoned in 2007 at an airport while attempting to leave the country to work in a foreign country with AIDS patients.

*In 2011 FDA agents raid an Amish milk farm with guns drawn to intimidate and scare the owners for selling healthy unpasteurized milk. The same thing happened at Rawsome Foods in Venice, California and other raw milk farms, confiscating property and jailing owners. (One can go on the internet to see the actual video.) Although consumers sign a waiver stating that they want whole foods unpasteurized and unprocessed in order to join the raw food club, the FDA insists on controlling the foods people put in their own bodies in order to be healthy, even if it means jailing the owners of these establishments. There can only be one reason why the FDA would enter into a store with guns drawn: to deliberately terrorize the owners and the public. Intimidation and terror is part of the history of the FDA. Both the FDA and the Obama administration defend the agency's actions while their legal battle continues against these business owners.

These are only a small handful of hundreds of instances of our wonderful FDA protecting American citizens. But who will protect us from them?

A true life example of the persecution by the FDA for curing people of disease is Dr. William Koch. MD PhD in Biochemistry, who had developed a medicine that was curing cancer, viral infections and numerous other diseases beyond any effectiveness medical science had seen up to that point in history. When the AMA learned of it, they confronted Dr. Koch to sell to them the formula. He was willing to do so, on the condition that the medicine would be made available to anyone that needed it, not just the wealthy that could pay for it. The AMA refused this condition, and thus was not sold the formula, as they would then have complete control over its use and dispensing. As a result the AMA brought the matter to the FDA who subsequently imprisoned Dr. Koch. Since they didn't have a case against him, the charges that were brought before him were "mislabeling" of a drug. As a result of that trial, Dr. Koch and the many doctors who were using his therapy on their patients, presented in court 20,000 successful cases demonstrating its effectiveness. This was never in question. However the FDA could not deny that his therapy was working, and could not find a legal way of stopping him from curing his patients. The FDA was determined to stop Dr. Koch at all costs, as his medicine was reducing the need for other cancer drugs at the time that were far less effective, and would have replaced not only those drugs, but the entire system that was built to siphon medical costs from patients and insurance companies.

Because of our government's persecution of Dr. Koch, he decided to no longer make it available to the public, was eventually forced out of the country, and never revealed its exact formula. That is why you have never heard of him. Two of his colleagues were murdered, as Dr. Koch himself was eventually murdered by poisoning. An interesting side-note about Dr. Koch's story was that in spite of the circumstances wherein the government was seeking to stop Dr. Koch dead in his tracks by prosecuting him in court, Dr. Koch had noticed a cancerous growth on the neck of the prosecutor, and had actually offered to help him by giving to him his cancer-cure medicine. Instead, Dr. Koch was ridiculed by him. Several months later that very prosecutor died of his cancer. It seems that sometimes Providence brings justice sooner than later.

This sounds like a story out of some made up movie, or that might take place under some evil dictator persecuting his own people. Yet stories such as these are filled in the annuls of the history of medicine with the FDA. The FDA is not your friend. But like the wolf that deceived little red-riding hood, they are deceiving naive Americans to this day.

Approximately a quarter of a million Americans die from FDA approved drugs and procedures each year, while at the same time they are trying to convince you that you need their healthcare coverage. Why? So that the entire legal syndicate the FDA has created can become even more expanded to control the liberties of Americans and their doctors. This is not a conspiracy that is being covered up. It is happening in plain sight and functioning as standard procedure in this country every day.

For example, the FDA is warning the public against using a product that is so highly effective against all kinds of pathogenic infections (and even cancers) that it could replace most antibiotics. Yet it could supply you with enough medicine for years for only $20. It is called Sodium Chlorite which has been activated with a small amount of citric acid. This produces chlorine dioxide gas which is very stable in liquid. It has been used in other countries against malaria. It has been reportedly used successfully against 75,000 malaria victims, with far greater effectiveness than any anti-malarial drug. Yet you will never here of it from your doctor, and its safety is not in question in the manner in which it is used. Yet the FDA has warned Americans not to use the product due to safety concerns, even though not one dangerous or toxic affect has directly been shown to occur from its use.

They will never cease to try to deliberately withhold the truth from you when it comes to medicines and substances which exist which are known to be effective against specific diseases and other medical conditions, if it is not part of their "approved" system. And part of the deception they will use is to tell you "there are no scientific studies demonstrating its effectiveness for that purpose." Now doesn't that sound convincing! As if to say that something does not work unless a scientific study proved it works. That is how they trick you. Like a magician with slight of hand, they try to distract you from the truth by making it sound logical. If you believe they have good intentions, then you may one day become a victim yourself.

So what if there are medicines out there that are very inexpensive, and are at least as effective, if not far more effective than prescriptions medicines for certain infectious diseases, but are not offered by your doctor? If this is news to you, then at least now you have the opportunity to stop being a victim.

A WARNING LABEL ON DOCTORS

This leads us to understand how conventional medicine has been manipulated and controlled by a much greater "medical establishment" as determined by the FDA which sets guidelines and approves what medicines are allowed to be used. The FDA is an organization of two faces. With one face they lead the public to believe they are looking out for their welfare by setting guidelines and policies that will insure the effectiveness and safety of the foods and drugs we use. With the other they approve poisonous drugs that do not cure; they harass or intimidate doctors that use therapies that have genuine healing potentials; and they mislead the public about the benefits of natural and non-drug therapies by prohibiting sellers of these alternative products from making claims as to how their products may be beneficial. Quoting Herbert Lay M.D., former FDA Commissioner:

"The thing that bugs me is that the people think the FDA is protecting them. It isn't. What the FDA is doing and what the public thinks it is doing are as different as night and day." San Fransisco Chronicle 1-2-70

And perhaps the greatest crime of the FDA is when they approve drugs that later are determined to cause serious side effects and even deaths, but then accept no legal responsibility for having done so, and actually have the audacity to hold the drug companies responsible for their own lack of over-site. I doubt little mercy will be shown to this organization on judgment day. The truth of the matter is, your doctor has the right to practice legal medicine, but not necessarily healing medicine.

It is no secret that drug companies are given free reign and actually encouraged and protected by the FDA. It is also no secret that profit and power are the motivations. But even with this being the case, one wonders how they are being allowed to get away with this at the expense of the health and the very lives of the people that they are supposed to be protecting. Here is how the public is being misled.

Within the paradigm of the legal system, without evidence a person cannot be prosecuted. But it doesn't mean they are actually innocent, any more than having some evidence that they may have committed a crime means they are truly guilty. In a court of law, that paradigm isn't truly interested in the actual truth, only what is considered *legally* true. People are in prison today that are *legally* guilty, but are in fact innocent. As real people living in a real world, what is considered true and *legally* true **should** be the same thing. But they are not. The FDA wants us to live in *their* legal world instead of a real world. In fact, given that so many have been falsely prosecuted for crimes they never committed, or others have been set free who were in fact guilty, the truth, and what is legally true often are opposites. It is no secret that the FDA, by its very policies has a special abhorance for natural and non-drug healing therapies. They deliberately set the laws to prevent natural cures from being made known by prohibiting them from making health claims, stating health benefits, and in some cases persecuting doctors using natural medicines. Even though Americans by the millions are dying due to these policies, they have no shame.

"The Lord has created medicines out of the earth; and he that is wise will not abhor them." -Ecclesiastes 38:4

Medical doctors are taught to live in a world of "legal medicine" not true medicine. Legal medicine can hurt people, or at the very least interfere with true healing since drugs do not cure illnesses, only manage them, or cover them up. (Yet the FDA tells us that only drugs can cure.) The ironic inconsistency with conventional medicine is how they will often cite the lack of evidence supporting a particular non-drug therapy as proof that it doesn't work. Did you read that right? No evidence (according to them) is evidence. Yet conventional medicine is guiltier of giving "proven" medicines to patients that not only do not work for them, but end up killing them to boot! Beware that this is the paradigm that conventional medicine works from.

Note: It is important to make clear that we are not saying that scientific studies are not important for natural medicine. On the contrary, verification of, and understanding the mechanisms as to how certain natural substances work is extremely helpful. But just as a person can learn to drive a car without knowing how it works, so medicines from the earth can heal without understanding how they work. The double standard and hypocrisy of conventional medicine however is obvious. Often they do not work at all and even kill. Yet conventional medicine prides itself in its ability to explain the modes of action of drugs.

Ultimately, there is only one way to know for certain if a medicine is going to work for someone. And whether taking a conventional or natural approach, only the subjective observation of improvement has the final say. Ultimately a therapy will only be known to be "safe and effective" if it is so *for you.*

TWO DIFFERENT APPROACHES

Evidenced-based medicine is based upon the idea that before a medication can claim benefit, there must be some objective scientific-based standard or test by which to gauge its safety or effectiveness. The guidelines that are set determine whether or not a medicine or drug is "legitimate", or whether the benefits outweigh the risks. Only drugs which demonstrate evidence proving it does what it says it can do are approved. This is the basis of FDA approved medications. These approved drugs then become the only "tools" allowed in the doctor's toolbox.

In contrast to evidence-based medicine, results or outcome-based medicine generally describes herbal and non-drug substances which cannot be patented for profit. Although some off-label use of drugs may be described as results-oriented, this approach recognizes the incredible disadvantage and limitations of evidence-based medicine. Evidence-based medicine requires a huge financial outlay due to the extreme requirements of testing.

The extent of testing done with results-oriented medicine however is very limited due to lack of financial incentives. Therefore the applications for and extent of their potential uses is limited to whatever in vitro studies are done, or "anecdotal" observations are made in patients using them. These medicines however have a much longer track record of success since many of them have been used for even thousands of years for all sorts of ailments. Their safety has been generally much more established due to their long history of use. Additionally there is much less concern of interactions as can be a potentially deadly result of certain drug combinations. Natural substances rarely ever hold this danger since they can more readily be combined to have a synergistic effect, without the toxicity usually associated with drugs. Although the specific doses and effectiveness are sometimes not quantified for specific applications or conditions due to the lack of testing done on herbal products, their possibilities are almost endless using the results-oriented approach.

One approach says, "we will only use medicines which have been scientifically put to a certain test that has demonstrated effectiveness against certain conditions at the exclusion of medicines that haven't been put to the test." The other says, "We don't know everything, but we know that such conditions have been healed without the use of drugs, and have observed prior effectiveness in similar applications." The one toolbox is highly controlled and limited. The other contains many tools that can be used to empower the individual to find healing much more safely and oftentimes much more effectively.

"Plant based medicines were designed by the Creator to work synergistically with the human body to heal. Drugs were designed to make money."

Personally I would rather open my world to possibilities that go beyond the limited scope of what some researcher or drug company has arbitrarily determined should or shouldn't work for me. Because even his "evidence-based" approach to medicine cannot prove any particular drug will work for me, anymore than he can prove that some other therapy outside of his approach won't work for me.

Having a limited scope within an evidence-based medicine paradigm creates impossibilities. In other words, the medicines that are available within this paradigm may not cure your condition, or address your problem. So, within this paradigm your condition would be considered "incurable" and leaves you without hope. For instance many cancers, infections, or allergies are considered "incurable" within this conventional evidence-based medicine paradigm. However once you leave that paradigm and enter into another that says, "we don't know everything, but we know these maladies are curable because we have seen them resolved in others," then, rather than live in arrogance and condescension we humble ourselves before the Universe that possesses all knowledge outside of our limited minds, and opens the possibilities for cures that are not available in another paradigm. So, **modern FDA-controlled conventional medicine actually "creates" incurable illnesses by limiting the medicines that are available to treat them.** Your paradigm will determine your possibilities. Choose your weapon.

Science becomes a false religion

We live in a time when drugs and drug-based treatments rule as king. We have always been lead to believe that only drugs were considered "science-based" medicine. This deception is based on the fact that non-financial incentive-based substances do not provide the "science" behind their use, and therefore have no scientific basis *proving* their effectiveness. Thus a stigma was unjustly attached to natural products, that being, "if they were effective, why are they not tested and used by doctors like drugs are?" Therefore they were relegated to the category of "snake oils" (whatever that is supposed to be) and became associated with charlatans that deliberately attempted to take advantage of the uneducated and ignorant. The reason for so many being deceived was due to the admittedly brilliant manner in which this was deliberately orchestrated. The fact is that the legal structure was designed to set "scientific standards" as a kind of false religion. If the FDA could convince enough people that scientific studies are the gold standard by which to determine the medicinal value of a substance, they could then instigate and establish laws which would prohibit the use of anything other than drugs as proven medicines, and the people would accept that hook, line, and sinker. This is what has happened.

Because drugs were given legal protection by laws that were designed to actually promote their use over natural medicines that had been traditionally used for thousands of years, no longer could the non-drug modalities be promoted as having a specific health benefit. Thus by default they have no efficacy, and can not make a claim unless supported by scientific research; hence the catch-22. In a sense, science became misused to support the new "religion" of medicine. And that religion was run by the Pope called the FDA and the AMA who made the decisions of what was truth and what wasn't truth, even if it meant lying in doing so.

No longer could the benefits of those substances given to man by God be espoused as having efficacy without the threat of persecution by the false religion that had taken over medical science. It would have been one thing to recognize both forms of medicine as having their own place, but to deny the reality of thousands of years of healing was tantamount to trying to convince mankind that the holocaust never happened. It's one thing to say that a medicine has not been put to the same tests as drugs. It is something else altogether to say that a medicine does not work or is a snake oil, just because it has not been put to a test to prove its effectiveness, when there are no requirements to do so.

This is the "guilty until proven innocent" syndrome. Ironically the the FDA has not found a drug to cure its own illness.

Many non-drug modalities are effective even though they have not been tested in a formal manner. Many, on their own merit have stood the test of time. For example silver has been known to be a preservative for thousands of years. Even though in early history they didn't know how it worked, they knew it kept certain things from spoiling. By consistently observing this action, then repeatedly observing the same thing, they came to certain conclusions, even though no formal "scientific research" was done. However in order to be able to make such precise observations, a highly technical mind that required years of keen study had to be acquired. And there was a difficult to pronounce scientific term used to describe the process used to come to such conclusions. It was called common sense. The forefathers of our modern doctors relied upon their own empirical observations, and served their patients well. They applied the rule of systematic consistency through the process of observation and repeatability—which by the way is the very definition of science.

Common sense and traditional science had its foundations in the merits of time tested observation and repeatability. For five thousand years the Chinese have had a form of medicine that has been highly effective, but until this past century has never been put to the testing rigors of modern day "scientific research". Yet it has been used in the treatment of diseases before modern medicine ever become known. The same could be said of Ayur Vedic medicine in India. It has only been recently that many of the phytonutrients and compounds being laboratory tested have been discovered to possess many properties that explain their effectiveness, which have been true all along. It is interesting that a substance can be a snake oil, until it is tested. Then magically it becomes a medicine! (They use to call this alchemy, or the conversion of a valueless substance into one of value. Seems the FDA's false religion has incorporated alchemy into its doctrine.)

It is interesting that the FDA's stated motivation is for the protection of the American people. Even if this means stopping the sale of so-called useless snake oils. Yet that same FDA's history has been to stop at all costs any non-drug substances that demonstrate effectiveness against serious diseases. For example laetrile and 714X are two non-drug cancer medicines which are essentially outlawed in the US. Yet, a rigorous study has been done by researchers to determine the over-all effectiveness of *approved* chemotherapy drugs against cancer. In the US the 5 year survival rate was only 2.1%!! Another dissenting opinion disagreed and felt it was much higher, 5-6%! [2] And these are the results of only one class of anti-cancer drugs. Imagine what would be learned if the whole truth about the FDA and their support of drug companies ever became known.

How can any competent human being take this organization seriously? Contrary to their stated legal definition, drugs do not in fact cure diseases. (When was the last time you heard of a drug that actually cured a disease?) To make matters worse, Americans are then forced to pay additional costs by being required to see their physicians in order to get a prescription for something that not only does not cure them, but virtually guarantees they will remain with the condition as long as they are taking the drug. Then we wonder why healthcare costs in this country are out of control. That is because there is a deliberate effort to force consumers to have to rely on drugs since the FDA, working in conjunction with the FTC has placed strict guidelines on the sellers of natural substances. They prohibit them from making any claims about their products that would imply health benefits, for the direct purpose of preventing the public from being made aware of their healing potentials that would directly compete with drugs. It is more than just a smear campaign. They actually establish policies wherein a business can be shut down and have their products confiscated or fined if they are violated—truth be damned!

An example of this was when the manufacturer of a product called Vitamin O, also called stabilized oxygen, was forced to pay a $375,000 settlement for claiming their product increased oxygen levels in the body, and the subsequent health benefits as a result. They were also told they could no longer make those claims. Several years later a scientific study was done on that product which conclusively proved that the product did indeed increase oxygen levels as claimed. However even today one can do a Wikepedia search and find that Rose Creek Health Products, the makers of Vitamin O are still being deliberately smeared as no mention of this study is made which in truth exonerates them from the false charges brought by the FTC. [3]

Americans are deliberately having their freedoms stolen from under them by the FDA by creating policies which inhibit, and whenever possible prevent information of natural health products and their benefits from being made known. We were finally forced to fight back with the passing of the Dietary Supplement Health and Education Act of 1994 (DSHEA). However efforts have repeatedly been made which seeks to either repeal or weaken the legislation to once and for all give the FDA complete control over what is a persons God-given right over his own health decisions. Americans are having this freedom infringed upon by having road-blocks put in place which limits information about the benefits of natural health products. Even most second and third world countries still have this freedom. Thomas Jefferson once said, "If people let government decide what foods they eat and what medicines they take, their bodies will soon be in as sorry a state as are the souls of those who live under tyranny." He was right since although it has often been said that we have the most advanced healthcare system in the world, we as a people are sicker and are required to spend more money on healthcare than almost all other industrialized countries. Under the FDA, the very medicines people are taking for their illnesses will often virtually guarantee they remain sick.

CONVENTIONAL MEDICINE LEADS TO ISOLATION

Within the evidence-based medicine paradigm, drug companies often seek to isolate chemical properties found in nature, then they try to artificially reproduce them in the lab to make a drug. As is part of their philosophy, conventional medicine then matches that drug to fit a particular disease state: one drug to match one disease. That in and of itself is not necessarily a bad thing. But we know that the primary reason for this is so that drug companies can patent a substance to profit from it. It makes no difference whether there are already natural substances that can do the same thing, oftentimes cheaper and more effectively.

However, from a philosophical standpoint, the problem with seeking to isolate a substance that is aimed solely at treating a specific ailment is that by trying to isolate a single chemical property it ignores the synergy of all nutrients and phytochemicals in a plant that would normally work in harmony to produce an end result. It also ignores the inherent intelligence, sychronicity and balance that all immune, endocrine, hormonal, neurotransmitter, biochemical systems etc, of the body interplay with each other. That is why so often herbal medicines work better, and in many cases, far better than drugs in many applications because they have many beneficial properties working together to affect the body chemistry on many levels, and *almost always* in a non-toxic manner. However we never hear of this because it is illegal to claim so in any specific applications and diseases. Whereas drugs are deliberately altered chemicals designed to have their molecular structures manipulated and to varying degrees become a poison to the body which must be monitored to prevent damage or death. And that is the real reason why so much scientific testing must go into conventional medicine, not because it is a superior form of medicine, but because it can do almost unbelievable harm if not explicitly controlled.

So the philosophy that has become a part of conventional medicine unfortunately is usually at odds with the need to address the overall and underlying health condition of the patient which led to the problem in the first place. This misguided system has now evolved to the point where the driving force is not the motivation to heal the underlying problem, but seeks to profit from it by creating drugs which chemically alters the body chemistry temporarily in order to, in turn, alter the symptoms of a deeper problem. That then places the patient in a position of having to depend on symptom-altering drugs much like a drug addict. In other words most drugs were deliberately designed to force users to remain dependant upon them, since they do not actually heal the underlying condition. And the users are being lied to since now names are given to symptoms as if the symptoms are actually the disease itself. By covering up the symptoms, one is being lead to believe that the "disease is being controlled". Add to that the side effects that contribute even further to the decline of health. Unfortunately the unsuspecting patient doesn't realize this is taking place because he doesn't understand that this is the way the game is rigged. There is a virtual deception underlying the entire system, but it is taking place under the guise of "science". In this manner, it is not just some government agency such as the FDA, or a medical board that is complicit, but doctors that deliberately push drug-based medicine on to their patients when natural alternatives are available are part of the problem.

Obviously not all doctors have the underlying motive to profit from their patients illnesses by participating in this game that has become part of conventional medicine. Many protest "under duress" by silently practicing medicine in a responsible and conscientious manner. These practitioners rather seek to identify underlying causes and whenever possible seek to find natural ways to balance their patient's health with every means possible. Yes that includes when necessary appropriate drugs when circumstances require the addressing of acute conditions for temporary management of an illness where no non-drug treatments are known to exist. Many doctors find themselves at odds with their own overseeing medical boards and government agencies which sometimes act with Gestapo-like vigor to intimidate in order to maintain this corrupt system.

Stated in a general way, what conventional drug-based medicine has done is taken observation and repeatability, or science, which has been used for thousands of years, and systematized it for the purpose of exploiting chemical substances for profit, *at the expense of natural healing*. Rather than attempting to understand the nature of true healing, it seeks to artificially manipulate the chemistry of the body to alter by chemical force, what the body seeks to correct on its own when all systems are balanced. This would be possible if the natural symbiosis of man and nature were allowed to be expressed by understanding the wisdom of plants and natural substances, and how they can work together to do what artificial manipulation and poisoning the body could never do.

This is not to suggest that taking of drugs does not have its place. They have excellent application in the area of emergency medicine, or where temporary manipulation for severe pain would be called for. But their overuse and attempts to replace natural medicine for every malady has truly risen to a false religion. Scripture says "He that is sick has need of a physician". Remember however, the only medicine that existed at that time was natural medicine. It did not say, "He that is sick is out of luck until the 20th century when artificial drugs come into existence." In fact, the original Greek word in the New Testament for "sorcerey" and "witchcraft" is "pharmakia". This is a reference to the abuse of a substance whose end was not for purposes of harmony and health, but to alter their mind or body to experience a temporary feeling wherein they were no longer in control, but given over to the substance (exactly what takes place when a person is given over to alcohol.) Certain aspects of that philosophy have crept into conventional medicine in that oftentimes drugs are actually preventing true harmony and healing from taking place, by allowing the underlying condition to remain, yet temporarily allowing the condition to become altered from a poisonous man-made drug that does not work with the body, but seeks to control it, and over time can throw the entire body out of homeostasis and lead to further problems. That is not to say that pharmacists are sorcerers. What is being said is that these two systems were even at odds 2000 years ago. And they are still at odds today.

I had a friend I use to work with on many of the construction jobs we did. He was as strong and healthy as a horse. He was in his mid-70's at the time and was always taking natural substances to keep himself healthy. However he was an absolute workaholic. He loved to work. He was loved by everyone who worked with him, and was a very caring individual. But we always wondered in amazement how a man of his age could out-work those of us 20-30 years younger than him often working 70 hours a week to complete a job.

Then one day he apparently pushed himself too far and had a mild heart attack. However his doctors put him on so many drugs (7 if I recall correctly) that within months that strong bull of a man had dwindled down from a 220lb man, to some 145lbs. He looked like a scarecrow. He could barely walk. He had absolutely no energy whatsoever. He looked like he was a 100 years old. We all worried about him since he kept coming to the jobsite wanting to work. (You can't keep a good man down!) We kept on hinting to him he needs to stop or at least significantly reduce his medication. But he said his doctor told him he would need to be on his medicine for the rest of his life. And we of course were not medical doctors and felt out of place making suggestions outside his doctor's authority obviously. This went on for nearly a year. Clearly whatever happened to him, it was not his mild heart attack that did this to him, since he healed very quickly after his surgery.

Then one day we heard he had died in his rocking chair at home. We were shocked (but not surprised.) We learned that the medical examiner determined that he died from the drugs the doctors had given to him. They simply destroyed his body, and his will to live, compliments of the great American medical system and with the blessings of our FDA. Multiply this story by 10,000 times, and you get a small idea of what drugs do to people. In *Death by Medicine* by Gary Null PhD, a group of researchers detailed incredible statistics that were gathered to study the effects of allopathic medicine.

> *This fully referenced report shows the number of people having in-hospital, adverse reactions to prescribed drugs to be 2.2 million per year. The number of unnecessary antibiotics prescribed annually for viral infections is 20 million per year. The number of unnecessary medical and surgical procedures performed annually is 7.5 million per year. The number of people exposed to unnecessary hospitalization annually is 8.9 million per year. The most stunning statistic, however, is that the total number of deaths caused by conventional medicine is an astounding 783,936 per*

year. It is now evident that the American medical system is the leading cause of death and injury in the US. [4]

Of those, between 100,000 and 200,000 are directly from drugs alone. We are not talking about drug abuse. We are speaking of side effects from prescription drug use. This means that more Americans have died under the oversight of the FDA and their irresponsible and pernicious policies than any other killer in the history of our country.

An article in Naturalnews.com titled, "The lawlessness of the FDA, Big Pharma immunity and crimes against humanity" cites,

> *In the preamble of the FDA's new "Final Rule" to take effect on June 30 (2006), the agency asserts that FDA approval of prescription drugs—and their implied safety—may no longer be second-guessed by consumers or organizations of any kind. The FDA's stamp of approval, the agency claims, is an absolute declaration of safety of all such drugs, for any use whatsoever . . . The FDA's new "Final Rule" would allow drug companies to operate with impunity, shouldering absolutely no responsibility for the harmful (even fatal) side effects of their prescription drugs, many of which we are now learning were only approved under highly suspicious circumstances that smack of fraud, corruption and outright criminal intent. Consumers harmed or killed by toxic prescription drugs—even drugs that their manufacturers knew were extremely dangerous—would have no recourse whatsoever.* [5]

It is beyond belief that this is happening in the so-called "land of the free". That means the FDA can approve any drugs they want, 200,000 people or more can die from those drugs, and we as Americans can do absolutely nothing about it. Period! And as disgraceful as that may be, that is apparently perfectly acceptable to us as Americans because we have been brain-washed to believe the FDA guidelines and policies must be based upon sound scientific reasoning and that they have our best interest in mind.

However in spite of the fact that this kind of practice is non-existent in the natural health arena where compared to conventional medicine harm being caused from natural medicines is virtually non-existent, they are labeled as "dangerous, unscientific, unproven snake oils". Yet it is interesting that if practitioners of alternative medicine practiced in the same manner as allopathic (drug-based) medicinal practitioners, it would never be acceptable, and many would have been imprisoned long ago. On top of all this, sadly it has also become commonplace for those unfortunate enough to have some sort of an "incurable" illness to try natural or alternative medicine as a last resort, when it is sometimes too late. Then alternative medicine is blamed for lack of success.

What does any of this have to do with Lyme disease?

There will be many that strongly disagree and hold dissent with what I am about to say, as it hits at the heart of a long-term belief system you may have held. Regardless, whether you agree or not, keep an open mind since your primary goal in the reading of this book is to gleam something that can aid you in your search for healing. Everything else is secondary.

There is a lot of resistance in some to the idea of herbal and non-drug treatments with any condition, let alone Lyme disease. Some believe that "real" medicine must be drug-based. Non-drug based medicine is therefore inferior at best, and snake oil at worst. The paradigm that you accept will determine which path you take. To have an intelligent discussion about the merits of whether or not a certain product works, it must be done not from a legal definition which is dishonest. After all, anything can be declared to be legal, even if it isn't the truth. But rather should be from an honest and objective viewpoint.

There is a general misconception that drug-based antibiotics are superior to herbal and non-drug substances. Of course it depends on which antibiotic and which non-drug product you are comparing to each other, and for what microbes you are testing them against. Remember however that one of the things we have become acutely aware of is the terrible consequences that have resulted from antibiotic development over the years, and the super-bugs that are now developing as a result.

Interestingly this same observation cannot be said of non-drug therapies. Nature was designed to maintain a balance, not to isolate.

The administration of antibiotics has not only lead to super-germs, but their side effects can include kidney and liver failure, nausea, hearing loss and ear damage, severe intestinal and abdominal cramps, systemic fungal infection, dizziness, headaches, to name a few. And in the case of some fluoroquinolone anti-biotics, some of which are prescribed for Lyme disease, very serious tendon ruptures and other serious side-effects have been life altering. But nobody thinks twice of this common practice in conventional medicine, even when these effects happen on a regular basis. And that's just with short term use. Multiply that by months and sometimes years in the unending administration of antibiotics to chronically ill Lyme patients who never are cured, the destruction they have on their health by damaging the gut, candidiasis and other parasite overgrowth, food allergy development, the killing off of good bacteria, and not to mention the weakening of the immune system since some 80% + of the immune system resides in the intestinal tract.

Herbal antimicrobials generally speaking have a distinct advantage over drug-based antibiotics in that many, if not most of them do not have nearly the same capacity to weaken intestinal flora as drugs. While most antibiotics are non-discriminating against all bacteria, good or bad, beneficial bacteria are generally helpful to both animals and plants/soils alike. However certain antimicrobials have broad antibacterial activity, which can in turn lead to a deeper problem.

The immune system has a difficult enough time as it is trying to gain a foot-hold against Lyme-related infectious microbes. Not only do they overwhelm immunity, but these germs have the capacity to deliberately down-regulate immune cells. By taking bactericidal substances that are meant to aid immunity, the gut becomes weakened, which has the unintended consequence of further weakening immune cells even more.

For a Lyme patient, relying soley on the immune system to battle against Bb and it's various co-infectious germs may be likened to requiring a 10 year-old little girl to lift 200 lbs. over her head. She may be able to handle 20 lbs. But 200 are just not within her capabilities. You can feed her all kinds of vitamins and protein shakes, but until you can whittle the weight down enough until it is within her capacity to lift, it just "ain't gonna happen." So Bb infection overwhelms the immune system. Although we can do everything within our means to enhance immunity, it is generally beyond the natural capacity of human protective cells to effectively battle against the Lyme pathogen without outside help. But this help, particularly as it relates to antibiotics, although may aid by the killing off a large number of bacteria, can also impede the immune system from taking over once the bacterial load becomes reduced to within a range when the body's immune system would normally take over. Unless the intestinal floras are maintained to a level that can strengthen the immune system, the body's own defensive capabilities will never adequately be able to be restored. This is another reason why the taking of antibiotics alone will seldom address the needs of the Lyme patient. Antibiotics indirectly damage the immune system not only due to its toxicity, but because impairing beneficial bacteria leads to a weakened immune response. This is a primary reason why so many patients relaspse. Their immune system is further weakened by antibiotics.

However on the flip side, some may say that the trade off is that drug-based medicine is much more potent, and that is the price we must pay to be able to have access to such medicine. That may in fact have some merit when one considers emergency medicine and the life-saving drugs and procedures that are used. In fact that is where conventional medicine excels. However when one balances the long term costs, side effects, and effectiveness of herbal and other alternative substances, that cannot be said of most other areas of drug-based medicine when it comes to efficacy. And it is especially not true when it comes to the area of antibiotic and anti-microbial therapies. If the same research were done in the area of herbal medicines, and the same double-blind studies were applied comparing antibiotics with non-drug therapies, it is my personal belief that the non-drug therapies would be far superior to most antibiotics, hands down. However that is an argument that is not likely to find an arena any time soon, since the exploration of herbal and other inexpensive non-drug based therapies does not attract financial incentives to fund such research to demonstrate comparable effectiveness as drugs, because that is the way the game is rigged. This "game rigging" however cannot fool or hide the truth from those of us that know the truth. *Lack of scientific evidence will never constitute proof that alternative non-drug based substances are ineffective. It just means they have not been studied.* In fact in some cases they are even far more effective.

For example, a highly drug resistant form of Staphylococcus aureus called MRSA is now resistant to most antibiotics, and has increasingly become a danger and threat of death to its victims. (Some forms of Staphylococcus, as well as other members of a group of bacteria sometimes called "flesh-eating bacteria" cause a condition called *Necrotizing fasciitis* in some immune-weakened individuals and diabetics which can be life-threatening. These bacteria emit toxins sometimes referred to as "super-antigens" which lead a person's own immune system to attack the infected tissues in an effort to control the rapidly spreading infection.) However a number of plant-based essential oil diffusions such as lemongrass oil and tea tree oil have been able to inhibit its growth, or kill it altogether when all other antibiotics have failed.

Chemical properties in a certain specie of tea tree have been discovered in a particular honey harvested in New Zealand called Manuka honey which is known to kill MRSA in studies.

Moringa, a tree with superior nutritional properties to virtually any known plants was studied and discovered to have equivalent anti-biotic activities as tetracycline in certain applications.

Kalmegh, a shrub that grows in northern India was studied and found to kill leptospira, another spirochete infection.

Citric acid activated sodium chlorite produces a gas called chlorine dioxide, and is proported to have more consistently cured malaria than any pharmaceutical drug known.

Many such examples can be sited, and will be explained later. However the notion that prescription antibiotics have a general superior activity to plant based extracts or other non-drug applications against Lyme disease has not been proven by science! What is supported by science is that they are studied and used more because they are profitable. And what has also been proven beyond a doubt, is that as a curative modality against chronic Lyme disease antibiotics are an almost complete failure. That's not to say that many do not find relief from them. But looking to antibiotics to cure chronic Lyme for the vast majority of Lyme patients has thus far been a pipe dream. As a matter of fact, due to the failure of antibiotics to adequately address chronic Lyme disease, many conventional lyme-literate medical doctors are now preferring natural antimicrobials over pharmaceutical drugs due to their effectiveness and lack of toxicity. There will always be the occasional exception. But to those critics that say natural or non-drug therapies against chronic Lyme have not been proven, neither have drugs.

As we proceed and later begin to discuss the various alternative Lyme therapies, keep in mind that it is especially true with Lyme disease that the responses that people have to any particular treatment vary widely from patient to patient, whether drug-based or otherwise. The Lyme patient must understand that he is about to embark on a journey of the unknown insofar as what will work for him/her, and for how long. There is no one plan that works for everyone, or perhaps even for most people as there are many variables in this disease—many strains of Borrelia, morphology (form of the bacteria), which co-infections you have, how long you are on a therapy, what combinations you apply, your own particular health challenges, your unique immune response, detox capabilities, etc. And it is up to you, working with your healthcare provider to determine what path to take, and what options to choose.

Therefore, as you begin to formulate your approach to the therapies you will employ, keep in mind this chapter. Your paradigm will determine your outlook and ultimately your decisions that will lead to your results. Use your own common sense and listen to what your heart tells you is right. What you are about to learn has been used by others in the past to find help, which gives you hope that whatever path you take has been walked before. However in the end, it is your journey and no one else's.

ENDNOTES

1. *How does the law define a drug?* From FDA website: http://www.fda.gov/cosmetics/guidancecomplianceregulatoryinformation/ucm074201.htm Retrieved Feb. 3, 2013
2. *Cancer: The Shocking Truth About The Effectiveness of Chemotherapy* Chris Teo PhD http://ezinearticles.com/?Cancer:-The-Shocking-Truth-About-the-Effectiveness-of-Chemotherapy&id=347096
3. *Proving the Existence of Oxygen in a Liquid Nutritional Product (Vitamin O) Through Blood Gas Analyses of Therapy/Placebo-Supplemented Hutterites* by John Heinerman, Ph.D http://www.brunnerbiz.com/vitamino/vitamino-2001study.pdf
4. *Death by Medicine* By Gary Null, PhD; Carolyn Dean MD, ND; Martin Feldman, MD; Debora Rasio, MD; and Dorothy Smith, PhD Life Extension Magazine March 2004 http://www.lef.org/magazine/mag2004/mar2004_awsi_death_01.htm
5. *The lawlessness of the FDA, Big Pharma immunity, and crimes against humanity (opinion)* Mike Adams Editor Naturenews.com June 29, 2006 http://www.naturalnews.com/019497_FDA_drug_the.html

CHAPTER 2

The Origins of Lyme Disease
(or Don't you Lyme to me!)

THE THREE STAGES OF LYME

Lyme disease generally unfolds in three stages. This book deals with the last two. It is generally accepted that the first stage is curable if caught early enough and treatment is aggressively administered. Stage one is of course the initial infection. The different vectors will be discussed in more detail later. However, whether from a tick bite, mosquitoe or other insect, contracting it from another person, or whether it emerges from a stealth form in an already infected individual, the spirochete form can suddenly incite a severe immune response. This reaction can lead to acute onset symptoms which are often exhibited as fever, muscle pain, headache, lethargy, chills, and if bitten, sometimes the erythema migrans (bull's eye) rash. Stage 2 Lyme, sometimes called "early disseminated" occurs when the spirochetes begin to multiply, spread throughout the body, and establish infection systemically. Generally in this stage, any number of symptoms may be present such as: joint pain; neurological symptoms—facial twitching and/or numbness in the extremities, meningitis, dizziness, restless leg or muscle twitching, sensitivity to light; brain and cognitive functions impaired such as severe depression, anxiety, rage, foggy concentration, sadness; sweats particularly at night, knee inflammation, skin rash or itching, chronic fatigue, heart palpitations or fluttering, sinus infection, swollen glands, sore throat, pain or swelling around eyes.

Of course there is no distinct set of symptoms exclusive to a particular stage. The symptoms likely are more a measure of the degree and progression of the infection both in regards to location in the body, as well as the manifestation of the morphology of the bacteria.

By stage 3 most Lyme sufferers have already received some form of treatment. Although some improvement is experienced, this often results in the bacteria becoming intracellular, expressing pleomorphic forms, and begin to develop biofilms as a defensive maneuver. This can further symptoms with low back pain, stiff neck, chronic skin problems, deep joint pain, sight problems or reduced field of vision, old injuries becoming arthritic. Stages two and three are often indistinguishable. However the longer this chronic form of Lyme lasts, generally the more difficult to eradicate as pleomorphism, intracellular L-forms and biofilm forms become entrenched in the body representing the extreme resistance that this stage is well-known for.

This is also the stage of the disease that many doctors are in denial regarding. The basis of their argument is that continued antibiotic treatments beyond the intial month or two do not improve the condition further. (This is like saying a person can no longer have cancer because the cancer drugs they took would have cured it. Or that a person can't truly be in continuous pain because their pain medicine would have stopped the pain if in fact they were truly in pain.) As a result, these physicians hold that the patient's condition must either be based upon some auto-immune aspect of the disease, or is attributed to some other underlying cause. In other words their entire position is based upon a false assumption that antibiotics would have completely cured the patient of the disease, and therefore any ongoing symptoms cannot be from unresolved infection. The interesting thing about these doctors that hold these positions is that they virtually never find or discover another cause that is treatable that can support their belief. They end up spending their patient's money on continuous tests until the patient finally gives up and moves onto another doctor. If they do find another underlying cause that is treatable, that does indeed prove that that particular patient did have another condition, but leaves the vast majority of Lyme patients with no help.

Many studies have verified the persistence of spirochetes even after multiple treatments of various antibiotics. [1, 2] As subjective evidence that unresolved infection is the cause of chronic Lyme, many patients have utilized therapies specifically designed to address the more difficult to treat drug-resistant aspects of the disease, and have found success, such as the Marshall protocol, salt/c and others which are designed as longer-term therapies. However biofilms are still going to plague many since our understanding of Lyme-based biofilms is so new that therapies resolving this problem are still in the early stages. Nevertheless, the chronic Lyme model is much more supported by scientific evidence than any other, when one considers that the entire basis of post-lyme syndrome is based almost entirely on an assumption that is not supported by science. [3]

> "Post-Lyme syndrome" is what some medical doctors are calling the symptoms experienced by Lyme patients generally following a course or two of antibiotics. The assumption is being made that the abx's worked, killed the infection, and now damage done to the body from the now-eradicated bacterial infection is the aftermath of the disease. They no longer, according to these doctors, have Lyme disease. They have "post-Lyme syndrome".

I would also like to give you a brief personal view regarding the origin of Lyme disease. Much of the evidence is already available from other sources. So I will not take much time reviewing their details, but only to highlight them and put them in a proper perspective. We have all at one time or another heard a story told, or were given the details of circumstances that lead someone to come to a certain conclusion, and said to ourselves, "something is just not right about that", or "there are just too many inconsistencies in that story for that to be believable". When we make decisions based upon false conclusions, or inconsistencies, then we can't make the right choices. Such is the story of Lyme disease.

Here is the false religion what we have been told to believe in the past. *Lyme disease is a tick-borne illness.* (Therefore it is not contagious and cannot be contracted by any other known means.) *It is found primarily in the Northeastern US.* (Therefore if you live in another part of the country, it is extremely unlikely you could have contracted it.) *It is like most other bacteria, except with its own unique set of symptoms.* (Therefore a course or two of antibiotics will kill it.) *Tests have been established by way of CDC guidelines to determine if you have the bacteria living in you.* (Therefore if your tests are negative, you do not have Lyme disease.) *There is no such thing as chronic Lyme disease, since abx kill the bacteria.* (Therefore any ongoing problems must be attributed either to some other condition, or you have emotional issues.)

If you are currently seeing a doctor that holds to these ideas, you may want to consider finding another doctor. Why? Because when one looks at the preponderance of evidence, "something is just not right about that", and "there are just too many inconsistencies in the story for that to be believable". This is "old-school" thought that has been slowly dying as more pieces of the puzzle are coming together. And your doctor is going to base his medical and treatment decisions based upon those old ideas. One can see the results of this false religion of Lyme disease being played out in the Northeast where these ideas are mostly accepted. Some medical doctors are not treating their patients beyond a course or two of antibiotics since legally a definitive positive lab test result is required in order to put a patient on long-term abx. Insurance companies are refusing to pay for ongoing therapy in the absence of a definitive conclusive test result and diagnosis, leaving patients with no way to pay for treatments. And many doctors have been sued by the state and even imprisoned for medical malpractice who decide to continue to help their patients because they do not follow certain guidelines of "standard" practice. This is all because some have accepted the false religion of traditionally accepted ideas about Lyme disease. But once you learn the world is not flat, how you view and live in that world changes forever.

Other vectors of infection exist that seem to be being blatantly ignored. Dr. Lida Mattman PhD in Immunology, long time researcher and professor, and Nobel Prize nominee in medicine wrote a ground-breaking book identifying microbial cell-wall deficient forms called Stealth Pathogens. As heretofore unknown sources of illness, these forms are known to morph or change from their classic forms, into sometimes a myriad of forms which have the potential to elude virtually every avenue used by human immunity to combat them. Dr. Mattman also became well-known for the development of a unique culturing method which allowed her to culture numerous forms of Borrelia Burgdorferi including the CWD (cell-wall deficient, aka "variant") form. This enabled the expansion of our knowledge of this pathogen enormously. Dr. Mattman was able to culture Bb and its various forms which had been previously challenging or impossible. Up to that time, it had been thought that arthropods or ticks were the only vectors or source of Bb bacterial transmission. However Dr. Mattman discovered many other sources of infection previously unknown. She was able to culture Bb and its various forms from not only ticks, but also from flies, mosquitoes, and fleas. Even tears. Her pioneer work in this area brought her notoriety in that she began to throw wide open the door to many critics whose ideas about Lyme disease had to be completely rewritten.

However European research began to reveal similar conclusions as it became known that mosquitoes in Europe are carriers of Borrelia. [4] So it is not just a tick-borne illness. If that is true, then the amount of infected people can only be described as staggering. One of the explanations as to why ticks are often demonstrated as inducing the bull's eye rash is that the spirochete, generally accepted as the most virulent form, is readily disseminated from the gut of the tick. That means that the most virulent and immune reactive form of the bacteria is disseminated into the body at the time of the bite, and is immediately detected by the immune system. This highly reactive response is extremely unlikely to occur with immediate exposure to other forms of the bacteria since the spirochete is the form that readily expresses the highly toxic lipoprotein outer surface antigens not generally expressed by other forms.

The well-known EM rash is rarely seen with the bites of other insects as Dr. Mattman had demonstrated that a high percentage of L-forms, which do not readily express these proteins, exist in these other insects. Thus cell-wall deficient forms are not nearly as virulent as spirochetes, and would likely not induce such a reactive response as spirochetes. In addition to that, the preponderance of evidence suggests that the northeastern strains tend to be more virulent and affect more bodily systems than other areas of the country and Europe. This is another contributing factor in the high incidence of EM rash reports in the northern US. We will later however learn of at least one other Borrelia specie other than the Burdorferi sensu stricto variety that does in fact commonly induce the bull's eye rash.

To those not familiar with the book *Lab 257*, very credible evidence that germ-warfare experiments were done on ticks on Plum Island. It is no coincidence then that the first reported case of what came to be known as "Lyme Disease" came from this area. Lyme, Connecticut is right across the waters from Plum Island where a 14 year old boy became infected. He was playing near the ferry dock which was the only way to and from the island. Deer and other small animals are known to travel to and from the island thru the water. The island was actually patrolled by armed guards in order to keep animals from traveling across the water. This would explain why Lyme symptoms from that northeastern part of the country are more virulent, has spread like wildfire in the northeast, and now has spread massively to other parts of the country.

Now Lyme disease is being reported in nearly every state. It should also be pointed out that similar disease states coinciding with Lyme symptoms have been recorded over a hundred years ago, particularly in Europe [5] (see Alfred Buchwald 1883, Arvid Afzelius 1909) although it is known that European strains are not as aggressive, nor do they affect as many physiological systems as American strains. [6]

We have been told that Lyme disease is not contagious, since it can only be caused by the bite of a tick. It has already been definitively proven scientifically that there many vectors of Lyme disease, other than tick bites. That is a truth that will die hard as it was also difficult to finally accept that the earth wasn't flat. But let's look further at some supporting evidence.

As early as 1985 a study was presented to determine the level and duration of infectivity of spirochetes thru several forms of direct inoculation in deer mice. The infection was observed by the development of antibodies as determined by indirect immunofluorescent (IFA) antibody titer. As controls, 5 uninfected mice were placed in the same cage as the infected mice. In time, each of the 5 uninfected mice developed antibodies to Borrelia Burgdorferi, and 42 days later Bb was isolated from one of the mice. This meant that direct contact was all that was necessary in order for Lyme pathogens to become infectious. The researchers concluded "These findings show that *B. burgdorferi* can be transmitted by direct contact without an arthropod vector." [7]

In 1986 an experiment was done on 3 dogs to see if Bb infection could be transmitted thru direct contact. One of the dogs was not inoculated, but allowed to play with the others. On day 21 after the initial contact IFA antibody titer indicated infection with Bb in the non-inoculated dog. Again, these researchers concluded "These results indicate that, contact transmission of B. burgdorferi may occur between dogs, dogs can be subclinically infected with B. burgdorferi and have persistent infections." [8]

An interesting document provided as a Biosafety sheet on Borrelia burgdorferi from the Canadian Office of Biosafety in 1997, edited and provided by the Colordo State University, indicates that even prior to 1982, the year of the "official discovery" of the agent of Lyme disease, there were 45 cases and 2 deaths from laboratory-acquired infections of Bb. The source of transmission was determined to come from "blood, cerebrospinal fluid, urine, skin scrapings, retinal and synovial specimens; naturally or experimentally infected mammals, their ectoparasites and their infected tissues." One of the primary sources of infection listed as an accidental hazard—infectious aerosols. This indicates that not only contact infection is possible, but mucosal transmission. [9] But even more interesting is that these reports indicate that Borrelia Burgdorferi was being experimented with and known about even prior to 1976 since the reports of infection came prior to that time. This means the gov't was aware of Bb and its dangers prior to its "official" discovery by Dr. Burgdorferi.

The Yale Journal of Biology and Medicine cited references that reported erythema migrans (skin legions from European "Lyme" disease) has repeatedly been observed to be transmitted from person to person. The etiological agent or source is determined to be from spirochete infection. [10, 11] Acrodermatitis chronica atrophicans (European EM rash) is also known to be caused by American strains of Bb. [12-14]

Spirocheteal forms of bacteria are notoriously a highly contagious form of bacteria. And this becomes another factor that makes the theory that only tick bites can cause Lyme disease have little credibility. There are many types of spirochetal infections. One such well known example that we are all aware of is Treponema Pallidum, the spirochete that causes syphilis. One of the unique features of spirochetes is that they are difficult to culture. They require very specialized conditions and culture mediums. Treponema pallidum, the spirochetal infection causing syphilis has been considered to be impossible to culture. Yet ironically is highly contagious, meaning it can't be grown in the laboratory, but can very easily be disseminated from the culture of human blood or bodily fluids. Many parallels have been made in research regarding the syphilis spirochete and Borrelia spirochete. It doesn't take a rocket scientist to understand that Lyme spirochetes, which comparatively speaking are much easier to culture than the syphilis spirochete, could also be transmitted in this same way. There have been reports of spouses giving Lyme to each other. [15]

According to an abstract presented by Dr. Gregory Bach DO at the International Scientific Conference on Lyme Disease, April, 2001, PCR/ Western Blot testing was performed on semen samples of male Lyme patients, and one female sexual partner. It was trying to be determined the potential for sexual transmission if only one partner had Western Blot or PCR determined Lyme disease. The results: "ALL positive semen/vaginal samples in patients with known sexual partners resulted in positive Lyme titers/PCR in their sexual partners." [16]

But the idea of Lyme being contagious thru sexual contact is immediately dismissed by most doctors because they have been trained to believe that ticks are the only vector of transmission. However, patients are known to have "incubating syphilis" in which they are infected long before any manifestation of disease, [17] just as Borrelia infections are. So a connection would not immediately be made. Hence these kinds of stories tend to be suppressed by doctors and governmental agencies which either don't take them seriously, or (in my opionion) are deliberately suppressing this information to prevent public fear.

(Another reason doctors discount the ability for Bb infection outside of tick-borne transmission is that tick bites often bring on an almost immediate onset of symptoms; while most other forms tend to be incubating, then brought on later due to immune-compromising or stress related factors, as well as the eventual interaction that prior viral, parasitic or co-infectious bacteria incite. More on this later.)

It has been suggested by the American Lyme Disease Foundation that the comparing of Lyme and syphilis spirochetes is not applicable due to Bb spirochetes having limited capacity to survive on the surface of the skin. [18] The forgone scientific studies have proven this to be untrue. But even if it were true, it is irrelevant since kissing and sexual intercourse goes beyond the "surface" of the skin to mucosal transmission. Even if that were true, Lyme spirochetes have demonstrated remarkable adaptability by morphing into a form that that would ensure their survival. Again, we refer to studies demonstrating that contact has caused infection.

Also, Dr. Ray Jones M.D. speaking of Lyme infection says "Of the 5,000 children I've treated, 240 have been born with the disease" indicating a congenital origin. Particularly in areas of the country where the more virulent strains are suspected such as the northeastern US, members of entire families have been known to have developed Lyme disease where no other explanation can be found, other than somehow internally transmitting the disease to one another. [19] Again, Dr. Mattman has even cultured Borrelia from tears. [20] So to say that even casual contact is not a possibility is ignoring scientific evidence.

Certainly no one doubts that the guts of ticks are an attractive culture medium for spirochetes, and particularly Borrelia Burgdorferi. As we said, spirochete lipoproteins express highly virulent antigens. Spirochetes do not like living in the body fluids where immune cells thrive since they are easily identified and induce an almost hyper immune response. And it explains why spirochetes almost always evoke severe illness in the beginning stages of the infection.

It has been believed by some researchers that other forms of Borrelia Burgdorferi besides the spirochete, (forms which do not express the highly toxic outer surface proteins) are unlikely to induce such a severe immune response. This is a likely reason why only a percentage of tick bites induce erythema migrans since spirochetes are known to be readily transmitted. Other forms, although perhaps transmitted as well, may lie in wait until they are challenged, only to later morph to express these proteins. This appears to be the primary factor in its ability to become infective. As proof of this, researchers removed certain Bb plasmids known to be necessary in order for Bb to alter its lipoprotein structures. They learned that in their absence Bb became non-infectious (would not induce an immune response.) So Bb utilizes these plasmids, or switches them on, in order for it to express variations and ultimately invoke an immune response. [21] Again, more on plasmids later.

Given what we now know of Bb's capacity to infect as any other bacteria do, why would anyone come to the conclusion that ticks are the only vectors of transmission? In fact the idea that any microorganism can only be vectored by one source is scientifically unproveable. That means you must have examined everywhere that it could be at the same time, and found it to not be there, which is of course just not possible. It may be accurate to state that Lyme disease is vectored by ticks, but it is deliberately misleading and untrue to imply that it only comes from ticks.

An interesting test that was made available several years ago was the patented Bowen QRIBb test developed by Dr. JoAnne Whitaker who has treated many Lyme patients. It utilizes the Direct Specific Flourescent Antibody Method enabling one to visibly see the microbe, not measure antibody titers. The fluorescencing stain technique is able to identify the cell wall deficient and cyst form in the blood of infected patients. Dr. Lida Mattman worked closely with Dr. Whitaker to confirm thru culture what they were finding thru the QRIBb test. From Bowen research literature, "Of 316 same draw blood samples, 316 cultured specimens grew out the organism Bb, and our Bowen Q-RiBb test was positive on all 316. The culture method is considered the 'gold standard' for making a definitive diagnosis of an infective disease." [22] Dr. Whitaker comments on why there are no negatives. "We believe this indicates the magnitude of the problem. We believe the problem is not only endemic, but may also be reaching epidemic proportions." [23]

This test has received a lot of criticism due to its high number of positive results. In fact I know of one doctor who sent in his blood sample for testing who did not even have Lyme disease or any illness, but wanted to see what kind of response he would have. The test did show positive for Lyme L-forms. One can therefore see why this would receive little diagnostic credibility. I can also recall one time reading on

Dr. Whitaker's website, that in some 1,700 tests, only two were negative for Bb—"a man from Germany, and a dog".

One interesting note regards a test that has fallen into some ill-repute with regards to its reliability for Lyme testing, the Elisa test. Many LLMD's now consider this to test to be virtually worthless as a diagnostic tool. According to one Lyme medical doctor, when the test was first developed for Lyme disease they were having problems in that an unexplectedly high amount of people were testing positive. [24] It was assumed at the time that Lyme disease was in fact a rare disease. But low and behold, many test subjects who were not displaying Lyme symptoms were testing positive. As a result, the test sensitivity level or set point was raised to exclude many borderline and marginally positive subjects. However the level was somewhat arbitrarily determined. What that now meant was that although many subjects may have been testing positive, they were excluded from a positive outcome and referred for other testing, Western Blot. Perhaps this was done in order to maintain some credibility, as a test that yielded mostly positive results, even in those that were not displaying symptoms, would be of little diagnostic value. This seems rather consistent with the QRibb test which was also finding the majority of patients positive for Borrelia infection.

Now before I make a point I would like to make an observation. One would have assumed that in order to have a non-infected standard control group (aka negative controls) by which to compare antibody levels, there would be a way to check for this. After all, if you are going to make a comparison of infected vs non-infected individuals, it would be necessary to be certain that the non-infected group was in fact—non-infected. But instead, patient symptoms and history were used as the determining factor, and an assumption was made that since this group had no history of specific predetermined symptoms of Lyme, they must be clear of infection. However the problem with this approach is that it makes several flawed assumptions: 1) That every infected person is going to display symptoms, which we now know is not the case. 2) That some of the individuals may have had past Bb exposure, but their immune system was able to control it. 3) That some of the individuals did in fact display symptoms of infection that were not included in the criteria. For example, low level generalized brain fog, fatigue, lymph swelling or headache, but were not (yet) displaying the major Lyme syndromes such as severe joint pain, neurological symptoms, heart palpitations, etc. 4) That the bacterial infection is in fact a rare occurrence.

As a result of this, many negative controls were not actually negative, and were producing positive responses to the test. Since it was assumed these were false positives, they adjusted the set points higher. Doing this meant that there was now an overlap zone wherein some negative controls that may have been reacting positively to the test who were displaying no predetermined symptoms were excluded, while some who had distinct Lyme symptoms were now excluded since their titer levels were below the set point.

In my opinion, this same faulty testing has filtered its way down to Western Blot testing. These tests are given almost random sensitivity guidelines which are supposed to be used to help determine a positive or negative outcome. In my opinion, most Western Blot tests start off on the wrong foot right from the beginning because the test usually utilizes only a few highly reactive strains called Bb 31 and Bb 297. Although the lipoproteins used to determine the band reactivity levels are supposed to be representative of most pathogenic Borrelia strains, they are not necessarily equal in their level of reactivity. Nor will any particular individual's immune cells react the same to each lipoprotein. Therefore the sensitivity of these tests must by their very nature be set arbitrarily. Not only will how each person react be different, but some less reactive strains in infected individuals will also render different responses in testing, since they are not the same strain used in the test, nor have their antibodies become sensitive to those particular lipoprotein expressions.

Let's put it another way. A rather obvious puzzling question is, although there are considerably fewer than a hundred known infectious strains of Bb, why would one give undue credence to a test that deliberately only uses two of the more highly sensitive strains that consequently would result in significantly lowered positive test results in patients who may be infected with a less sensitive strain? A false assumption is being made here which is rather obvious and yet seems to be the elephant in the room that no one is mentioning: everyone's immune cells will not react the same to all strains or their lipoprotein expressions. Therefore how can a definitive test based upon these criteria be used to fundamentally diagnosis Lyme disease?

Add to that the CDC also inexplicably, and to the disbelief of many medical doctors, set the guidelines for positive test results so high it was difficult to not think that this was done deliberately to mask the scope of the epidemic, and to fool the public from believing that Lyme is far more prevalent than they want you to believe. The sensitivity levels were set so high that it excluded many infected individuals, even those manifesting obvious clinical symptoms. (Incidentally and a little off topic, one may also ask why the CDC did not originally scrutinize Plum Island government biological research laboratories when the first outbreak occurred in Lyme, Connecticut once it was learned that the source of Lyme disease was a bacterial agent? Plum Island would have been a prime suspect to interrogate as an obvious source for the spread of an infectious disease, because it is their job to do so by looking at all possibilities to protect the public.)

Culture testing is the single most reliable testing available, as it is able to confirm other kinds of tests. This QRIBb test was confirmed to be accurate by culture testing. So we therefore know that those who were tested were in fact actually infected by Borrelia L-forms, but does not necessarily tell us if all those infected did in fact have the actual disease, that is, the expression of symptoms. As we said earlier, Lyme spirochetes do not like to live in the blood stream because they are wide open to immune system attack. So they tend to hide intracellularly, as well as burrow deep into tissues out of range of macrophages. They can also morph into the L-forms and return to or remain in the bloodstreams and other bodily fluids in these stealth forms since they don't have a normal cell wall as spirochetes do. That is one reason why spirochetes are not commonly found florescencing in these blood tests as are L-foms, and it is also why many who test positive for these tests may be asymptomatic in the absence of the spirochete expressive form of the illness.

What tests such as QRIBb and other such tests imply, particularly given they demonstrate a very high number of positive test results, even in those that do not exhibit Lyme symptoms, is that many, if not perhaps even most people may be infected with the CWD form of Borrelia! Let me say that again. I personally believe that many more people are in fact infected with some Borrelia strain than is currently believed. It is not only my own personal viewpoint, but the viewpoint of many researchers and Lyme cognizant doctors, that some CWD forms of Bb have existed in a symbiotic relationship with man and beast for millennia.

"Nick Harris, Ph.D., director of the International Lyme and Associated Diseases Society (ILADS), states 'Lyme is grossly under-reported. In the U.S., we probably have about 200,000 cases per year.'" [25]

This is a personal viewpoint that may have no relevance in a person's personal journey for healing from Lyme. So whether it is true or not, makes no difference except that it offers a logical explanation why so many develop Lyme disease who were never remotely exposed to ticks.

Until Dr. Mattman's work, the shear magnitude of Lyme disease was not known to the general public. That's why the Attorney General for the State of Michigan ordered her to stop providing assistance to doctors with her culture testing. Her work uncovering the extent of cell-wall deficient form infections of Bb led many to realize that Lyme infection is being harbored in many people who do not yet even have Lyme symptoms. When one realizes that for hundreds of years humans have co-inhabited America where these bacteria were infecting not only ticks, but other insects, it was inevitable that humans would soon themselves become carriers. Since our modern learning has taught us that spirochetes are much more virulent, we assumed spirochetes were the only source of illness. With our current understanding that Bb is pleomorphic and that benign forms can change into disease-producing forms, we now know that almost anyone anywhere can develop Lyme disease. This is why Dr. Joanne Whitaker's work using Bowen testing revealed that virtually everyone they tested had the CWD form living in them. Even in those that had no Lyme symptoms. This makes perfect sense. It is my belief that Lyme is a disease that is being carried by most people in one form or another. It is NOT just a tick-borne illness. I am not unique in that I personally developed Lyme disease, not from a tick-bite, but from an injury that stressed the body to react to a microbe that had already been infecting me long before who knows when. That is another reason why so many have the illness in one form or another who do not even suspect Borrelia Burgdorferi infection. It is a very common infection. It just doesn't always make itself known.

Remember, we know that Lyme disease has developed in people who have never been bitten by a tick, and whose illness was vectored by no known cause. And yes, even in those that have never even visited the northeastern and far western United States. Even an emotional stress has been identified as a cause, since we know that stress places the immune system on high alert, and would therefore bring about a condition of hyper-sensitivity to microbes previously tolerated.

In 1998, a study conducted in Switzerland demonstrated that only 12.5% of the patients that tested positive for Borrelia developed clinical symptoms confirming that Borrelia burgdorferi infection is often asymptomatic. A report from Germany outlines the case of a 12 year old boy that developed Lyme Arthritis 5 years after being bit by a tick. The case indicates that the latency period between tick bite and onset of Lyme Arthritis may last up to 5 years. All asymptomatic carriers of Borrelia are at risk of developing Lyme disease at some point. Stress, an increasing health concern for physicians worldwide, may have been the trigger that activated Lyme disease in a patient in Sweden. The case is reported of a 26 year old woman with latent Lyme borreliosis that was concurrently activated with a herpes simplex virus type 1 infection. Immune suppression by stress may have caused activation of both infections. [26]

If in fact there are many vectors of transmission, such as flies, mosquitoes, congenital, sexual, and even casual contact, then it stands to reason that Borrelia infection is a significantly more widespread and common bacteria than has previously been believed. However this should not come to a surprise. There are many other pathogens that are also known to be infecting most people and that have been around for millennia. For example, herpes simplex virus is said to infect most people, [27] yet only a small percentage of the population develops cold sores. The same can be said of Epstein Barr virus, [28] which years ago was identified as being a source of chronic fatigue syndrome. Candida albicans are ubiquitous yeast living in a symbiotic relationship in the gut of animals and humans. Yet Candidiasis, an illness manifesting itself as a systemic overgrowth has only recently in the past 15-20 years been understood to be an iatrogenic or "doctor-borne" illness due to the overuse of antibiotic drugs. That means that Candida must rise to a certain level that triggers sensitivity symptoms and illness. This is exactly what can happen in those infected with some forms of Bb, and sheds new light on what we have come to understand about Lyme disease. Many are carriers who do not display symptoms.

Until Dr. Mattman's research few questioned that only ticks were carriers of Borrelia. Why? Because that is the only place they were looking for it. That is where it reared its ugly head and shouted "hear I am". But as she began to uncover more and more vectors of infection, and realized that she could culture the bacteria from even people who weren't even exhibiting symptoms of Lyme disease (yet), the entire story of Lyme disease had to be rewritten. What many doctors had been saying all along was true. Lyme could even be contracted by simply developing an injury or accident because that set off the immune system to set to repair the area, and low and behold what was found lurking in the injury because it was in the body all along—Borrelia Burgdorferi! Only it was there in its L-form which is a stealth form hiding from the immune system. Then when the worker cells from the immune system examined the injury closely to repair it, they uncovered the bacteria. Upon attempting to extract and kill them, the bacteria defended themselves by turning on gene-like plasmids which altered them to activate a spirochete form in order to be more mobile. This way they could not only move quickly to evade macrophages, but could express proteins which were highly poisonous to immune cells. This is not science fiction. This is a fact that is occurring in thousands of people every day.

A distinction therefore needs to be made and understood between simply being "infected" with a bacterium, and the actual manifestation of symptoms. Bb may remain in a benign form without ever reverting to disease-inducing spirochetes. So that simply being infected with a microbe doesn't necessarily translate into the "disease". This is the important distinction that creates such confusion as well as controversy. Lyme disease is the actual manifestation of symptoms being caused from the presence of Bb infection. It develops when the bacteria have activated specific plasmids which induce an immune response. This is important to distinguish since it would be unrealistic to label Lyme disease with everyone that has been determined by one test or another to have the actual bacteria living in them.

Others would disagree with this. But if so, where is the line drawn? Perhaps Lyme is similar to HIV and AIDS. We say someone is either HIV positive or negative. But being HIV positive does not necessarily mean they have developed AIDS (yet). Just because someone has the flu or cold virus doesn't necessarily mean they have the flu or a cold. So Lyme disease may not necessarily mean that a person has the bacteria living in them, but the manifesting of an actual disease.

The problem that some have in accepting this is that they think of Borrelia as any other pathogen. They do not understand the implications and the seriousness of its pleomorphic capabilities. However when the conditions are right and the immune system is challenged thru a stress or injury, it can "see" once latent or benign stealth germs as a threat, and attack. Thus the battle begins.

Knowing what we do of Borrelia Burgdorferi, these and/or other spirochetal strains of bacteria have been suspected to be either the source of many different illnesses, or certainly has shown good cause to be a contributive factor in Alzheimer's disease, MS, ALS, fibromyalgia, Bell's Palsy, Ankylosing Spondylitis, and a whole host of "mysterious" illnesses and conditions that have gone undiagnosed in many people. If in fact Borrelia is much more common than we thought, it changes everything we have known and believed about Lyme disease.

So what then is the truth? How is Lyme truly vectored, how common is it, where did it originate? The bottom line is that it doesn't matter how one developed Lyme disease, or what the theories might be as to the origins of the bacteria or illness. What is important is recognizing the signs, and seeking proper treatment, whatever that treatment is. The problem however is that in the absence of a positive test result, or with those doctors that don't use clinical diagnoses as their primary determinant, the patient is left vulnerable through no fault of their own. It is bad enough to have become a victim of Lyme disease. But to become a victim of a doctor's ignorance or prejudice that further undermines the patient is inexcusable. Fortunately they are in the minority. In such a case, you the patient must empower yourself, and remember that you are the doctor of your own decisions. You must do what is in your own interest and look out for yourself. It is hoped that these new insights will brush away some of the confusion that has long overshadowed this disease, and give to the reader a new perspective to help him/her make more informed choices along the journey.

ENDNOTES

1. *Detection of Bb by polymerase chain reaction in synovial membrane, but not in synovial fluid from patients with persisting Lyme arthritis after antibiotic therapy.* Ann Rheum Disease 1998 Feb;57(2):118-21, also *Persistence of Bb sensua lato in patients with Lyme Borreliosis* Epidemiol Mikrobiol Imunol 2001 Feb; 50 (1): 10-6, also *Serronegative Chronic Relapsing Neuroborreliosis* Eur. Neurol. 1995;(2):113-7

2. *Chronic Septic Arthritis caused by Bb.* Clin Orthop 1993 Dec(297): 238-41

3. *Chronic Lyme—An Evidence Based Review* Steven Phillips MD http://www.ilads.org/lyme_research/chronic_lyme.html

4. *Detection of Borrelia burgdorferi sensualato in mosquitoes in recreational areas of the city of Szczecin.* Kosik-Bogacka, D., Bukowska, K., Kuzna-Grygiel, W. Annals of Agricultural and Environmental Medicine, (2002) 9(1), 55-57.

5. Vanderhoof-Forschner, K. *Everything you need to know about Lyme Disease.* Hoboken, NJ: John Wiley & Sons, p. 39. (2003)

6. *Immunochemical and immunological analysis of Borrelia burgdorferi strains* Wilske, B., Preac-Mursic, V., Schierz, G., & Busch, K.V. (1986). Zentralbl Backeriol Mikrobiol Hygiene, 263(1-2), 92-102.

7. *Experimental Inoculation of* Peromyscus *Spp. with* Borrelia Burgdorferi: Evidence of Contact Transmission Elizabeth C. Burgess, Terry E. Amundson, Jeffery P. Davis, Richard A. Kaslow, and Robert Edelman Am J Trop Med Hyg March 1986 35:355-359

8. *Experimental inoculation of dogs with Borrelia burgdorferi.* Burgess EC. Zentralbl Bakteriol Mikrobiol Hyg A 1986 Dec; 263(1-2): 49-54

9. *Section 1 - Borrelia Burgdorferi* Lab Animal Resources—Colorado State University website: http://web.research.colostate.edu/ (S(q1o4w355ebxdjs45bqaufu55))/LAR/ams/borrelia.aspx?AspxAutoDetect CookieSupport=1 Retrieved Feb. 3, 2013

10. *ExperimentelleUbertragung des Erythema Chronicum migrans* Binder, E., R. Doepfmer, and 0. Hornstein von Mensch zu Mensch. Hautarzt 1955 11:494-496.

11. *Acrodermatitis chronica atrophicans Herxheimer als Infektionskrankheit.* Gotz H: Die Hautarzt 5:491-504, 1954; 6:249-252, 1955

12. *Identification of three species of Borrelia burgdorferi sensu lato (B.burgdorferi sensu stricto, B. garinii, and B. afzelii) among isolates from acrodermatitis chronica atrophicans lesions.* Picken RN, Strle F, Picken MM, Ruzic-Sabljic E, Maraspin V, Lotric-Furlan S, Cimperman J Source: J Invest Dermatol 1998 Mar;110(3):211-4 Organization: Research Service, Hines Veterans' Administration Hospital, Maywood, Illinois, USA.

13. *Late cutaneous Lyme disease: acrodermatitis chronica atrophicans.* Authors: Kaufman LD, Gruber BL, Phillips ME, Benach JL Source: Am J Med 1989 Jun;86(6 Pt 2):828-30 Organization: Department of Medicine, State University of New York, Stony Brook 11794-8161.

14. *Spirochetes in atrophic skin lesions accompanied by minimal host response in a child with Lyme disease.* Stephen E. Gellis, MD, Miguel J. Stadaecher, MD,PhD, and ALLEN C. STEERE, MD Journal of The American Academy of Dermatology Volume 25-Number 2, Part 2 August 1991

15. *Human to human transmission* Blog posting http://lymetwistontherocks. blogspot.com/2011/01/human-to-human-transmission.html Retrieved Feb. 3, 2013 see also *A most unusual case of a whole family suffering from late lyme borreliosis over 20 years.* Gasser, R., Dusleag, J., Reisinger, E., Stauber, R., Grisold, M., Pongratz, S., Furian, C., Feigl, B., & Klein, W. (1994) Letter to the Editor, *Angiology* **45**(1):85-??. http://ang.sagepub.com/cgi/ pdf_extract/45/1/85 Retrieved Feb. 3, 2013

16. *Recovery of Lyme Spirochetes by PCR in Semen Samples of Previously Diagonosed Lyme Disease Patients* Dr. Gregory Bach, Do.O., P.C. 2415 North Broad Street, Colmar, PA 18915 http://www.canlyme.com/sex.html

17. Gruber, J. (2005). *Lyme Disease: Statistical evaluation of a symptom lag and an empirical theory of flare cycles.* Retrieved July 26, 2005, from Lyme Net Website: http://www.lymenet.de/symptoms/cycles/statistics.htm Retrieved Feb. 3, 2013

18. *Misinformation About Lyme Disease* http://www.aldf.com/Misinformation_about_Lyme_Disease.shtml Retrieved Feb. 3, 2013

19. Rowen, Robert (2003). *If you have ANY chronic debilitating disease, you could be the victom of a Monster Epidemic!* Second Opinion Vol X111 No. 11 November 2003

20. *Stealth Pathogens* "Recovering from Chronic Disease" Presentation by Lida Mattman at the Autoimmunity Research Foundation March 12, 2005. http://www.youtube.com/watch?v=WozrCFW0mRM Retrieved Feb. 3, 2013

21. *Genetic variation of the Borrelia burgdorferi gene vlsE involves cassette-specific, segmental gene conversion* Zhang JR, Norris SJ Infect Immun. 1998 Aug;66(8):3698-704

22. Schaller, J. (2005). *Amazing special darkfield images of tick diseases using fluorescent antibodies.* Retrieved July 26, 2005 from Personal Consult. Website: http://www.personalconsult.com/articles/bowenresearch.html Retrieved Feb. 3, 2013

23. Whitaker, J.A. (2003). *New test for identifying morphing menace: Quantitative rapid identification of Bt (Q-Ribb).* Nutra News: New Thinking, New Discoveries in Nutraceutical Research, Oct., 2003, pp 8-11.

24. *Lyme antibodies revisited* LymeMD blogsite July 15, 2008 http://lymemd.blogspot.com/2008/07/lyme-antibodies-revisited.html Retrieved Feb. 3, 2013

25. *Pilot Study Reveals New Weapon Against Lyme Borreliosis* Article on NutraNews pg. 4. October 2003 http://www.samento.com.ec/nutranews/pdfs/nnutranews1003_high.pdf Retrieved Feb. 3, 2013

26. Ibid. pg. 3.

27. *"Good" Virus/"Bad" Virus The Truth about HSV-1 and HSV-2* Article on Herpes You Are Not Alone website. http://www.herpes.com/hsv1-2.html Retrieved Feb. 18, 2013

28. *Epstein-bar: Scientists Decode Secrets of a Very Common Virus That Can Cause Cancer* Article from "Science Daily" material from Duke University Medical Center Dec. 15, 2010 http://www.sciencedaily.com/releases/2010/12/101215121905.htm Retrieved Feb. 3, 2013

CHAPTER 3

A Few of My Own Efforts

If you have been suffering from Lyme disease for any length of time, then you are well aware of the battle for the search for answers that is involved. And it is truly difficult for those that have not suffered to understand what you are going thru since by all appearances, "you seem to look fine". It's almost like an invisible illness at times since there are often very few external symptoms to observe. But the agony, pain, fatigue, and emotional disturbances can be almost intolerable. This is what becomes the huge motivational factor in our quest for relief, which non-Lymies do not understand. The myriad of products, devices, therapies, gadgets, drugs, and long list of practitioners becomes almost comical as we look outside the box for anything that will render relief. My life has been no exception.

In 2006 I completed my first book called *Lyme Disease, Energy Medicine, and the Biochemistry of Borrelia*. This had been very in-depth research since I was attempting to be as comprehensive as possible looking at Lyme disease from every angle. I must have read several hundred research articles of every nature in an effort to learn everything I possibly could to understand what made this illness so difficult to overcome. That meant having to study not just what people were saying about it, but also important to know was what was not yet understood. Since virtually all of the research that was being done was being examined from an allopathic/conventional paradigm, the solutions (or lack of them) were being addressed from that level. Einstein once said "You can't solve problems by using the same kind of thinking we used when we created them." And I could see from the general lack of lasting healing that was taking place using the conventional approach that I needed to examine different options.

So my focus went beyond the current seemingly unresolvable problems facing both allopaths and naturopaths alike, by exploring the possibilities of using some of the newer advances in the fields exploring quantum energy medicine. I shared a bit about this in an earlier chapter. Some examples of these are NAET developed by Dr. Nambudripod, Bioset by Ellen Cutler, and CranioBiotic Technique (CBT) by Dr. Tony Smith to name only a few. After all, I had tremendous success in my own healing using these methods for other applications. So I knew they worked. And the science behind how they worked was in a completely different paradigm and much firmer ground than so-called conventional medicine. (It's not that I am against conventional medicine so much as that way that it is being used. In my personal opinion conventional medicine excels in emergency medicine, or diagnostics, but mostly doesn't have a clue resolving chronic diseases.)

Since allergic conditions manifested in the body as a result of energy blockages, hence a frustrated or over-reactive immune system, it was only a matter of identifying and releasing those blockages, and resolving individual allergic conditions. I had already understood the basic concept behind energy medicine, and had incredible success employing those therapies. My almost unbelievable healing led me to personally experience over a hundred "clearings" of allergens, or substances which my body was no longer having any kind of allergic reactions to. (You will not hear of these kinds of healings from your medical doctor. They will be scoffed at and ridiculed since he/she has not been trained to heal in this manner. This has become a very common occurrence as energy healing is now becoming more and more mainstream and accepted. You can deny the truth for only so long until at some point the public sees through the false denial from the allopathic medical profession, and their inability to maintain their image of god-like omniscience they hold over the public. Allopathy is slowly becoming like a house of cards they are trying desparately to maintain. I believe the saying "Those who say it can't be done, need to get out of the way of those that are doing it" applies well here.

With this in mind, my research began focusing on the possibility of identifying a specific Bb toxin(s) that might be acting in a similar fashion as other microbial toxins which can wreak havoc on the body, and the immune system's reaction to such substances. After all, I had already experienced a complete resolution to Candidiasis years earlier when my practitioner had identified Candida's specific toxin (acetaldehyde), and eliminated the body's blockage (allergic reaction) to that toxin which had manifested itself as a hyper immune response to Candida. This same principle was used by Dr. Koch when he identified that hyper allergic responses within infected cells to specific viral toxins were the causative agents of tumors and cancer in many of his patients, which he was able to resolve very quickly using his glyoxilide. So I knew this was a very sound and proven principle. The question now remained: could there be some specific identifiable toxin of Borrelia Burgdorferi that is the underlying source of Lyme disease?

After several years of research, I came to discover that no such toxin could be identified as the primary inciting agent in Lyme disease as it was known to occur in many other bacteria, e.g. as botulinum is the neuro-toxin of Clostridium. Working with several practitioners over a 2 year period, and making over 150 attempts at clearing a multitude of combinations of lipoproteins and adjuvants did not result in the elimination of Lyme disease in spite of my best efforts. I had come to learn that while some illnesses were actually based upon an allergy to a toxin, other toxicity effects seem inherently beyond the capacity of human cells to tolerate them. What I eventually came to learn was that certain kinds of intra-cellular infections did not respond to this approach.

So I was forced to try other approaches of energy medicine. The term "energy medicine" encompasses a broad field of research. And no one therapy describes how it is used. Essentially it is the use of modalities that tap into, adjust, modify, and alter, the underlying holographic energy field that gives rise to the physical part of the human body. For example the emotions are a part of that energy field. And when the emotions are affected, it has a direct effect on the physiology of a person. Thoughts can also give rise to changes in the physiology of a person as well. For example stressful thoughts can raise the blood pressure, increase the heart rate, etc. That is a simplistic illustration. Acupuncture would be one example of a kind of therapy that might be called energy medicine. But a completely different paradigm is addressed using energy medicine that addressing physical symptoms alone would not affect.

I soon learned of a practice called Advanced Cell Training being used by a Gary Blier in Rhode Island. He had been using his own special technique which was a form of energy healing. It worked by "retraining" immune cells to focus on the underlying response to the Lyme organism, and by clearing any emotional blocks that might be affecting or inhibiting a healthy and proper immune function. It doesn't use drugs or medicines of any kind. It merely helps the body to heal itself by supporting and restoring the natural flow of intelligence innate within the person that can in turn allow the body to address the infection and heal itself.

It apparently works to various degrees in different people, just like so many other therapies do. According to the testimonies of Lyme patients, its effects range from complete healing of their Lyme, to vast improvement, and in a small percentage of people they experience no benefit at all. When I learned of this therapy, I was intrigued since I was very much involved in this sort of healing already. So I tried it for several weeks, hoping I would be one of the fortunate individuals in the first group. If someone is going to experience improvement, it should start to be seen relatively quickly in the first week or two. It may not be dramatic, but you should see some benefit. If not, it is likely you are one of those that it simply doesn't work for. Unfortunately after several weeks, I couldn't tell it was helping me at all. (They give you a refund within a certain period if it doesn't help.) Over the next year or two I tried it again for a period, but again without benefit. So I had to move on.

> The scientific basis for such healing is explained in some of the newer revelations about how our own DNA can be reprogrammed using words and frequencies together. A Russian biophysicist and molecular biologist Pjotr Garjajev and his collegues, by combining certain radio or light frequencies with language, were able to alter cellular metabolism, as well as correct genetic defects. In one experiment they were actually able to reprogram cells of frog embryos into salamander embryos without gene splicing or using a scalpel. They simply communicated the information using language and frequencies. This explains what some "spiritual healers" and other esoteric forms of

healing have been accomplishing for perhaps thousands of years. Interestingly, the Human Genome Project, which was supposed to be one of the greatest collaborations of scientific research ever endeavored upon, discovered that only about 4 percent of our genes are encoded. What of the other 90+%? It has come to be known that our DNA possesses a language just like our own verbal communication. By using the correct frequencies or channels, DNA can be altered/influenced in ways that years ago would seem unimaginable. So what so-called "scientistis" have been laughing at and criticizing for years as being hocus pocus, or the false deceptions of charlatans, or even have put down as the placebo effect, once again have proven themselves to be closed-minded and unscientific thinkers themselves. A good source of reading is Lee Carroll's *The Twelve Layers of DNA*.

Still seeking to find something that would work, I soon read in the *Townsend Letter for Doctors and Patients* of a therapy that had been tried by a former Congressmen from Iowa, Berkley Bedell, called a *Universal Oral Vaccine*. [1] He had developed Lyme disease which was not being helped by conventional medicine. In short, the "vaccine" is actually oral colostrum from a heifer that had previously had her udder innoculated either directly with Borrelia Burgdorferi, or the infected blood is injected up thru the teat prior to giving birth to the calf. This in turn stimulates an immune response in the animal which causes it to develop antibodies to Bb. Once she gives birth to her calf, the first milk, called colostrum now contains antibodies to Bb and is collected. This colostrum acts much like a vaccine in that the immunoglobulins in the transfer factor confer immunity to the Lyme patient. The result of this is that the immune system learns to fight the bacteria on its own, and eliminates the disease. The Congressman had worked with a friend who was a rancher that was familiar with the procedure. The end result was that it cured him with no further symptoms, even with the complete elimination of his Lyme arthritis.

When I learned of this, I naturally wanted to try this myself. However since some of the people who were involved in trying this were arrested for so called "practicing medicine without a license", I simply couldn't find anyone anywhere that could help me. Due to legal reasons, I cannot explain what I did in the ensuing months that led me to see if this was a viable therapy that might work for me. I will only say that I became the owner of my first cow that I ever owned. I also later learned that the taking of antimicrobial herbs can reduce or even eliminate Lyme spirochetes from the blood, which are necessary in adequate numbers in order to sufficiently induce an immune response in the heifer. If enough of the infectious organism is not present, then the immunity of the animal will not develop a sufficient or effective enough antibody response to produce a proper or effective Lyme-specific colostrum. In the words of Forrest Gump, "And that's all I have to say about that."

Several years before this I had flown to Mexico to see a physician about some research they were doing using the placentas from sharks. They had been having some success using it on Lyme patients. (Apparently there are few reported cases of sharks developing Lyme disease after a tick bite.)

It's amazing the things we will do to get well. So many of us with Lyme disease end up spending years, even decades searching for anything that will relieve our symptoms, let alone cure us of the illness. I recall spending considerable time researching hyberbaric oxygen (HBOT), as my DO recently had installed a system in his office. (By now you know that when I research something, there is no stone left unturned in my attempt to get at the truth of a therapy.) I had a conversation with the director in charge of the unit. I later learned that he actually sells the units and sets them up for doctors in their offices training personnel to use them. I was curious as to what he could tell me of the effectiveness of hyberbaric oxygen for Lyme disease as I was hearing some good things about it, but hadn't heard of anyone that had experienced extended relief from its use. So I asked him his opinion about whether it should be considered as a viable option as a potential to cure Lyme disease. He told me that it usually helps to relieve the symptoms of Lyme disease, but that it won't cure the disease. Ironically, I learned that his own wife has Lyme disease, and has had it quite some time. She has had it for so long in fact, tried so many different treatments with no success, (including virtually unlimited access to HBOT obviously) she said that if she knew that drinking motor oil would cure her of the disease she would do so, she was so desperate for a cure. She is an M.D.

I spent a lot of time researching this therapy and learned that many have found it useful in alleviating symptoms and reducing inflammation. But I have personally never heard of anyone resolving their Lyme disease from its use. Dr. James Schaller MD, who has treated many Lyme patients, ran his own study to determine the effectiveness of HBOT on Lyme and other tick-borne infections. His conclusion was "After 120 treatments at 2.4 atmospheres for 90 minutes each, all participants still had clear and obvious positive findings for all four infections. It failed completely! So advertising that HBOT "kills" Lyme disease is nonsense".[2] Given it is cost prohibitive even as a symptom reducer, I moved on.

For years prior to that time I had become disillusioned by my experience with doctors who didn't seem to know much more about Lyme disease than it is was a tick-born illness, and required antibiotics to be taken for an undetermined period of time. I had already known that, and quickly learned that was a dead end, as relapse seemed the rule more than the exception.

However in the early days when I first began developing Lyme symptoms, like most victims, I didn't know what it was. But after studying my symptoms for awhile, I began to suspect Lyme. I didn't immediately see my medical doctor since I had grown accustomed to finding help for so many of my health problems from alternative practitioners over the years. Although technically speaking alternative doctors are not legally recognized as being qualified to diagnose infectious diseases, they have their own methods for getting a pretty accurate reading on what is going on based upon symptoms and kinesiology. And every one of them was telling me the same thing. But I knew sooner or later I would need to see an MD or DO to confirm my suspicions.

I eventually found myself seeing my DO (Doctor of Osteopathic Medicine, similar to an MD) who had given to me several of the traditional Lyme tests. PCR, Elisa, and Igenex Western Blot. Some of which were borderline positive, some were negative, but my IgM was screaming loud and clear positive. OspA which is not a cross-reacting protein (meaning it is not found in other microbes) and exclusive to Bb, is the most studied, well-known, and reactive of the Bb lipoproteins, also called kd31. And I was having a very strong response 3+ intensity to this protein. Although I had known that Lyme disease was a clinical diagnosis (a diagnosis based upon your history and symptoms rather than relying on lab tests), many doctors were still putting more weight on Lyme testing than patient symptoms. I had been reading the literature that most LLMD's were putting more weight on clinical diagnoses, and in fact my history and symptoms were classic Lyme. However my DO didn't seem to accept that I had Lyme disease since my tests according to him were not definitive. (I later learned that his assessment was incorrect since many LLMD's do not accept the almost ludicrous criteria first set by the CDC.) Also my co-infections came up negative as well. He told me he couldn't legally prescribe to me long-term antibiotics without positive blood tests. But he did start me on several short term doses of Doxy and flagyl, and several others as time went by to see if I would benefit.

It's difficult to place confidence in your doctor when he does not even accept that you have an illness simply because your test results do not fit into his narrow unrealistic view, in spite of the fact that it is actually quite common for Lyme victims to have test results which were not textbook definitive. And it is especially true when your symptoms are completely consistent with Lyme disease, and when other doctors who are specialists in treating Lyme would interpret your test results as being positive since a specific band that was specific to Bb was highly reactive. So I was put into a position of having to find another doctor and start the whole process over again, or find my way on my own. As the years went by, I ended up going to see many doctors of all kinds of specialties, in different states, and as I mentioned, went to Mexico twice. However I would periodically return to see my DO to discuss some new things that I had learned with him. But due to the fact that my symptoms were classic Lyme symptoms, and that most of the other common co-infections had been ruled out, I continued to proceed on the basis that I had Lyme disease. I continued my herbal remedies, which were giving to me good results.

According to CDC "guidelines" it was required that you have both positive IGg as well as IgM antibodies respond to a particular number of bands, as well as specific bands *for reporting purposes*. My classic Lyme symptoms and IgM was screaming loud and clear that I had Lyme. However my IgG were not. IgG antibodies are supposed to be the most numerous, yet second group of antibodies to respond to an infection, and are supposed to indicate the presence of a long-term infection. I say *suppose* to because in people that have a weakened immune system, they are going to create fewer and less responsive IgG antibodies, even if an infectious germ is present. And it has been the experience of LLMD's that certain co-infective microbes have the ability to inhibit the development of Borrelia antibodies altogether. The IgM antibodies are fewer in number, but are going to be the first responders. They generally indicate an active infection, which I of course had. Their presence combined with long-term clinical symptoms in the absence of IgG can indicate a chronic infection, with a weakened immune response. More on that later.

It is funny how things work out in hindsight. Because if I did have a definitive blood test, and my DO did in fact put me on long-term anti-biotics, and if I would have had an intial positive response from the antibiotics, I may have bought into the idea that abx were the answer I was looking for, and wouldn't have spent years searching for what ended being discoveries that have healed my condition. I would still be on the same road as many other Lyme victims hoping for a cure that would never come.

I had already known of many Lyme patients that had been on abx for many years who were still sick. From all that I had come to learn from years of studying Lyme disease, antibiotics were able to stabilize and improve the overall condition of some Lyme sufferers, but almost never offered lasting help for the chronic Lyme patient, as he/she almost always seemed to relapse, or the abx stopped working. Even if you are put on the best antibiotics for long term, your chances of being cured are slim to none. I have always believed in being realistic and honest with people, even if it wasn't what they wanted to hear, so that they could adjust themselves to reality rather than being taken in by false hope. Personally, learning that abx are not likely to cure Lyme disease wasn't a sentence of hopelessness, but a message that I had been knocking on the wrong door.

I will mention that my own experience with antibiotics was that compared to the natural or herbal products I had been taking, antibiotics were offering me little benefit. The herbal products were so effective and having such a positive killing effect, that switching to antibiotics showed little if any (sometimes no) further benefit. This was my own experience. There was however one antibiotic that seemed to show some short-term benefit. A short course of Cipro spontaneously knocked out a long-standing Lyme-induced inflammation in my knee that has never returned. But then Cipro stopped working after awhile, and had showed no benefits to my systemic Lyme symptoms. The herbs however had been consistently giving to me massive herxes, followed by noticeable improvement in my symptoms. So when I switched to abx, very little difference was noticed since the herbal products I was taking were obviously working at least as good, if not better, or even far better than antibiotics.

**There is a general belief that antibiotics are superior to herbal products in their antimicrobial effectiviness. You are not likely to find objective, third party, double blind scientific studies that have proven this to be true. Because it has been the practice of medical doctors to use antibiotics over herbal medicine does not constitute proof that they are more effective, depending on the application. In fact, two of the most respected medical doctors that have successfully treated Lyme disease, Dr. Lee Cowden, and Dr. Deitrich Klinghardt, use herbal and antimicrobial medicines often as their primary choice for Lyme disease. Ezekiel 47:12 ". . . and the fruit thereof shall be for meat and the leaf thereof for medicine."

Mine is only one story. And as you learn more and more about Lyme and hear the testimonies of others, you will hear similar and very dissimilar stories. Each is so different that one wonders sometimes if they all have the same disease. Of course that possibility is part of the equation as co-infective microbes need to be eliminated as a possibility before proceeding forward with your treatment decisions. But the good news is that most of the treatments listed later in this book are broad spectrum, and will likely benefit you even if it is something other than a Bb infection.

If someone were to say to me, "Craig, what do you now know about Lyme disease that you wished you would have known when you first began your journey to help those of us new to this to begin moving on the fast track to recovery?"

I would answer that by saying: get a firm understanding of the nature of this bacterium. There is a propensity to treat this like any other bacterial infection, which it is not. We are not just speaking of it in terms of its resistance to antibiotics due to its morphology, or its ability to alter itself into any number of its pleomorphic forms. It goes beyond that. Once you understand why Borrelia Burgdorferi is different, and what makes Lyme disease unique, then you will also understand why most of the approaches, not only of conventional medicine, but even those that take a more alternative approach, struggle to get beyond temporarily feeling better for awhile, only to eventually relapse.

Lyme disease, virtually never resolves on its own. In fact, it is at the very time when you feel like your immune system is going to take over from the medicines you have been taking, and you feel like the disease is finally being put behind you that you need to take even more aggressive steps to go further, and continue your therapies on an even deeper level. If you do not remain diligent and relentless far beyond the point when you are feeling better, based upon the pattern that is seen in most Lyme patients, it will almost always return with a vengeance. Just when you thought that you had beaten the disease, you find, "it's baaaack", and you never had completely conquered it.

There is one popular website that many Lyme patients have come to know about a lady who is touting teasel root as a cure for her Lyme disease. She has apparently had Lyme disease 8 times, and teasel root has come to the rescue 8 times. I don't deny the potential for very unique herbs to have a profound effect particularly on illnesses such as Lyme. In fact teasel root is mentioned later in this book. The problem is that it is difficult to accept that most people are never cured of Lyme, while one person claims to have been beaten it 8 times! To me, this illustrates the point that often times Lyme was never completely resolved to begin with. The overt symptoms can go dormant for a time due to a therapy that addresses the killing of the virulent spirochete forms, whether using prescription anti-biotics, or a product such as teasel root. But in fact it is only hiding until ready to reemerge with a vengeance. This is why it is important to understand the nature of Bb and how it manifests the disease.

Certainly each person will take a different approach and will need to find therapies that work for them personally. But understanding the nature of Lyme disease and the bacteria that causes it will put you way ahead of the game by knowing what to expect ahead of time. It will help you to better understand how to develop protocols when you understand what you are up against. And if you are not clear on that, then you will be wandering aimlessly from one treatment to another. Take deliberate steps toward the solution based upon how you know Bb is going to act, not timid ones. Bb is not timid. You and your approach need to be forceful and with confidence that you will get well. I am not talking about the placebo effect here. I am speaking of the prolific manner in which you approach the therapies you decide upon. They need to be consistent and aggressive within the confines of your ability to detox, that is—not overdoing it. And you must be resolved to remain that way as long you are dealing with this illness.

But perhaps nearly as important as understanding the nature of the Bb, I think any person who has had the disease for any length of time at any level of experience will tell you the same thing: there is no fast track to recovery. I don't mean to sound pessimistic. In fact I truly believe that you will save years of pain, suffering, and cost by what you are about to learn because you are learning not only what to avoid, but more importantly, what your focus should be on.

Don't be taken in by what you read of claims to have a fast and reliable way to a cure. These are ads designed by people who do not themselves understand the nature of chronic Lyme disease. If something works and is real, it will certainly spread like wildfire on its own merit. But if these important points are not understood, that is, the prolific and often deceptive nature of Lyme disease, then you will find yourself having false expectations and drastically reduce your chances to find lasting healing.

ENDNOTES

1. *Universal Oral Vaccine: The Immune Milk Saga!* by Anthony di Fabio Parts 1-4 Townsend Letter For Doctors and Patients' Archives http://www.tldp.com/ Retrieved Feb. 3, 2013
2. *The 18 Reasons Lyme Treatments Fail: Tick-Borne Infection Medicine for the New Millennium* by Dr. James Schaller, M.D. http://www.publichealthalert.org/Articles/jamesschaller/18_reasons_lyme_treatments_fail.htm

CHAPTER 4

Borrelia Biochemistry

With all the different kinds of treatments that I had already tried that either didn't work, or whose benefits were nominal, as well as reading of the experiences of others who were also finding little success at what first sounded promising, I felt very discouraged. Yet I also knew that somehow what I learned would not be in vain, although as yet I couldn't see how it could be used.

With all that I learned about Borrelia Burgdorferi and its related strains, it seemed like the perfect organism. It seemed like it was created or designed in such a way that nearly every possible contingency had been planned with careful forethought not only for it to survive, but to thrive even in the presence of all of man's seemingly insurmountable technology and the higher intelligence advantages that we possessed. It also occurred to me that it simply couldn't be possible that such a microbe could have no weaknesses. Everything has a weakness. Even the most sophisticated machines designed by man, or the natural world of creation created by God has a weakness. It seemed to me that all I needed to do was to find that weakness and exploit it. But what was its weakness? What had I learned about Bb that I could take advantage of that had thus far been overlooked?

A proper understanding of the underlying biochemistry of Borrelia Burgdorferi is key to formulating anti-Lyme strategies. Once you understand what it is that allows Bb to do what it does, and how it functions, it gives to us the upper hand. Knowing your enemy is the key to defeating him. Treatments specifically designed to thwart Bb will be introduced later. But this chapter becomes the basis from which these therapies will form.

THE RESEARCH

Several aspects of Lyme disease caused by Bb infection have been examined in detail by others. There are so many trails to travel down and examine, each having very valid potentials.

But when I first began studying the biochemistry of Bb, I did so not knowing what I would find. So I didn't know what to look for along the way. It was only after my work was complete was I able to make a simple yet rather obvious observation.

But I'm getting ahead of myself.

Early on in my research, it occurred to me that the development of Bb both genetically and morphologically was so perfect, it was looking more and more like the genetically manipulated and altered microorganism of Plum Island fame. Apparently the Texas star-backed tick is not native to this northeast region of the United States where a great prevalence of Lyme disease has occurred. But it was found there being a carrier of Borrelia burgdorferi, yet was not found in any of the states in-between! [1] This appears to be no coincidence either. Significant evidence points to another microbial-based disease outbreak having been born in this same area for instance: West Nile virus. [2]

It is also interesting that the northeastern strains tend to be much more virulent. Far more cases have been reported of erythema migrans and severity of symptoms from this area of the country. This makes sense if in fact Plum Island gave birth to genetically altered strains.

But I realized that although an interesting story which very well is likely true, focusing on whether the government Plum Island experiments were true or not played no bearing on my end goal—to be healed of this condition and to get well.

Regardless of how it occurred, this organism is so innately intelligent, that it has acquired from our own cellular information (either by man's manipulation or mutation) an understanding of human immunity so as to completely evade it. It's almost as though it knows what the body is thinking and adjusts itself accordingly. It has the ability to grasp onto host immune cells and deactivate them. Then it uses them as a kind of camouflage—particularly the cell-wall deficient form. Since this form has no surface wall to attach to as in most other bacteria, this becomes a perfect form of evading immunity which naturally utilizes receptor sites on the cell surface. Morphing from the spirochete form to an un-attachable and undetectable L-form enables it to down-regulate immune response. One example of this is a surface protein of Bb termed *Bb CRASP-1* (Compliment Regulator/Acquiring Surface Protein.) It "actively binds to and down-regulates factor H and factor H-like protein of the compliment immune system". [3] Additionally, Borrelia spirochetes are known to attack, invade, and kill human B and T lymphocytes. [4] It would therefore seem logical to assume that many more yet undiscovered Bb capabilities allow it to regulate or evade human immunity.

Borrelia infection is also known to down-regulate a specific cytokine called Interleukin-10, which is an anti-inflammatory cell-signaling messenger used to aid innate immune responses. By elevating IL-10, Bb is able to establish infection by lowering and inhibiting communication responses such as macrophages, MHC antigens, and other cytokines.

Bb has been called a pleomorphic microbe, and each of the various morphological forms seems to have their own function. Although the most notorious is the spirochete which is the focus of most research, the cyst, for example is more like a kind of incubation pod which is highly resistant to most antibiotics. In fact, antibiotics actually push spirochetes into the cyst form, where they lie in wait until the coast is clear, later to reemerge. The L-forms, also known as cell-wall deficient forms, are probably the most advanced stealth form of all the bacteria as it relinquishes its cell membrane in order to remain invisible to the immune system. They often tend to be intracellular pathogens.

The bleb forms are round sphere-like in shape. They can develop upon being stressed by immune agents. Spirochetes have been observed as folding their membrane to form a bud which is then completely pinched off and released from the spirochete to be an independent entity containing the same lipid and protein expression as the mother spirochete. It is believed that this may be a defensive maneuver acting much like a decoy to draw immune cells away from the larger infective cells. These blebs are more resistant to treatments than spirochetes, and allow for a much longer-term infection to reside. [5]

Granular forms are perhaps the most resistant of all Bb forms.

Most antibiotics have traditionally been chemically designed to attack the cell wall of bacteria. Since the cell wall form of Bb is the spirochete, which is the form that is most susceptible to antibiotics, is it any wonder that the recurring relief/relapse cycle experienced by doctors with their patients seems to be the norm? Or that antibiotics simply stop working altogether? It is not difficult to ascertain that these other forms of the bacteria are only temporarily inducing less aggressive symptoms, while the underlying infection is still present. This is the reason why patients never really get completely well.

Borrelia has a special knack for developing antibiotic resistance far beyond the capabilities of other bacteria. Here is why: Bacterial DNA contains the genes that allow them to code for the expression of proteins, for RNA transcription, reproduction, as well as traits which characterize the building blocks or structure of the bacteria. These are inherently part of the bacteria. They encode information that allows them to proliferate and survive.

Plasmids possess similar properties. However plasmids are separate and distinct from bacterial DNA or genes, and are sometimes referred to as extra-chromosomal genes. Although they also encode information, one of their characteristics is that they hold the ability for self-replication, and can reproduce themselves along with host daughter cells. They are like viruses which have no life of their own, except when they are incorporated into a cell and govern its functions. They appear to possess a similar symbiotic relationship to the host bacteria they infect as mitochondria do to human cells, in that they are separate and distinct entities, yet carry out functions which are mutually beneficial.

Different plasmids have the capacity to encode different kinds of information. One such example is the ability to resist certain antibiotics. Since not all plasmids encode the same information, not all host microbial cells have the same defensive capabilities. Different bacteria, even of the same strain within a particular infected individual, may not possess the same survival potentials. For instance, sometimes only 1 in 5,000 plasmids may contain a particular informational transformation capability. As germs are then exposed to a particular antibiotic, and millions die, the ones that contain the plasmid-encoded antibiotic resistant information survive, and then reproduce allowing subsequent generations to also resist the drug. It only takes one to develop this capability, which will ultimately allow an entire colony within an infected individual to become antibiotic resistant. Then as subsequent onslaughts of various drugs threaten the bacteria, and even one or two learn to develop defensive strategies, they are stored in the plasmid information system, and called upon when future attacks necessitate evasive action. In time, a virtual library of defensive strategies can be drawn upon from which to defend itself from a multitude of various drugs.

However, in addition to encoding antibiotic resistance, plasmids encode information that allows Bb to evade many avenues of human immunity as well. One might describe plasmids as possessing a kind of "genetic sheet music", the transductional outcome of which instructs and directs a molecular pathway to externalize bacterial protein expressions and/or variations which ultimately brings about the necessary conditions in the microbe that allows it to elude specific immune responses that it has learned. So for instance, certain T-cell mediated antibodies may have been manufactured against a specific outer-surface protein of Bb. As an evasive response, plasmid information may be transcribed which allows that protein to change its protein expression which is no longer responsive to that particular antibody. That is the reason Bb has been able to develop variable proteins. As such it may be necessary for the body to develop new antibodies to what is perceived as a different protein. Or, as response to threat, another plasmid or groups of plasmids may be called upon to vary an entire group of lipoprotein molecular configurations which may ultimately lead to a change in morphology or the changing of its form altogether. And due to the high number of plasmids in Bb, its evasion from immune cells seems almost limitless, and explains why natural immunity is almost non-existent in Lyme disease. (Interestingly, the highly resistant HIV and mycoplasma also possess variable proteins.)

This may also explain in part the varied antibody responses observed in Western blot testing, and how they can change over time.

So plasmids hold the key to the ultimate survival information necessary for physical expression (*phenotype*) called upon for evading immunity. It is no surprise then to learn that this same microbe which is perhaps more highly advanced in its ability to adapt to host immunity as well as virtually all known natural and pharmaceutical based treatments, also possesses more plasmids than any other known bacterium to date. [6]

Certain plasmids have been identified as possessing specific information that governs Bb's overall ability to be infective. Lp28 and Lp25 (linear plasmids) are known to be absolutely vital for infection to occur. These plasmids in vitro are unstable, and after several generations of growth, can become lost. This must mean that they require at least some challenge from the immune system in order for them to remain active, since in vitro they would experience no external threats from the immune system. Once these plasmids are lost, the bacteria can lose their abiliiy to be infective, even when they are reinocculated into an immunocompromised host. [7] (Again, this explains why so many people are infected with a form of the bacteria that have not yet turned on or expressed these plasmids.)

One study demonstrated a direct connection between Lp28 and a certain externally expressed lipoprotein site which allows for antigenic variations called VlsE (Expressive variable lipoprotein site). This site is able to rearrange Bb's proteins in order for it to adapt to direct immune responses. Studies have been done that point to a direct connection or correlation between Lp28-1 and this VlsE. [8] That means that plasmids are not only responsible for encoding evasive information, but also can change and alter the proteins to affect the way the immune system sees it. This VlsE is a highly vulnerable site which may explain why it has developed this capacity to alter itself for protection.

However it has also been observed that these variable proteins can only maintain one expression at a time, meaning they cannot change simultaneously. [9] This has very important implications as it gives to us an understanding of the underlying ways in which Bb defends itself. Bb alters its proteins in order to adapt. One research study concluded, "This novel adaptation mechanism could be a critical step for *B. burgdorferi* to proceed to chronic infection, as the pathogen would be cleared at the early stage of infection if the spirochetes failed to undergo this process." [10]

Remember I said that this microbe must have a weakness? We have been aware of its ability to constantly morph to evade the immune system and antimicrobials for a long time. But this gives to us an explanation as to why so many Lyme treatments fail. When Bb is exposed to any particular antimicrobial, it is vulnerable to that antimicrobial's mode of action. So when any one therapy is used for any length of time, those specific plasmids are going to be sending information to variable proteins, and enzyme expressions that allow for it to defend against the manner in which that particular antibiotic works, since it can only express one plasmid instruction at a time. Therefore, the ideal plan of action, taking into consideration this microbe's weakness, is to use not only multiple therapies, but to constantly change those therapies in order to short-circuit the microbe. Like a fortress that does not have enough soldiers to defend against all four fort walls at the same time, the others are left unguarded or vulnerable.

It has been mentioned in a previous chapter that conventional medicine prides itself for its ability to match one drug with one disease. You see the implications? Where has this gotten conventional medicine in its battle against Lyme disease? And even in alternative treatments where a one or two antimicrobial approach is taken, the disease process is prolonged. However by taking an approach that takes into account the weakness of Borrelia, we can design a therapy that can dramatically not only put the odds of success on our side, but can also speed the healing process perhaps even exponentially.

THE LIPOPROTEINS

Bacterial lipoproteins or BLP's are known to be significant immune activators, some acting as neurotoxins, and each having their own pathway of activation within various human cells. A lipoprotein is basically a fat that has joined together with a protein to form a covelant or chemical bond. It is the lipoproteins which have been at the center of most research to discover a way to possibly neutralize the affects of their neurotoxic activities.

Although many proteins make up the organism, there are particular lipoproteins which have been identified as being particularly immune reactive. Many are used in Western Blot testing, and are identified by their molecular weight. The following is a list of some of the commonly known American strain lipoproteins as cited by Karen Vanderhoof-Forschner in her book, <u>Everything You Need to Know About Lyme Disease</u>.

9kd—cross-reactive for Borrelia
12kd—specific for Bb
18kd—unknown (now is known to be specific for Bb)
20kd—cross reactive
21kd—unknown
22kd—specific for Bb
23/2—outer surface protein C, specific for Bb
28kd—unknown
30kd—unknown, probably an outer surface protein
31kd—outer surface protein A, specific for Bb
34kd—outer surface protein B, specific for Bb
35kd—specific for Bb
37kd—specific for Bb
38kd—cross-reactive for Borrelia
39kd—major protein of Bb flagellin, specific for Bb
41kd—flagellin protein of all spirochetes; this is usually the first to appear after infection and is specific for all Borrelia
45kd—cross-reactive for all Borrelia
50kd—cross-reactive for all Borrelia
55kd—cross-reactive for all Borrelia
57kd—cross-reactive for all Borrelia
58kd—unknown, but may be a heat-shock Bb protein
60kd—cross-reactive for all Borrelia
66kd—cross-reactive for all Borrelia, common in all bacteria
83kd—specific antigen for Lyme bacterium, probably a cytoplasmic membrane.

93kd—unknown, probably the same protein as 83, just migrates differently in different patients.[11]

Here is an example of specific lipoproteins used in testing for some European strains:

93 kd chromosomal protein highly specific of the Borrelia genus; the antibody response is mostly IgM and appears in the course of chronic infections; bands at 93 kD are strongly associated with advanced stages.

62-72 kd heat shock proteins; these bands are not specifically associated with a Borrelia infection and are found in several bacterial infections.

60 kd common bacterial antigen; non-specific.

41 kd flagellin; this protein is not specific to the Borrelia genus but is useful in the test interpretation; cross-reaction with other spirochetes are common; a flagellin positive reaction may occur at early as well at late stages.

39 kd a protein highly specific of the Borrelia genus.

32.5 kd OspA: surface protein highly specific of Borrelia garinii.

28 kd surface protein.

22-23 kd OspC: surface protein highly specific of Borrelia garinii and a marker for early infections.

18 kd the specificity of this protein has been recently established; excellent marker for late infections. [12]

The subject of Borrelia Burgdorferi lipoproteins is quite extensive, and the research is voluminous. We will only do an overview and examine important points.

Some evidence has been presented in research that specific, as yet unidentified proteins are in fact the toxins emitted by Bb. [13] But many of the known lipoproteins are so highly antigenic and immune evoking, that they are considered toxic in and of themselves. This is what makes Bb so much different from other bacteria which often have limited antigenic factors. Of these proteins, 20kd, OspA, B, C, 39kd, 83kd and 93kd are considered to be most reactive. And each one has been discovered to induce its own unique responses from different immune cells in the body.

One of the most researched of all the lipoproteins is OspA, kd31. One study showed that OspA had the affect of causing certain brain and spinal cord cells called astrocytes to be become diseased and were induced to commit suicide (apoptosis). The function of astrocytes is in a supportive roll to help form the blood-brain barrier, for nutritive support, and for the sending of signals to support inter-communication of cells which involve brain and central nervous system signaling. It's no wonder that neurological symptoms as well as depression and emotional agitation are some of the most significant symptoms of Lyme disease. And that's just from OspA.

What is important to know about the lipoproteins is that although a lot of research has gone into identifying specific proteins and the role each seems to have in its capacity to incite specific immune cells, the end purpose of that research was mostly towards the development of a Lyme vaccine. However there were some problems using that approach. For instance a study at the University of Shizuoka, Japan's Dept. of Microbiology, demonstrated that three groups of Borrelia strains, although were able to be distinguished from other strains, "were divergent from each other in the molecular masses of putative outer surface protein A (OspA) and in the sequences of the ospA gene." [14] In other words, although they were the same outer surface protein, they differed greatly from one strain to another, which in turn would affect how antibodies and immune cells responded to them (which is what we previously pointed out in the weaknesses of Western Blot testing). Also, an interesting observation regarding the efficacy of OspA-based vaccinations was that they appeared to be highly strain-specific. Apparently OspA molecules for the American sensu stricto strain differs from at least 2 other European strains which would necessitate the development of separate vaccinations for each of those specific strains. [15] How then, given that Bb possesses so many immune invoking proteins which are so highly strain specific, do the developers of antibody testing believe that using only a few strains will accurately be representative of the many different lipoproteins expressed by so many different species of Bb enough to lend credibility of these tests over clinical diagnoses?

So in time of course a vaccine was developed for Lyme disease. However a problem developed. There is a phenomenon known to occur in certain microorganisms called "molecular mimicry". This occurs when certain pathogens deliberately alter their outer surface protein molecules to resemble the proteins of their host. In this way, the host immune system is fooled into thinking they are part of the "self", and fail to exhibit a full immune response. The result is that sometimes only a limited immune response is made such as cytokine release that can damage tissue, but not do much harm to the mimicking organism. Such became the problem when it was learned that spirochete flagellum proteins resembled myelin sheath proteins covering human nerves such that it was feared that a vaccine based upon certain proteins might also invoke a Multiple sclerosis/auto-immune-like response. Eventually the vaccine project was abandoned. However it is interesting to note that one of the most famous studies done in the early 1930's involved a direct connection between Multiple sclerosis patients, and spirochete infections. [16] MS of course is thought to be an auto-immune disease wherein the body's own immune system attacks the myelin sheath or insulation surrounding the nerves. It appears they may be blaming the wrong source.

Although one study demonstrated that in vitro OspA induced a strong monocyte response, it was not as strong as the whole bacterium.[17] So one cannot isolate certain proteins to develop a practical vaccine any more than any one particular antibiotic can address each aspect of a bacterium whose very lipoproteins are "variable" or changing constantly.

VARIABLE PROTEINS

Borrelia burgdorferi is made up of well over a hundred different lipoproteins. Together they are grouped by what are called "variable small lipoproteins", and "variable large lipoproteins". They comprise an entire antigenic system called VMP or variable major proteins. Other bacteria and even viruses are known to possess variable proteins. But what makes Bb so unique is the shear volume. Variable proteins are proteins that have the ability to change the way they express themselves on the outer surface. One particular region on Bb called VlsE was discussed under the heading of plasmids. An interesting observation was made of this expression site in one study. VlsE gene recombination is known to take place within its hosts, but does not take place within spirochetes in vitro, lending support that VlsE is intended and utilized specifically for immune evasion. [18]

It was mentioned under the section on plasmids that variability in protein expression can potentially be an enormous problem with Western blot testing. This in my opinion is one of the primary reasons for the unreliability in test results. Given that any particular variable protein is going to possess its own epitope or antibody coupling site, these will deliberately change as the protein changes. That's why is it often observed in other bacterial infections that the longer the infection resides, the more IgG antibodies will build up and be present to indicate either present or past infection. But clinically this is not often seen in Lyme disease. [19] If these proteins are constantly changing to whatever degree, then the ability to accurately measure IgG antibodies may erode over time. This is also a primary reason why IgM antibodies are often showing positive bands (chronic infection) while IgG bands can often be negative in Western Blot testing for Lyme disease.

Conserved Proteins

Not all Bb proteins are variable. It has been discovered that other regions on Bb do not alter or change, but remain constant, also known as 'conserved'. These are called *Invariant Regions 1-6*. They do not evoke immune responses or the development of specific antibodies, except one. IR-6, or C6 peptide, which although remains constant, is considered an immunodominant major protein as it does in fact induce a strong immune response. As such, it crosses Borrelia specie lines by evoking a specific antibody known as C-6 antibody. C6 peptide is highly specific to all known Bb strains and its antibody has been used as a marker to detect IR-6 in infected patients. This becomes an important tool in testing because it is not only a protein which is possessed by all known Borrelia strains, but because it doesn't vary. This will be discussed more in the chapter on testing.

TOXINS

A lot of discussion has been made surrounding what some have termed "Lyme neuro-toxin". Lyme infection has frequently been called *neuro-borreliosis* due to the neurological symptoms being affected that some have attributed to this neuro-toxin. This is a description of how Bb can affect the central nervous system as its primary target and is sometimes in contrast to or in conjunction with Lyme arthritis, depending on which system or systems are being affected.

Neuroborreliosis describes neurological symptoms such as neuritis or inflammation of a nerve or series of nerves, ringing in the ears, mental and emotional disturbances, lymphocytic meningitis, headaches, Bell's Palsy-like symptoms, lack of coordination, or even the feeling such as electrical shocks in the brain or elsewhere. A conclusion has been drawn by some that a toxin must be attributed to these conditions since neuroborreliosis resembles the affects of a toxin.

The problem is that researchers have not been able to discover a distinct definable toxin being released from Bb infection as one would find from Clostridium and its botulinum toxin that causes botulism. The only thing that comes close to an identifiable toxin was when Sam Donta MD and his collegues at Boston University Medical Center were able to isolate a new toxin by amplifying DNA extracted from Bb strain 2591 to identify genes that exhibit proteins comparable to other known bacterial toxins, namely diphtheria and pertussis toxins. In testing of mice and rats, exposure to this toxin, which he named Bbtox-1, induced cell death in C6 and Y1 cells. It apparently functions similarly to a botulinum toxin. [20, 21] However this "toxin" does not appear to have had much follow-up, nor has it been demonstrated to be able to be detected or measured in an infection as are other known bacterial toxins, and thus appears to have little practical relevance.

Although a toxin per se has not been specifically discovered that one may classify as such which can be demonstrated to exhibit properties similar to other known toxins, it is believed that specific glycolipids which are contained within the bacterial membrane may act similarly. Recently two new glycolipids were discovered in Borrelia:

"cholesteryl 6-O-acyl-β-D-galactopyranoside (B. burgdorferi glycolipid 1, BbGL-I), and 1,2-di-O-acyl-3-O-α-D-galactopyranosyl-sn-glycerol (BbGL-II)." [22] They have been observed to elicit antibody response in rodents, as well as the sera of known Lyme patients. These glycolipids are classified as *cholesteryl galactosides*. Since Bb has no detectable toxic lipopolysaccharides (LPS) which are the main composition of many other bacterial membranes, it is thought that GL-1 and 2 act in a similar manner as LPS due to the structural make-up and high lipid content of its membrane (over 36% of the Bb's total mass). [23]

Some doctors believe that these glycolipids act as toxins and due to their chemical make-up, can become stored or built up in the body much like fats. Along these lines, one MD, a Dr. Ritchie Shoemaker has used a novel therapy taking off on the idea that if indeed toxins abide in this cholesteryl galactoside, it reasons that the body would be continuously reprocessing the toxin thru the gut. Utilizing a cholesterol-binding drug called cholestyramine he has had remarkable success in lowering patient toxin load and significant reduction of symptoms by binding the toxin-containing lipid and at least lowering the immune load from that angle. [24] Some doctors and patients are incorporating the natural product beta sitosterol as a substitute.

In all likelihood, Bb lipoproteins act much like toxins since they are so highly reactive against immune cells. So no matter whether an identifiable toxin exists or not, Borrelia is highly toxic and its lipids found in the proteins possess properties which act nearly like poisons. Later, zeolites will be discussed which also have been used to reduce Lyme neurotoxicity.

Remember this chapter when beginning your Lyme therapies, as it forms the basis upon which to develop treatment protocols. Unless you vary your therapies and are constantly exposing Bb's vulnerability to multiple substances at the same time, these bacteria are going to outsmart even the most deadly of weapons.

ENDNOTES

1. *Plum Island, Lyme Disease And Operation Paperclip - A Deadly Triangle* Paper by Patricia Doyle, PhD 8-21-5 http://www.rense.com/general67/plumislandlyme.htm Retrieved Feb. 3, 2013

2. Carroll, M.C. *Lab 257.* New York: Harper Collins Publishers, p. 28-34. (2004)

3. *Lyme Disease: Burgdorferi CRASP-1 protein characterized.* (2004). Retrieved July 26, 2005, from News Rx Website: http://www.newsrx.com

4. *Invasion and Cytopathic Killing of Human Lymphocytes by Spirochetes Causing Lyme Disease* David W. Dorward, Elizabeth R. Fischer, and Diane M. Brooks From the National Institute of Allergy and Infectious Diseases, RockyMountain Laboratories, Hamilton, Montana http://home.pon.net/caat/lyme/killing_lymphocytes.pdf

5. 2010 *Metamorphosis of Borrelia burgdorferi organisms - RNA, lipid and protein composition* Al-Robaiy S, Dihazi H, Kacza J, Seeger J, Schiller J, Huster D, Knauer J, Straubinger RK. J Basic Microbio 2010 Oct 21. (Epub)

6. (2003). *Adaptation of Borrelia burgdorferi in the vector and vertebrate host.* Utpal, P., & Fikrig, E. Microbes and Infection, 5,(2003) 659-666.

7. *Development of Vaccines to Infectious Diseases.* Biology 160 2005. http://www.brown.edu/Courses/Bio_160/Projects2005/lyme_disease/history.htm. Accessed April 30, 2010

8. *Effects of VlsE complementation on the infectivity of Borrelia burgdorferi lacking linear plasmid.* Lawrenze, M.B., Wooten, R.M., & Norris, S.J. Infection and Immunology, 2004 72(11), 6577-6588.

9. *Plum Island, Lyme Disease And Operation Paperclip - A Deadly Triangle* Paper by Patricia Doyle, PhD 8-21-5 http://www.rense.com/general67/plumislandlyme.htm Retrieved Feb. 3, 2013

10. *Molecular Adaptation of* Borrelia burgdorferi *in the Murine Host* Fang Ting Liang, F. Kenneth Nelson, and Erol Fikrig J Exp Med. 2002 July 15; 196(2): 275-280.

11. Vanderhoof-Forschner, K. *Everything you need to know about Lyme Disease.* Hoboken, NJ: John Wiley & Sons. (2003)

12. *Borrelia IgM Blot Immunoblot for the confirmation of Borrelia burgdorferi sensu lato specific IgM antibodies in human serum* http://www.novatec-id.

com/fileadmin/user_upload/Product_Insert/LYM110____Borrelia_IgM_
Blot.pdf Retreived Dec. 2012

13. Travis, J. (1999). *A toxin at the heart of Lyme Disease.* Science News, 155(24), p. 377. http://www.sciencenews.org/pages/pdfs/data/1999/15524/15524-13.pdf

14. *Determination of members of a Borrelia afzelli-related group isolated from Ixodas nipponensis in Korea as Borrelia valaisiana.* Masuzawa, T., Fukui, T., Miyake, M., Oh, H.B., Cho, M.K., Chang, W.H., Imai, Y., & Yanagihara, Y. (1999). International Journal of Systematic Bacteriology, VOL(4), 1409-1415.

15. Hoppe, H. (2000). *Recombinant glucocerebrosidase and Lyme Disease vaccine made by genetic engineering.* Journal of Biotechnology, 76, p. 263.

16. 2005 Presentation in Chicago by Lida Mattman PhD Autoimmunity Research Foundation's Chicago Conference http://www.youtube.com/watch?v=WozrCFW0mRM

17. *Borrelia burgdorferi induces chemokines in human monocytes.* Sprenger, H., Krause, A., Kauffmann, A., Prien, S., Fabian, D., Burmester, GR., Geemsa, D., & Rittig, MG. (1997). Infection and Immunity, 65(11), 4384-4388.

18. *Analysis of Borrelia burgdorferi VlsE gene expression and recombination in the tick vector.* Indest, K.J., Howell, J.K., Jacobs, M.B., Scholl-Meeker, D., Norris, S.L., & Philipp, M.T. (2001). Infection and Immunology, 69(11), 7083-7090.

19. *The IgM question: Is it chronic Lyme disease?* Lymeblog LymeMD 2-14-2010 http://lymemd.blogspot.com/search?q=IgG Retreived Feb. 3, 2013

20. Travis, J. (1999). *A toxin at the heart of Lyme Disease.* Science News, 155(24), p. 377.

21. Cartwright, M., Martin, S., & Donta, S. (1999) *A Novel Toxin (Bbtox1) of Borrelia Burgdorferi.* Abstract for 1999 Lyme Disease Conference. http://www.lyme.org/conferences/99_abstract.html Retrieved Feb. 3, 2013

22. *Newly discovered cholesteryl galactoside from Borrelia burgdorferi.* Meachem, B., Kubler-Kielb, J., Coron, B., Yergey, A., & Schneerson, R. (2003). Proceedings of the National Academy of Sciences, USA, 100(13), 7913-7921.

23. Ibid.

24. *A new diagnostic tool and a new drug therapy provide major weapons against the surging epidemic of post-Lyme sydrome.* (2005). Retrieved July 26, 2005, from Chronic Neurotoxins Website, http://www.lyme.org/conferences/99_abstract.html

CHAPTER 5

Biofilms

For a long time it has been thought that the main reason Lyme has been difficult to treat was due to its pleomorphic capabilities which allows it to be so evasive. If it were to remain in the same form, its weaknesses would also remain exposed and obviously be made vulnerable to both immune and antimicrobial actions. No doubt this has been true. However whether someone has been fortunate enough to have found success using antibiotics or non-drug treatments, as there are many varied therapies listed later in this book, even those crafty and evasive pleomorphic forms eventually can succumb to the overwhelming onslaught of varied therapies. For those of us fortunate enough to have remained diligent in our battle against the disease who have reached a point where the systemic infection has been repelled due to the wearing down and eventual killing off of planktonic (free-swimming) bacteria, there is left one major battle that is the most difficult of all to conquer—biofilms.

In fact it would not be incorrect to state that there exist two primary resistance factors of chronic Lyme disease: Simply stated, pleomorphic Lyme, and biofilm Lyme. Although both overlap, it is the latter that seems to hold on even after the first has been mostly eradicated. The one form that is a last refuge is also the one that is the most difficult to defeat. And if left unresolved, can become a base from which the disease could potentially repeatedly reemerge over and over again. A brief overview will be made of what biofilms are, how they are formed, and why they are difficult to destroy.

Traditionally bacteria have been understood to exist as individual entities floating around independent of one another creating havoc as either focal infections, or spreading systemically throughout the body infiltrating virtually every area. And that has been the basis upon which anti-bacterial agents have been used. Even though in time, these independent bacterium are often able to develop resistance to particular antibiotics, an even greater defensive mechanism that was developed in bacteria was biofilms:

> *In modern clinical microbiology, the establishment of bacterial biofilms is often considered a pathogenicity trait during chronic infections. Biofilm formation is an example of microbial community behavior. Both Gram-positive and Gram-negative bacteria have been found to coordinate this behavior through cell-to-cell communication mediated by small, diffusible signals. This phenomenon has been termed quorum sensing and is prevalent among both symbiotic and pathogenic bacteria associated with plants and animals. Many of the phenotypes regulated by cell-to-cell communication are involved in bacterial colonization and virulence.* [1]

These signal molecules have been identified and given names: Auto-inducer 1 (AI-1) and auto-inducer 2 (AI-2). AI-1 refers primarily to same or intra-specie communication. However of greater importance is AI-2 which crosses specie lines and is sensed on a more universal basis. In other words bacteria of other species are able to exchange information with one another, a kind of universal language. The source of AI-2 appears to a metabolic or waste by-product of the bacteria [2] and in some cases a specific gene-expressed enzyme referred to as "LuxS". [3]

These auto-inducers afford planktonic bacteria a means of communicating with each other. The way it functions is that by coordinating their efforts and using auto-inducer molecules as a means of communicating, free-swimming bacteria form a "quorate" which in time allows the entire population to sense that it is ready to make a group-based decision. The decision "is thought to afford pathogenic bacteria a mechanism to minimize host immune responses by delaying the production of tissue-damaging virulence factors until sufficient bacteria have amassed and are prepared to overwhelm host defense mechanisms and establish infection symptoms." [4] This description helps us to understand the process that occurs immediately prior to the development of disease symptoms that have not yet arisen to the point of an immune response in those that have an infection. In other words, they are not yet sick. Once the communication takes place on a universal basis, the bacteria then, as a united group will simultaneously alter gene or plasmid expression to affect virulence factors which in turn are sensed by certain immune cells and cytokines. Hence the illness or disease process begins or advances.

But this is only the beginning, as it only explains the process of communication. It also tells us something of the intelligence that bacteria possess. Somewhere in their genetics is a universal or invisible understanding that while in their host they are in a foreign land, and a prime means of defense is in their ability to communicate as a whole, and work together for survival purposes.

DESCRIPTION

Essentially, biofilms are shelters often observed as slime which are formed by the bacteria themselves to establish colonies in which can dwell various forms of either the same specie, or mixed species of microbes. In general we may describe biofilms as bacterial excretions used for the development of structures that act as adhesions as well as protective capsules made up of what are called *exopolysaccharides*. These are structures formed from sugar molecules excreted for various purposes.

Bacteria generally produce their own unique polysaccharide, e.g. cellulose is produced by Acetobacter xylinum, N-acetyl-heparosan from Escherichia coli, xanthan from Xanthomonas campestris, and hyaluronic acid from Streptococcus equi, etc. These exopolysaccharides possess properties which allow them to retain water and other fluids, and function similar to a regulatory system in which the environment on the interior can be maintained and managed. Biofilms are thought to be formed for various purposes, such as protection from oxygen radicals from the environment, from immune cells and other offensive measures within the body, in times of nutrient depletion wherein their metabolic processes may slow down, antimicrobial protection, and others. So biofilm growth enables both conservation as well as protection of the colony. It has been observed that many exopolysaccharides are not necessarily immunogenic of themselves. Hence may not induce a specific antibody response. No doubt this is done by design in order to avoid attracting attention from immune cells. As the bacteria continue to grow and proliferate, they will obviously seek to maintain and balance their environment, and therefore they are not truly in a state of "hibernation", although the metabolic processes are slowed down. EPS's are able to absorb many times their weight in water, hence are highly water soluable.

Biofilms form in various stages. Bacteria utilize adhesive properties to initially attach themselves to surfaces, as well as to each other. This initial attachment to a surface is the first stage of their growth. In Bb some of these adhesion molecules have been identified called *decorin-binding proteins*. First they use these adhesion molecules to attach to a surface or membrane within the body. Then using hair like appendages they permanently bond to the surface as well as to each other. They then excrete exopolysaccharides into the immediate invironment which allows for the development of structures to form. These are the characteristic slimes or goos that biofilms are known for. Then fibrin or proteins are used to form structures within the exopolysaccharide slime. Cationic (positively charged) calcium, magnesium, and sometimes other metals are used in the cementing process. As the bacteria inside proliferate, they would naturally shed proteins, which would become incorporated into the structure, thus increasing the level of toxicity in the environment. They will then incorporate dead host cells as a camoflage within the matrix. Inevitably however the accumulation of bacterial debri, dead proteins and toxic accumulations become a part of the biofilm, making it a chronic target of inflammatory cells. This becomes the source of quintessential chronic Lyme disease.

Exopolysaccharides are well known for their ability to hold many times their weight in water within the biofilm structure. The existence of channels and conduits inside the films have been observed, which allows for fluid exchange, and gives an outlet for toxins, as well as an intake for nutrients, but also makes them susceptible to very limited antimicrobial attack. And as the biofilm grows, it would eventually reach a critical point where quorum decisions within the colony would signal for the biofilm to disperse, perhaps releasing thousands of individual bacteria into the environment.

Although biofilm research has been done on many bacteria, we are only in the very beginning stages of this research for Bb, as very little is known of the actual chemistry of Bb biofilms. Dr. Alan MacDonald made the first remarkable presentation on Borrelia biofilms at the University of New Haven in 2008 called "Biofilms of Borrelia burgdorferi and Clinical Implications for Chronic Borreliosis". [5] In his research he has developed a way to cause the proteins of Bb to fluoresce. Under a microscope it can be observed that not only do spirochetes, cysts and circular forms fluoresce, but the entire biofilm mass can be seen fluorescing, indicating that the biofilm is either actually made out of proteins, or proteins are incorporated in its formation. This suggests that Bb biofilms are more than just a structure in which they hide, but are in a sense being called a morphology or "form" of the bacteria.

Current active research is being done on Bb biofilms by Dr. Eva Sapi Ph.D, Associate professor of the University of New Haven who is a Lyme disease victim herself. She has observed live active Bb biofilms and found that all of the pleomorphic forms can be seen in and around the biofilm. Spirochetes, L-forms, bleb, granular, and others in various stages of growth can be seen entering and leaving. Although this observation is being made in a live culture, it likely represents similar activity as one might expect to see in the body. And it does illustrate that Bb does in fact function in this manner as do other bacteria, and likely explains why antibiotic resistance is so prevelant in Lyme disease. [6]

Observations about biofilms from the NIH (National Institute for Health):

- Biofilms can increase antibiotic resistance by up to 1000% over planktonic bacteria.
- They allow a greater opportunity for genetic exchange to occur between various forms, and can increase virulence in less virulent bacteria.
- Some biofilms are known to be occupied by several different kinds of microbes. This leads to an even higher pathogenicity since many infectious microbes are in fact toxic to one another, and may turn on even more virulence factors than single specie bacteria.

- Bacteria deep inside biofilms are capable of resisting further immune attacks since those bacteria near the surface may possess different antigens than deeper embedded bacteria.
- Phagocytes which normally engulf a bacteria are not able to engulf biofilms. In response they release pro-inflammatory enzymes and cytokines which can lead to the destruction of nearby tissues. [7]
- It is now believed that some 80%+ of bacteria form biofilms. [8]

For more study on biofilms, the following websites are provided: Medscape.com/viewarticle/441355_6; and http://www.quantafoods.com/downloads/08%20Spring%20QM%20Newsletter.pdf

So biofilms may represent the last stand for Borrelia infections. As your Lyme therapies kill off your systemic infection over time, you may find your symptoms subsiding to the point where they may be imperceptible, and you think you have beaten the disease. However if they return in time, the culprit may be the biofilms. They can harbor infection for a long period of time with no symptoms until such a time when the colony has matured and dispersed, beginning the process anew.

Due to the lack of historical research and understanding of biofilm development in Lyme disease, and that biofilm studies are still in the early stages, doctors are only now beginning to explore the possibilities of finding substances that hold the potential of dissolving biofilms. While drug companies are seeking ways of creating "anti-pathogenic" drugs by developing drugs with quorum inhibiting properties, some research has been done that discovered that specific enzymes have the capacity to reduce biofilms in certain bacteria. And although these enzymes often appear to be exopolysaccharide-specific for each particular bacterium, some physicians have begun to utilize varied enzyme cocktails along with anti-microbials to work synergestically to, over time, reduce biofilms and their habored bacterial infections. Based upon the evidence thus far, there are good reports showing some effectiveness over using antibiotics alone. Later you will hear the remarkable success I have personally had using these therapies.

Biofilms, once formed are very resistant to attempts to dissolve or penetrate them. So attempts to find substances that can accomplish this are paramount to finally resolving Lyme disease once and for all. Although difficult to eradicate as a whole, the most difficult part of the problem may not necessarily be because we have a lack of substances that can remove, inhibit, or dissolve them, but because the places they tend to form are so far out of reach from anti-biofilm substances, that the volume or concentration levels needed to resolve them completely can be difficult to attain. They can form inside blood vessels, the urinary tract, and the intestinal tract. And in theory these would be relatively easy to remove since anti-biofilm herbs and enzymes can readily reach and contact them in sufficient volume to have an effect. But the most common refuge for Bb such as in the brain, joints, connective tissue, and even bone are areas much more difficult to reach, and would likely require long-term and/or aggressive therapies to acquire sufficient biofilm reduction that would lead to their ultimate elimination. Later we will explore and examine specifically targeting biofilm inhibiting, slowing, and perhaps even dissolving substances that take a multi-pronged approach to this most resistant form of Lyme disease.

OBSERVATION

One of the most important observations I have made during my years of Lyme treatments was that as I continued to aggressively target the bacteria thru antimicrobials of all sorts, even though my systemic symptoms gradually over time would decline, there seemed to be an almost commensurate spreading and deepening of chronic pain. The pain I am speaking of is not the typical systemic or migratory joint pain generally associated with acute Lyme disease that is often observed to decline following antibiotic treatment. I am speaking of injury sites that although healed long ago, became a nest for the entrenchment of infection that not only was not resolved with antimicrobials, but almost like the spreading of a cancer, expanded and deepened. We have often been told by doctors who strictly accept conventional medical paradigms, that auto-immunity or arthritis is to blame for these chronic conditions. And especially to those that have previously been treated for Lyme disease, these might be termed "post-lyme sydrome". However

I personally never accepted or believed that view. It has been observed that the condition seemed to worsen as my Lyme treatments became more successful. The more my treatments were working (i.e. the more my systemic symptoms were decreasing), the worse these areas of pain seemed to deepen. In fact I could actually feel stiffness associated with the pain as if some structure was growing.

This instinctively told me that biofilms must be growing in response to the treatments in an effort to further evade the ongoing therapeutic efforts. Besides the occasions when I would take antibiotics, I had always incorporated natural antimicrobials and non-drug products as part of my antibacterial therapies. And I was well aware of the potential for these substances to force spirochetes into cyst forms. But not being "biofilm-literate" in my earlier years of treatments, I never paid attention to this fact, nor was I incorporating therapies that would address biofilms since it was not yet a commonly known phenomenon in Lyme disease. However as the awareness of biofilms was growing, my thoughts began to naturally suspect this may be happening. It perfectly fit all the models that were illustrated for the development and proliferation of biofilms. And it has been known that biofilms form in response to environmental threats. However I had not yet understood another connection that soon become apparent.

I have personally known quite a number of Lyme patients over the years. One observation I have made is that old injuries seem to be a common, yet highly resistant location where biofilms love to grow. In fact several of these patients had nearly completely eliminated their Lyme except for a few areas where injuries had occurred. It is known that injured cells can lose their capacity for cellular respiration which is necessary for the burning of sugars. This leads to not only significanly reduced energy levels, thus inhibiting cellular communication with immune cells, but also lowers ph levels, oxygen levels, as well as induces cytokine production, making these injured cells ideal targets for opportunistic pathogens.

The secondary injury is the infection itself. Colonies of bacteria proliferate around injuries. One research study, *Biofilms in Chronic Wounds* cited,

Molecular analyses of chronic wound specimens revealed diverse polymicrobial communities and the presence of bacteria, including strictly anaerobic bacteria, not revealed by culture. Bacterial biofilm prevalence in specimens from chronic wounds relative to acute wounds observed in this study provides evidence that biofilms may be abundant in chronic wounds. [9]

Dr. Dietrich Klinghart MD, PhD who has successfully treated many Lyme patients says in an article Lyme Disease: A Look Beyond Antibiotics says, "The microbes often invade tissues that had been injured . . ." [10]

Here is what happens. In time as the body naturally seeks to repair the injury, and fibrous tissue and adhesions develop, bacteria and their biofilms can grow as part of the fibrin and intermingle with the internal scar adhesions such that it seems to never truly heal. Over time the fibrous tissue can continue to expand within the focal area (and biofilms along with it) since the body is continuously receiving cytokine signals that the injury is not healed. The infected cells releasing cytokines signal for more immune cells to come to the rescue. Since the infection is now guarded by biofilms, they hinder immune cells from penetrating. (*Phagocytes,* or immune cells which engulf and dissolve bacteria, mostly do not have the capacity to engulf biofilms, thus making it sometimes impossible for the body to resolve biofilms without outside help.) But in response the bacteria naturally reinforce and strengthen their internal barracade to resist further immune attacks, and the process continues. Thus old injuries become a hot bed for the proliferation of biofilms.

Injuries would obviously not be the only lodging for biofilms, but opportunistic bacteria such as Bb seem to naturally be drawn to injured cells and tissue. Biofilms can theoretically grow anywhere, but seem to love both injured and more stuctural tissues, joints and bone. From the hypertextbook "Biofilms" chapter 3, What is the connection between biofilms and persistent infections?:

Biofilm infections form preferentially on foreign surfaces as well as dead or damaged tissue. These infections develop gradually and may be slow to produce overt symptoms. Once established, however, biofilm infections persist. They are rarely resolved by host defense mechanisms, even in individuals with healthy innate and adaptive immune reactions. Active host responses, such as invading neutrophils, can even be detrimental since those cells can cause collateral damage to neighboring healthy host tissue. Biofilm infections respond only transiently to antibiotic therapy. [11]

This is nearing the final stage and most resistant aspect of Lyme disease. Biofilms that develop can themselves become like an injury in that this constant signalling from the infected tissue cells drives more and more damaging immune cells to the site in an effort to remove the infection, which, in a cycle further damages surrounding healthy tissue. This is why it is so crucial to aggresively eliminate Lyme and its biofilms, not just stop your therapies when you are "feeling better". Yes, the systemic illness will have improved and you will feel "almost healed" by killing off of the planktonic bacteria over time. But unless the therapies you employ address these final bastions of resistance, biofilms may continue to expand over time, and entrench the disease even more so.

Do not be hoodwinked by the false teachings of the conventional medicine model. What has been called "post Lyme syndrome" is almost certainly understood to be an unresolved infection. Here, many doctors that have not accepted the true nature of Bb pleomorphism, its ramifications, and its propensity to form biofilms will say that your infection is gone. And all that remains now is an autoimmune condition left over from, or as a result of the infection. As proof of this they cite that continued or long-term antibiotic treatment does not improve the condition. This is because they are still living in an old paradigm that does not acknowledge biofilms as a contributing factor in the disease. This is where the true contraversey exists. This is the same contraversy that resides over a similar condition called rheumatoid arthritis. Rheumatoid arthiritis is believed by many doctors to actually be staph and other bacterial infections masquerading as auto-immune disease in the joints of their patients. Hands and finger joints are good examples of repetitive injury through over-use. Thus, injuries are ideal locations for biofilms to form. One can often see fingers and other joints become deformed over time as a result of the body attempting to heal the area, and the damage that results from chronic infection.

In an interview with Amy Proal of bacteriality.com, Dr. Randoll Walcott, a bacterial biofilm wound specialist says,

> . . . I have been reading several review articles that link autoimmune disease to chronic inflammation, and the more we've read, the clearer it's become that chronic inflammation is a result of bacterial infection. So we think there is a clear link between chronic inflammatory diseases and bacteria, and when we think, "chronic inflammation" we believe we are typically dealing with biofilm infections. [12]

In myself, as I turned to aggresively employ specific antibiofilm therapies, there was a rather pronounced reaction where no antimicrobial response was previously observed. The chronic and spreading inflammation in and around areas of old injuries and their biofilms began to reverse and slowly subside. Very strange and obvious feelings of localized herxing was experienced such that I knew it was the therapies attacking the biofilms and their harbored infections. The spreading of the area was now reversing, and several areas were now painful after many years of degenerating conditions. If in fact this was some autoimmune or arthritic condition as is often described by some "old paradigm" conventional doctors, then they will have a difficult time explaining why the combining of specific antibiofilm therapies with antimicrobials resolve such a condition that doesn't fit their medical model.

If you have found success in your Lyme treatments, but have areas of past trauma that have not healed, or chronic conditions that have not resolved, it may be due to the presence of highly resistant biofilm colonies that have formed. These may actually be used as a gauge to determine the success of any anti-biofilm therapies you may employ. These will be discussed under the chapter on therapies.

Discussion: It is my personal view that the planktonic or free-swimming bacterial infection is the first stage and major battle that is fought in Lyme. Even in many who are aggressive and persistent in their therapies, coming to the point where they get a handle on this aspect of the disease can sometimes take years. And to those of us who have, we have been rewarded by conquering it to the point where all, or the vast majority of systemic symptoms are gone. In essence, we have beaten the major battle of the disease. However many still have some unresolved lingering pain or symptoms that are only a fraction of their previous condition. No doubt some of this is due to damage that was done from the years of infection that may take years more to heal. Just as measles can leave scars that can be seen far after the disease is gone, so perhaps Lyme may leave some yet unresolved healing that will take time to resolve completely if ever.

However, perhaps even in the majority of patients who have reached this advanced level of healing, what is really still plaguing them are the very deep biofilms that have formed that are being misinterpreted as "unresolved damage", or damage left over from the infection. If the disease was completely gone, there would be no need to continue taking antimicrobials, which is what is often seen in some that have beaten the systemic symptoms, and are "hoping" they are cured. But they continue to treat themselves as a precaution, not against re-infection, but re-emergence of an unresolved old condition. Many battles have been fought and victories have been won. But unless these biofilms are addressed and completely eliminated, the war is not over.

We had earlier said that biofilms may represent one of the final stages in the progression of the disease that needs to be addressed. We have also described how biofilms seem to be preferentially drawn to sites in the body where injuries, lesions or even chronically stressed tissues (such as joints and connective tissue) reside. Although biofilms certainly play a major role in the resistance factor for Lyme disease, and later antibiofilm substances will be illucidated, the problem with this form of chronic infection is that it can in turn lead to an even deeper problem.

In order for biofilms to begin their initial attachment, bacteria must first have a means to initially attach themselves to host tissues and cells. In Borrelia a relatively new understanding as to how this is done is coming to light. We have described how that fibrin is often a component of biofilms.

Fibrin is an insoluble protein which is converted from a soluble protein called *fibrinogen* in the body. As it relates to injuries and wounds, fibrinogen is first deposited into the site of the injury as part of the coagulation process wherein the body attempts to stop initial bleeding, and begin to repair the wound. Another enzyme protein called *thrombin* then converts fibrinogen into the insoluble fibrin. However in order to adhere the cellular matrix together, a substance called *fibronectin* is incorporated into the mix along with *laminin* and *collagen* formation. Fibronectin (FN) also aids in the growth of the wound tissue by connecting the cells together in the immediate injured area called the "extra-cellular matrix". FN then expands and forms small fibrils, which are thin fibers used to further attach tissue cells together and rebuild the injured site. FN can be distributed in any area where inflammation due to injury occurs. But it is also found in certain membranes in the body and in the plasma. FN is involved in the granulation process which can replace fibrin with permanent scar tissue once the healing process is finished. This is what doctors call *primary intent healing*.

In *secondary intent* wound healing however, often lesions do not properly heal due to infection as bacteria can become trapped in tissue. This is no accident however. Some bacteria, including Borrelia Burgdorferi possess fibronectin-binding proteins which specifically target fibronectin in the extracellular matrix of tissues. These have been identified as BBK3 and RevA outer surface proteins.[13] And although we are talking about injuries here, Lyme is known to gravitate especially towards any connective tissue and endothelial cells where it can infect fibrin, fibronectin and fibrils within the extracellular matrix.

> We examined the traversal of B. burgdorferi across the human BBB (blood brain barrier) and systemic endothelial cell barriers . . . traversal of B. burgdorferi across human BMEC (brain macrovascular endothelial cells) induces the expression of plasminogen activators, plasminogen activator receptors, and matrix metalloproteinases. Thus, the fibrinolytic system linked by an activation cascade may lead to focal and transient degradation of tight junction proteins that allows B. burgdorferi to invade the CNS.[14]

Particularly in infections such as Lyme disease where immune responses are deliberately down-regulated by the bacteria themselves, the infection cannot be cleared by macrophages and neutrophils. As a result, in a secondary effort to prevent the spread of the infection, the body can itself attempt to sequester or isolate the bacterial colonies which actually end up preserving them within the wound, thus aiding them. It's as if the body as an unintended consequence of its own healing process is actually providing its own biofilm factory ready-made for bacteria. As the infection persists, this may have the affect of over-stimulating the production of fibronectin and excess fibrin in chronic inflammation as the body is continually working towards clearing the infection.

But it's not just trauma or injuries which can draw Bb infections. Anyplace the bacterial colonies or infection forms however can induce further injury by the immune system itself. As the infection persists, inflammatory cytokine messages are continually being leaked into the tissues and cells, drawing tissue-damaging immune cells and complexes into the matrix. Since these phagocytic and innate immune cells are not effectively able to remove the infection, their activity actually promotes further inflammation. In effect, it is not the bacteria themselves that are as damaging as our own immune system's attempts to clear the lesion. As a result, this further damage is in turn followed by the body's attempts to heal what it inflicted upon itself, and draws more fibrinolytic activity to repair the damage. As this cycle continues, scar-like lesions can accumulate on top of the infection, and create masses of fibrin, or increased levels of fibronectin thus allowing the infection to spread even more.

Thus, we come to understand how chronic Lyme disease can develop. Spirochetes and perhaps other forms preferentially are drawn to and bind to the fibronectin the body is laying down in order to heal the damage that was created by the inflammation in the first place. We can therefore understand how important anti-inflammatory herbs and non-drug remedies can be in reversing this disease process. And in fact, if inflammation is not controlled and reversed, this chronic accumulation of fibrin can act by impeding the healing process since it acts by blocking immune cells from clearing the infection.

We have been aware of the need for fibrinolytic and proteolytic enzymes to aid in the dissolution of fibrin that is incorporated into biofilms. However the tissues themselves can expand into fibrous and granulated cell masses which become an ongoing source of inflammation as long as the bacteria remain trapped within this extracellular matrix. These can continue to be plaguing even long after much of the surface biofilms have been resolved, since they represent the deepest source and substrate upon which the infection initially sprang up. These may also require even longer term more intensive therapies.

By reducing the excessive non-productive inflammation, the immune system won't have to work as hard against itself, and thus the disease process has the potential to reverse.

The good news is that some studies have demonstrated that berberine has been used in some bacterial infections to inhibit or block the microbe from attaching to fibronectin, or reduce excessive fibronectin expression under certain conditions. [15, 16] These are only studies, but they hold potential benefits. Berberine will be discussd more later.

ENDNOTES

1. *Pharmacological inhibition of quorum sensing for treatment of chronic bacterial infections.* Hentzer, M., & Givskov, M Journal of Chemical Investigation, 2003 112(9), 1300-1307.
2. *The Lux S gene is not required for Borrelia burgdorferi tick colonization, transmission to mammalian host, or induction of disease.* Blevins, J., Revel, A., Caimano, M., Yang, X., Richardson, J., Hagman, K., & Norgard, M. (2004). Infection and Immunity, 72(8), 4864-4867
3. *Lux S-mediated quorum sensing in Borrelia burgdorferi, the Lyme Disease spirochete.* Stevenson, B., & Babb, K. (2002). Infection and Immunity, 70(8), 4099-4105.
4. *Pharmacological inhibition of quorum sensing for treatment of chronic bacterial infections.* Hentzer, M., & Givskov, M. Journal of Chemical Investigation, (2003). 112(9), 1300-1307.
5. *Biofilms of* Borrelia burgdorferi *and Clinical Implications for Chronic Borreliosis* Dr. Alan MacDonald MD University of New Haven Lyme Disease Symposium New Haven New Connecticut May 17, 2008 http://

www.molecularalzheimer.org/files/Biofilm_New_Haven_ppt_Read-Only_. pdf Retrieved Feb. 3, 2013

6. Interview with Eva Sapi PhD: Professor of Cellular and Molecular Biology University of New Haven August 28, 2009 Interviewed by Richard Longland—Youtube posted April 3, 2010 Bacterial Biofilms and Lyme Disease http://www.youtube.com/watch?v=AmvgOfIN_8c

7. "Research on Microbial Biofilms" From NIH website.Release date: December 20, 2002 PA NUMBER: PA-03-047 http://grants.nih.gov/ grants/guide/pa-files/PA-03-047.html Retrieved Feb. 3, 2013

8. Ibid.

9. *Microscopic and physiologic evidence for biofilm-associated wound colonization in vivo* Davis SC, Ricotti C, Cazzaniga A, Welsh E, Eaglstein WH, Mertz PM. Wound Repair Regen. 2008 Jan-Feb; 16(1):37-44. Epub 2007 Dec 13.

10. *Lyme disease: A Look Beyond Antibiotics* Dietrich K. Klinghardt, MD, PhD Explore Magazine, Volume 14, No. 2, April 2005 http://www.samento. com.ec/sciencelib/4lyme/beyondantibiotics.html Retrieved Feb. 3, 2013

11. *What is the connection between biofilms and persistent infections?* Biofilms Hypertextbook Chapter 4 Biofilms in Health and Medicine Section 2 Biofilms and Chronic Infections http://biofilmbook.hypertextbookshop. com/working_version/contents/chapters/chapter004/section002/blue/ page001.html Retrieved Feb. 3, 2013

12. Interview with Dr. Randall Wolcott, bacterial biofilm wound specialist By Amy Proal Bacteriality April 13, 2008 http://bacteriality.com/2008/04/13/wolcott/ Retrieved Feb. 3, 2013

13. *Borrelia burgdorferi RevA Antigen Binds Host Fibronectin* Catherine A. Brissette, Tomasz Bykowski, Anne E. Cooley, Amy Bowman, and Brian Stevenson Infect Immun. 2009 July; 77(7): 2802-2812.

14. *Borrelia burgdorferi, Host-Derived Proteases, and the Blood-Brain Barrier* Grab DJ, Perides G, Dumler JS, Kim KJ, Park J, Kim YV, Nikolskaia O, Choi KS, Stins MF, Kim KS. Infect. Immun. Feb. 2005 vol 73 no. 2 1014-1022

15. *Berberine sulfate blocks adherence of Streptococcus pyogenes to epithelial cells, fibronectin and hexadecane.* Sun D, Courtney HS, Beachey EH Antimicrob Agents Chemother 1988 Sep, 32(9): 1370-4.

16. *Berberine reduces fibronectin and collagen accumulation in rat glomerular mesangial cells cultured under high glucose condition.* Liu W, Tang F, Deng Y, Li X, Lan T, Zhang X, Huang H, Liu Mol Cell Biochem. 2009 May; 325(1-2):99-105. Epub 2009 Jan 14.

CHAPTER 6

The Infectious Process

This chapter is an interesting side note that helps to explain how the infectious process takes place. Based upon what we now know of the biochemistry of Bb, we can draw some conclusions as to how the disease actually unfolds in the body. We already understand how it develops when a tick bites because we know that the spirochete form, which is the most immune provoking form, is already in the gut of ticks and incites the wound site upon initial infection. This is "classic" Lyme disease. It is the way most people understand it to originate, and is the way most doctors were trained to think.

However authorities have maintained that the disease can develop from many other sources. We have already cited Dr. Mattman's research that demonstrates that other vectors such as flies, fleas, mosquitoes are carriers and potential sources for the spread of infection, that it can be congenitally transmitted, sexually, and even thru contact. One of the plaguing questions has become why these other sources of infection do not commonly display the same severity of symptoms with the rapidity of tick bites? For instance, why is the EM rash rarely witnessed when being bitten by mosquitoes, or flies? Or why are the acute symptoms of Lyme not witnessed with the same severity and contagious reputation as syphilis if in fact they are both infectious spirochetes? Why are there few reports of this?

However a person becomes infected, that initial infection obviously does not always translate into a full blown disease. Bb can be latent and dormant, just as is possible with the treponema spirochete in syphilis. Many people have even tested positive and had elevated IgG antibodies to Bb with no visible simples (yet). [1]

Since only about 50% (depending on the source you read) of those being bitten by a tick develop the EM rash, it is impossible to know if a person's Lyme disease came from a tick bite or from some other source, as obviously many if not most do not ever remember being bitten by a tick. Therefore, a tick being the causative agent for any particular person's Lyme disease development cannot be quantified.

What we do know is that tick bites seem to be the one form of transmission that immediately precipitates the expression of disease. There are three primary reasons for this.

1. Ticks are known for being carriers of, and readily disseminate the spirochete form of Bb. However Dr. Mattman's work demonstrated that flies, mosquitoes and fleas were often seen as carriers of the CWD forms which are not as virulent.

2. Outer surface protein A (OspA) is a highly virulent antigen of Lyme spirochetes which receives a very rapid and strong immune response once inoculated into a human host. This spirochete protein is readily expressed in the tick gut. During the process of traveling thru the salivary glands and being injected dermally under the skin and subsequent blood contact, it rapidly begins to down-regulate this protein and expresses another protein, OspC (outer-surface protein C). OspC is not always an immune target. Only sometimes. If this conversion of OspA to OspC does not take place in time, OspA induces a very strong immune response wherein the EM rash can develop. It appears that the bacteria sense this change in environments and quickly seek to adapt by altering protein expression. This would explain why EM rashes are not always seen in tick bites. [2] This process of converting its protein during the transmission process would not be observed in other non-spirochete transmitted vectors such as human to human contact or insect bites because . . .

3. There is a salivary protein in ticks called *salp 15* which is known to bind to spirochetes and interact with OspC, thus protecting them from antibody response upon subcutaneous inoculation. [3, 4] This saliva protein would not likely be present in other vectors such as flies, mosquitoes, fleas, etc. This salp 15, by protecting Bb OspC would explain why such a strong immune response, but a lack of antibody-mediated killing exists upon initial infection from a tick bite. This is perhaps the reason why it is incorrectly assumed that ticks are the only carriers of infection. In fact, it

appears extremely likely that this salp 15 protein may be the primary trigger that initiates the disease process by protecting Bb spirochetes from being killed off upon initial infection.

However having stated this, there have been reports of some having known mosquito bites producing the EM rash followed by Lyme-like symptoms.

> One woman was certain her illness came from a mosquito bite. She recalled being bitten by a mosquito and woke up the next day with a target skin lesion at the bite site (same skin lesion as seen in Lyme Disease) and such profound weakness she was unable to get out of bed. Another woman recalled a target lesion at the site of a mosquito bite. Both women remain ill 20 years later. [5]

Testimonies from other individuals have been given which demonstrates that both mosquitoes [6] and spider bites [7] have been known to induce the bull'e eye rash.

We have been told by the CDC that EM (bull's eye) rash is all that is necessary to diagnose Lyme disease, even in the absence of laboratory confirmation. If that is the case, then by their own definition, Lyme disease is confirmed to be vectored from mosquito bites, and spider bites as well as ticks, confirming what Dr. Mattman was finding in the laboratory. Therefore, to state that ticks are the only carriers of infection is to deliberately ignore the evidence.

Bb is a much more highly evolved and adaptable bacterium than Treponema Pallidum in that it possesses a plasmid system. This syphilis spirochete does not. This explains Bb's ability to almost immediately adapt to a new environment. That Bb readily and easily responds to varying environmental conditions by turning on its plasmids is an established fact. It would therefore explain why the expression of disease symptoms would be delayed as compared to syphilis. Based upon what we now know of the infectivity of Bb, syphilis may not truly be a more contagious disease than Lyme, only that it more readily makes itself known, and that the expression of the disease is much more immediate.

Other than tick-vectored infection, compared to syphilis, Lyme on the other hand, is much more subtle.

Since research suggests that many people are carriers of infection without even knowing it, there is a high probability that the forms infecting these individuals are in fact the L-forms ("L" referring to the Lister Institute where they were first observed and named) which often do not induce pronounced symptoms since these forms do not express the strong immune invoking lipoproteins expressed by spirochetes. These lipoproteins are "turned on" or expressed as a defense mechanism when an immune cell is threatening the bacteria. Remember we said that scientific research revealed that expression of Lp28 and Lp25 plasmids are necessary for infection to occur. These plasmids are responsible for the conversion of non-virulent forms into the sickness-producing or pathogenic forms such as spirochetes, cyst, bleb and other pleomorphic or variant forms. So someone who is only a carrier may likely remain that way unless an immune response is ignited.

The process may go something like this. Whether thru sexual contact, tick, insect, or other means, Bb is exposed to a new host. At this point the person is only a carrier if his/her immune system does not react and begin producing antibodies. Perhaps it is a matter of semantics how you define "infected". To some, the actual presence of the bacteria in the host may be defined as an infection. To others, an actual infection does not occur until an immune response is initiated. In either case, once some aspect of the immune system threatens the bacteria, it can activate its gene or plasmid expressed lipoprotein system to begin actively taking evasive maneuvers thru its morphological variations and expression of toxic proteins. And as long as the immune system is reacting, it will threaten the bacterium, which will in turn cause the bacteria to continue to express defensive and offensive reactions. This back and forth exchange or battle continually perpetuates the disease, thus escalating the cycle. They in essence feed on one another. The immune system induces plasmid activation, which turns on immune invoking lipoproteins, in a never ending cycle.

Since the entire process began with the quorum decision to amass large numbers of bacteria, which led to an activation of plasmids to express a symptom-invoking immune response, then in theory the same thing may happen in reverse. Once bacterial loads have become reduced significantly enough by the killing off of vast colonies and planktonic bacteria thru the use of antimicrobial therapies, the immune response will also be reduced. In theory, at some point it is possible that not enough of the individual bacterium exist to maintain the need for the expression of those defensive plasmids. Hence, they may respond by, in essence, turning-off their expression since they are no longer serving a purpose. Once the immune system gains the upper hand, it may no longer feel threatened and significantly down-regulates its hyper-response in kind.

Therefore, in theory it is possible that eventually with continued therapies killing and reducing the over-all bacterial load, a point may be reached when so few individual bacterium are sensed by the body, that the immune system down-regulates its response to the infection. Then in kind, with the lack of quorum sensing auto-inducers present to maintain a defensive activated plasmid expression, Lp25, Lp28 or other plasmids may become lost or deactivated as is known to occur in vitro. At such a point, although Bb bacteria may still be present in the body, they may become non-infective, and remain such until conditions change that would renew the entire infectious disease process again. (This process may explain in part why so much relapsing occurs in Lyme disease.)

However, since so few people who develop chronic Lyme disease reach the point when their immune system is no longer reacting, the complete cessation of the disease is seldom seen. And the development of biofilms would insure that immune cells would forever be on high alert. Although not common, we have seen some people who have indeed defeated the illness who no longer express symptoms. They no longer take antimicrobial medicines either. It is my own personal view that they were able to reach this point not because every single bacterium was destroyed as a result of some therapy, but rather because they were reduced in numbers in both their planktonic and biofilm forms to the point that gene expression altered their virulence factors, which resulted in the turning off of the immune response, which is what induced the actual disease symptoms in the first place. For those with Lyme disease, it may not be possible to completely eradicate every single bacterium.

And in order to become "cured" of Lyme disease it may not be necessary to do so. Only that it is necessary to reduce the bacterial load to the point where the immune system is no longer stimulating the bacteria to maintain what I call "active Lyme disease plasmids". My personal view and theory is that when and if these plasmids are no longer activated, Bb may no longer possess the ability to remain infective. That is only a theory. But in the absence of another explanation, it seems difficult to believe that any Lyme therapy has the ability to destroy every bacterium in the body in all of its forms.

ENDNOTES

1. *Latent Lyme neuroborreliosis: Presence of Borrelia burgdorferi in the cerebrospinal fluid without concurrent inflammatory signs.* Pfister, H.W., Preac-Mursic, V., Wilski, B., Einhaupl, K.M., & Weinberger, K. Neurology, 1989 39(8), 1118-1120

2. *Expression of* Borrelia burgdorferi *OspC and DbpA is controlled by a RpoN—RpoS regulatory pathway* Hübner A, Yang X, Nolen DM, Popova TG, Cabello FC, Norgard MV. Proc Natl Acad Sci U S A. 2001 Oct 23; 98(22):12724-9.

3 *Antibodies against a tick protein, Salp15, protect mice from the Lyme disease agent.* Jianfeng Dai, Penghua Wang, Sarojini Adusumilli, Carmen J. Booth, Sukanya Narasimhan, Juan Anguita and Erol Fikrig. Cell Host Microbe 2009 November 19:6(5):482-492

4. *The Tick Salivary Protein Salp15 Inhibits the Killing of Serum-SensitiveBorrelia burgdorferi Sensu Lato Isolate* Tim J. Schuijt, Joppe W. R. Hovius, Nathalie D. van Burgel, Nandhini Ramamoorthi, Erol Fikrig, and Alje P. van Dam INFECTION AND IMMUNITY, July 2008, p. 2888-2894 Vol. 76, No. 7

5. *New Ideas About The Cause, Spread and Therapy of Lyme Disease* Dr. James Howenstine Townsend Letter for Doctors and Patients, July 2004

6. *Lyme Disease/Bull's Eye Rash From Mosquito Bite* Article by allexperts.com 8/29/2007 http://en.allexperts.com/q/Lyme-Disease-2911/Bull-Eye-Rash-Mosquito.htm Retrieved Feb. 3, 2013

7. Spider Bite Bullseye Article First Aid About.com http://firstaid.about.com/od/bitesstings/ig/Spider-Bite-Pictures/Small-Bite-Bullseye.htm Retrieved Feb. 3, 2013

CHAPTER 7

The Limitations of Testing

A thorough discussion on the topic of testing goes way beyond the scope of this book.

This is an area of incredible controversy. The controversy has been created due to the many views that doctors have about Lyme disease. But it is also caused by the many variable factors that come into play from the biochemistry of Borrelia and its many forms. That in turn plays itself out in the way the immune system reacts to the bacteria, which is different in every person. So creating a standardized test for Lyme disease that works in every person is nearly impossible.

Although we have discussed testing somewhat along the way, I hesitate to spend much time on this subject because it is so involved and would require undo time and space to adequately address all the variables. Lyme disease is a clinical diagnosis pure and simple. From the CDC's own Lyme report, "The diagnosis of Lyme disease is based primarily on clinical findings, and treating patients with early disease solely on the basis of objective signs and a known exposure is often appropriate." [1] Period!

However both patients and doctors often want a greater sense of certainty since other coinfective bacteria and even mycoplasma infections can resemble Lyme disease. So a laboratory serological test (a test based upon blood and other bodily fluids) that could give a definitive diagnosis would certainly be more preferable. Also, since chronic Lyme is often a permanent sentence, a higher degree of confidence would certainly give potential sufferers a sense of "knowing" what they are facing, rather than living with uncertainty.

Most people who acquire Lyme disease do not realize the quagmire and controversy they are about to engage in. The illness is difficult enough as it is. But the political battles that involve government agencies, medical societies, medical boards, doctors and their often controversial views and treatments are without a doubt more reflected in Lyme disease than perhaps any other illness. There is a real need to simplify the complex matters so you the patient can let go of the confusion to focus on what is important.

No discussion of testing could be complete without delving into the controversy to some extent. But rather than dealing too much with the controversy we will give a brief discussion of testing, and then some bottom line points to allow the reader to do his/her own research into the complexities of Lyme disease testing. After all, the purpose of this book is not to deal with the diagnostic aspects of Lyme disease, but to learn about what makes this disease so unique and offer real world solutions.

Many of the difficulties of Lyme are spawned by lack of reliable testing. Doctors walk a fine line between wanting to meet certain government or medical board guidelines, recommendations, or the criticism by their peers, and wanting to help their patients. Often this conflict ends up being a tug of war where the patient gets the short end of the stick. Some doctors value their reputations in higher regard than their patients needs. Often you will see that some of the most respected and loved doctors are the ones that champion their patient's needs at the expense of their own popularity. They don't care what their peers think, or what medical society standing they have. They want to help their patients, period. They are the true heroes.

My own delving into Lyme research was motivated in part by the frustration I experienced when my own lab results did not meet the early CDC guidelines. The problem that it caused is one that has been experienced by many Lyme disease patients. You wonder, do I really have the disease? Is my doctor going to be able to give me the necessary treatments? What about insurance? What else could it be? And so you sift thru all the confusing questions because you feel impotent to know how to proceed since you don't understand the complexities of the issues, what the test results mean, and who is telling you the truth. In my own case, although my symptoms were perfectly consistent with Lyme, my doctor diagnosed me with ankylosing spondilitis because he was hesitant to diagnose me with Lyme since I didn't meet pre-defined criteria. (This was ludicrous since I had more than 16 symptoms of classic Lyme, most of which do not parallel anything resembling ankylosing spondilitis.)

That leads you to wonder, what do those guidelines or criteria mean? How are they determined? Who sets the guidelines? Why do the guidelines seem to differ from one agency or organization to another? Why do they change sometimes from one year to the next? Why are test results so inconsistent? Why does one test say I have Lyme disease while the other is negative? Why would my doctor ignore my obvious Lyme symptoms when I even have Western Blot bands to support a clinical diagnosis? And on what basis does he make that decision when another doctor would have immediately diagnosed me with Lyme? And the list goes on. All these are legitimate questions to be asked, particularly by the patient that has clinical symptoms of Lyme disease, but who receives a negative test result.

It is not so important to know the answers to all these questions as it is to understand that these are the circumstances that Lyme patients face. It could require an entire book and a point by point discussion to answer each of the questions, as each will have a sub-point and sub-sub point under each explanation. I am not that smart, but it took me considerable study to help me to get to a point where I at least had a working knowledge of how not only the tests are performed and how they work, but then to understand how the results are defined. Add to that various Lyme and infectious disease societies and government agencies that come along and tell you how to interpret those tests, all being worlds apart in their conclusions. That is what you are facing.

Lyme disease is one illness you absolutely must do your own research and come to your own conclusions about. You must educate yourself and not rely solely on the advice of any one particular healthcare practitioner. It is important that you not only understand, but feel comfortable with what you are told, and have at least a competent understanding about what you are dealing with. You must have your hands on the steering wheel and not blindly follow someones advice. That is not to say, "Do not trust your doctor." It is to say, understand what you are being told and why. If you do not, ask questions until you are satisfied. Not only will this give you confidence to know what is happening, but that confidence leads to decisiveness in your decision-making. Your life changes when you learn you have Lyme disease. And you will need to become a strong and self-reliant person to steer thru the confusion. Even more so if your goal is ultimately to defeat the disease.

SEROLOGICAL TESTS

According to the CDC there are some 70 serological tests approved by the FDA for Lyme disease. Each of them works in a different manner. Direct assays are methods using either biopsy or culture testing, and are the most defining since they observe or grow the actual bacteria from your body. But these tests are seldom used in Lyme disease since Bb is so difficult to culture, and a test that doesn't grow the bacteria only means that it couldn't be grown, not necessarily that you don't have it in you. So for Lyme disease, several popular tests are often used. These are those mostly recommended by the CDC since they require the reporting of certain infectious diseases by your doctor, of which Lyme is one. Hence they have created criteria which a patient must meet in order to satisfy the requirements for reporting. In the early days, it was not made clear that the criteria were for reporting purposes. As a result, many physicians and insurance companies adopted the guidelines set for CDC reporting, and used them for diagnostic purposes.

The problem was that the criteria for a definitive serological positive test result were set so high, that an incredible amount of false negatives was the result. Many patients were having their western blots positively reacting on certain bands, and were even having classic Lyme symptoms in conjunction with living in endemic areas where high tick populations were known. Yet the CDC for some unknown reason arbitrarily determined that those patients were negative according to their guidelines. This made no logical or scientific sense whatsoever, except as it was previously mentioned, I believe the CDC has deliberately raised the standards for reporting such that many who have the disease are being left out of the reports to deliberately mislead the public. Most experts agree, and even the CDC itself admits that the actual numbers are far greater than are being reported, perhaps ten-fold.

When in 1994 the Centers for Disease Control and Prevention (CDC) and the Association of State and Territorial Public Health Laboratory Directors (ASTPHD) developed interpretive guidelines as to what constitutes a positive Western blot, activists, frontline physicians and many scientists criticized the criteria as too stringent and, in some aspects, unscientific. [2]

Later and subsequent Lyme conferences clarified that the guidelines set by the CDC were for reporting purposes, not for diagnostic. This only helped a little in that it clarified for insurance purposes that the diagnosis was to be made by the physician, not the guidelines. But that still didn't solve the problem since medical boards and governmental agencies often set rules and laws that wouldn't allow a physician to administer long-term antibiotics in the absence of a serologically defined infectious agent or diagnosis. That meant that doctors could not treat patients accordingly even though they were able to clinically diagnose them with Lyme disease.

One example,

Texas State Sen. Chris Harris, who was ravaged by the effects of undiagnosed Lyme disease, is now working to get the House and Senate committees to pass two bills that target the gap in proper treatment for Lyme disease . . . Harris said his doctor, fearing punishment from the Texas Medical Board, initially refused to treat him. The doctor believed a long-term course of antibiotics was required, he said, but the disciplinary board seemed to back treatment that limited antibiotic use to one month or less. [3]

This often appears to be the rule rather than the exception.

But an even further problem arises with the question of chronic Lyme disease. "Of patients with acute culture-proven Lyme disease, 20-30% remains seronegative on serial Western Blot sampling. Antibody titers also appear to decline over time; thus while the Western Blot may remain positive for months, it may not always be sensitive enough to detect chronic infection with the Lyme spirochete." [4] Many doctors rely heavily on lab tests for Lyme diagnosis, and believe that a course or two of antibiotics should kill the spirochete just as any other bacterial infection. When their patient's test results are negative, these doctors refuse to treat further, even though their patients continue to display clear symptoms consistent with late stage Lyme. Many doctors still do not accept that these bacteria can resist antibiotic therapy, and so they blame their patient's conditions on some other factors, even in the absence of any other identifiable underlying causes.

Both circumstances wherein doctors were not allowed to treat patients with antibiotics in the absence of positive test results, and when patients clearly manifested late stage chronic Lyme disease also in the absence of serological confirmation, placed the patient completely on his/her own with regards to finding help for their illness—meaning they simply couldn't be treated for their disease. This situation has been one of the most egregious violations of patient trust in the history of our country. And it is still going on today.

In 2006 the Infectious Diseases Society of America (IDSA) came out with guidelines which stunned many doctors and Lyme disease patients alike. From their manual:

> *There is no convincing biologic evidence for the existence of symptomatic chronic B. burgdorferi infection among patients after receipt of recommended treatment regimens for Lyme disease. Antibiotic therapy has not proven to be useful and is not recommended for patients with chronic (_6 months) subjective symptoms after recommended treatment regimens for Lyme disease.* [5]

Please note this statement is made by a medical doctor who reversed his positions after having received a multi-million dollar research grant funded by our government. This was proven to be the case by Steven Phillips MD in a report submitted to the International Lyme and Associated Disease Society (ILADS) entitled "Chronic Lyme: An Evidence-Based Review" wherein he definitively not only proves using multiple research sources the existence of chronic Lyme, but that long-term therapy has shown to be significantly beneficial to those sufferers. Additionally he cites many direct reversals of positions by the very writers of the original guidelines showing they contradicted their own conclusions. [6]

However even though these are only considered "Guidelines", and as such hold no legal or compulsory requirements that physicians must follow, such guidelines are used by insurance companies as supporting documentation to deny coverage to Lyme patients.

Also, it was stated earlier that the CDC, by placing reporting criteria so high that most Lyme disease sufferers would test negative according to their guidelines, are misleading the public by doing so. Given that the CDC is a branch of the U.S. Department of Health and Human Services (the government) one may also question the connection that the government plays in their involvement with IDSA given they were granted $76M Federal funds to study chronic Lyme disease. That same organization came to the conclusion it doesn't exist, even though most Lyme-cognizant medical doctors disagree. Additionally their conclusion has been scientifically proven to be false.

Due to the circumstances surrounding their receiving a huge grant and that their conclusion was obviously suspicious, the Connecticut Attorney General Richard Blumenthal launched an investigation against the IDSA charging conflict of interest that influenced their decision. (In other words the government paid them off to come to such conclusions, since the evidence was obviously to the contrary.) This was the first ever lawsuit against a medical society. The verdict resulted in the compromise to allow the IDSA panel to review their conclusions and allow contrary positions to be introduced. Yet they ultimately maintained their position. This was reported in an April 2010 article by Dr. Bransfield of the ILADS. [7]

By this it should be learned that corruption and the covering up of the seriousness of Lyme disease goes well beyond the illness itself. It shows the illness is so serious in its scope that even our own government is displaying evidence attempting to cover up and hide the extent of the problem from the people. If one ever reads that Lyme disease is easily treated with antibiotics, unless that source is referring to early detected Lyme, it is simply untrue. One additional observation that should be made relative to Lyme disease is that one research group cited that biofilms are caused by some 80% of all bacteria, and is known to be a factor in chronic infections. [8] Yet the IDSA did not mention biofilms once in their manual. This shows that they, in addition to distorting the facts of research, are using outdated information to come to such conclusions since biofilms would be a primary factor in chronic Lyme disease, and would perfectly explain why antibiotics would tend to lose their effectiveness over time.

LAB TESTS

It had been mentioned that various factors are involved which makes relying on lab tests for Lyme disease often unreliable at best, inappropriate at worst. From Lyme Federation, Inc: "Scientists believe a variety of reasons, including strain variation, the fact Bb is polymorphic (able to change the proteins on its outer surface, thus causing different antibodies to be produced) and the health of the patient's immune system are some explanations for this variability." [9]

One Lyme Disease Association conference report found that PCR testing (a method that necessitates capturing an antigen) is only 35% accurate for blood testing, and Western Blot only 50-60% accurate. ELISA was found to be below these levels. [10] And these are supposed to be the primary tests we rely on to help confirm if we have the disease! Even though these may have been improved over the past several years, they are notorious for failing to confirm the disease even in the face of positive clinical symptoms.

It is for this reason that the tide is finally beginning to turn giving help to Lyme sufferers. On June 21, 2009 Connecticut Governor M. Jodi Rell announced that she has signed a bill that would allow physicians to prescribe long-term antibiotics to those clinically diagnosed with Lyme disease. [11] This now allows a doctor to treat a patient that exhibits classical Lyme symptoms in the absence of laboratory confirmation in that state. It is hoped that other states will follow suit. This illustrates what has always been the case, but until now lacked a legal protection for practitioners: Lyme disease is a clinical diagnosis.

Perhaps this is part of the reason for some of the confusion surrounding test results. For those interested, a discussion is given that helps to explain why even the best Western Blot tests can be flawed.

It bears repeating that one of the fundamental flaws in this test in my opinion is that the primary strains that are used in testing are those which are mostly found in ticks in specific geographical locations of the country, but which also happen to be more highly virulent than strains in other parts of the country. That means that certain assumptions are being made that could affect the way these tests are interpreted.

There is simply no way to know of certainty that the individual lipoproteins in all strains of a particular genospecie will react the same as some standard you are using in testing. But that is the assumption that is used in test interpretation. One slight variation could mean the difference between a band forming or not.

Using only a few strains that are representative of only a small geographical area of the country truly makes no sense. (You don't go looking for a Bengal Tiger in the bogey woods of south Texas where there are an abundance of Bobcats.) That means if a strain of Borrelia differs enough from the highly virulent strains generally located in the northeastern area of the United States where there is a high likelihood of these being genetically modified strains, they will have compared that particular patient's antibody response to a bacteria that does not represent his/her infection close enough to render the test sensitive enough to make a definitive determination. *If you cannot know whether the strain of bacteria that is infecting a person is a close enough match to the strain used in the test, then the entire basis of the test becomes diluted.* To repeat, when tests are viewed and interpreted, if the strain of Borrelia and hence the protein virulence factors of that particular strain differ from the standard strains used in the test, there is a systematic inconsistency in the test factors.

If you were to take two rulers and lay them side by side, you could line up the inch marks on the rulers and they would be an exact match. If however you are using one standard ruler that uses inches, and the other ruler is based upon the metric system, you would not be able to line them up. Some marks may line up closely, a few almost exactly, but most would not line up at all since you are not using the same standards. This is what is happening in Western Blot testing. They are using a few strains that do not exactly match or accurately represent all strains close enough to render it a reliable comparison. That is the reason for such dramatic inconsistencies in these tests. Add to that, since Borrelia possesses variable proteins which can be altered over time and from bacterium to bacterium, it is not only like using two different kinds of rulers, but the marks on the rulers are constantly moving around. This illustrates how difficult it can be to find accurate results using these tests.

Additionally, these tests not only do not seek to differentiate between highly virulent and less virulent strains which could result in huge differences in test results, they do not seek to identify strains at all, as that is not the purpose of the Western Blot test. However it is assumed that within a given window of variance, all strains of Borrelia will have *the same measureable lipoprotein virulence factors*. Because this has not been consistently proven to be the case, the test results will be skewed, often dramatically.

However that is only one problem with the Western Blot testing. If the way that any particular lipoprotein expressed itself was always the same, there would be a consistent standard by which to compare antibody responses. But they do not. One example was illustrated when three groups of Borrelia strains, although were able to be distinguished from other strains, "were divergent from each other in the molecular masses of putative outer surface protein A (OspA) and in the sequences of the ospA gene." [12]

Not only can lipoproteins differ from strain to strain, but they can express themselves differently even within their own strain, depending on the host immune response.

Although Borrelia is not unique in its ability to alter protein expression, its capacity to do so is significantly greater than most other bacteria in this respect. (We are not just speaking of the ability of Borrelia to morph from one form to another, we are speaking of the ability of the protein structures, called epitopes, that make up the cell membrane and other structures to change to appear differently to the immune system in order to deliberately avoid antibody-coupling.) This affects the degree to which antibodies can react. Specific antibodies respond to specific antigens. The degree to which the antigen (or lipoprotein) varies, may determine the level of response of that antibody. So if a variable lipoprotein becomes altered enough, an antibody which was once highly reactive, may later become less responsive. Not only that, but one of the reasons some Western Blot tests are inconsistent is because the very process used in collecting and preparing the antigen alters or denatures it in such a fashion that certain proteins whose epitope (that molecular region on the surface of the lipoprotein that elicits an immune response) conforms to antibody sites becomes distorted. Therefore the very process that is used to collect protein samples can render the normal antigen-antibody coupling non-functional, or less responsive. Again, here is another inconsistency which can skew test results. And that is just the bacterial side.

The other side of the coin is that all patients immune responses can and do vary dependent upon a number of factors. For example a severely immune compromised patient that has had an infection for only a certain length of time may not even have developed enough antibodies to be responsive. This is yet another reason why test results can change over time. Western Blot testing is completely dependent upon the creation and normal distribution of antibodies to react to any given proteins introduced in testing. Pacific Frontier Medical made a list of 53 individual scientific research studies demonstrating the seronegativety in Lyme disease (false negatives), meaning that test results were negative while later they were confirmed to be positive to Borrelia infection.[13]

I personally heard of one lady that had a daughter with Lyme disease that had 8 tests done before she finally had a positive test result. She had been displaying classic Lyme symptoms, but her immune system simply was not creating a high enough antibody count sensitive enough to develop the necessary western blot bands. Without this understanding, this can create a great deal of frustration and conflict not only for you, but between you and your doctor, especially when your doctor is not doing his homework.

Sometimes what is taught about antibody functions does not always find its way in real life applications. For instance we have traditionally been taught that plasma cells make specific antibodies for specific antigen sites. If that is the case, then it would not matter how many different kinds of infectious organisms you have, the body would produce a sufficient amount for each one, and bind to those sites thus marking them for destruction by other immune cells. Thus it is assumed that any tests that measure immune responses to a particular pathogen will accurately represent that assumption.

However Bartonella infections for example are known to inhibit the production of immune factors. [14] This is because Bartonella significantly impairs immune cells due to its lipopolysaccharide which is known as an antagonist, or blocker of cell signaling. [15] This has translated into clinical observations for instance by some physicians that Bartonella infections can actually inhibit the formation of Bb antibodies. Thus it has been observed that oftentimes a patient will receive a negative Western Blot test for Lyme when it is accompanied by a Bartonella infection. Once the Bartonella infection is resolved, antibodies for Bb begin to show up. Dr. James Schaller MD, a prominent doctor having treated many cases of Lyme disease in children has cited in an article that his experience has shown that when he treated coinfections first his patients "began to make Lyme antibodies and became positive over time." [16]

Additionally, Bb spirochetes are known for attacking T-lymphocytes, which are responsible for signaling B-cells for antibody production. Thus the infection itself inhibits the production of antibodies necessary for its destruction.

Therefore one can readily and easily observe why many patients that have Lyme disease will very highly often respond negatively to tests which involve measuring immune response such as ELISA and Western Blot, which incidentally have historically been the two primary tests recommended by the CDC.

Summary: In Lyme disease, antibody tests are notoriously inaccurate due to:

1. Using a very small number of strains without knowing if the strains being used accurately represent the strain in the infected individual. The strains used in most popular tests are known to be both geographically specific, as well as more reactive than other strains.
2. Variable proteins are being measured which are known to change over time, and thus will not be uniformly or consistently measurable.
3. Each person's immune response will be different, and will affect the development of antibodies. Thus antibodies are not an accurate measuring tool to determine infection.
4. Coinfectious bacteria and viruses can inhibit immune cell communication and affect the production of antibodies. Bb itself can destroy the very immune cells necessary for signaling antibody production.
5. It is the very nature of Bb infections to down-regulate immunity. This is why natural immunity to Bb is virtually non-existent, yet ironically that is the very thing that western blot is attempting to measure.
6. Attempting to develop a standard by which to measure everyone is a dangerous practice wherein the patient is always the loser. Patients are individuals, not statistics.

Conclusion—Antibody assays can be extremely unreliable when being used as a diagnostic standard for Lyme disease. It may obviously be useful in those cases where a positive response is the outcome. But what purpose does that solve for those with negative bands yet clinically observed to have Lyme symptoms?

In spite of the inherent inaccuracy of these tests, patients and doctors still insist on seeing where they stand in regard to these unreliable standards. That is because the CDC criteria involve the recommendation of two common tests. They are ELISA (enzyme-linked immunosorbent assay) and Western Blot. Both are antibody tests. ELISA is performed first by taking Bb and breaking apart the proteins usually thru sound waves, then using the resulting compilation as antigen targets. Then using a medium, they are combined with the patient's blood to form antigen/antibody complexes. These are in turn exposed to another group of antibodies which react to human antibodies, to which are joined or "linked" a special enzyme. This ezyme then reacts with certain chemicals to produce a color change that indicates a positive reaction has occurred.

Bb is known to possess certain bacterial proteins which are similar to or common in other bacteria. Therefore often there is a positive reaction to a protein which may not have come from Bb. This is one reason for such a high number of false positives. Usually if a patient does not react positively to ELISA they are not recommended for further testing.

On the other hand, the developers of this test attempt to filter these high numbers out from a statistical or probability standpoint by raising the number of proteins or sensitivity levels that must react in order to be considered positive. Based upon what has already been described with Bb, there is no way to know if their false positive is truly false. Nor is there a way to know if by raising the sensitivity standards they are in fact screening out true positives that show low reactivity. This is why this test is seldom given much weight and why these are often followed by Western Blot tests. From the International Lyme and Associated Diseases Society, "The ELISA screening test is unreliable. The test misses 35% of culture proven Lyme disease (only 65% sensitivity) and is unacceptable as the first step of a two-step screening protocol. By definition, a screening test should have at least 95% sensitivity." [17]

However sometimes the WB only fairs somewhat better. Western blot measures the body's antibody response to a particular lipoprotein of Bb. Each protein expressed by the bacterium is going to invoke a different antigenic response to the antibody that corresponds to or that targets it. Each band represents a different protein, and is given a number rating that represents the degree of response to that protein. The higher the number, the higher degree of antibody response. The Western Blot was designed to differentiate between specific antibody protein reactivity. These proteins are identified by their molecular weight. Again however, some of these proteins are considered "cross-reactive" meaning they are found in other bacteria other than Bb. The following are considered specific proteins to Bb. Test results identifying these bands are very specific for certain Borrelia strains known to cause Lyme disease. These include: Bands 18KD, 23-25KD(OspC), 31KD(OspA), 34KD(OspB), 37KD, 39KD, 83KD and 93KD are specific for indicating Bb exposure. Bands expressing reactions to these numbers are considered to have come from Bb exposure.

Other bands are also identified in the test, but are either cross-reactive bands to other bacteria, or to other Borrelia strains not considered to cause Lyme disease. For example 41kd is a flagella protein (used for mobility) that is common in most spirochetes regardless of the species, and is not considered unique to Bb.

Here is where the simplicity ends (as if that was simple!) Different labs often use different antigen strains or processing methods. They can each interpret results differently, and put more importance on one band over another. This is where the CDC stepped in and tried to make things simpler. In fact, they made things not only far worse, but confused the entire playing field by requiring that in order for a person to be considered positive, they must exhibit a certain number of bands. But those bands even included proteins that were not even considered unique to Bb! It appears as though what must have been in their minds was to use statistical analysis to figure the probability of someone having Lyme based upon a minimum number of bands. It was obvious they were not thinking like doctors, but like statisticians. If a protein is specific for only one kind of bacteria, then any reaction your immune system is having to that protein is also highly specific. It is like notifying you that someone is at the door by pushing the doorbell. The question is: how many doorbells do you need ringing on your front door to know if someone is ringing it? One, three, five? The CDC said you need to have at least 2 IgM and 5 IgG doorbells ringing before they think someone is at the door. Do you see the ludicrousy of this?

The following were the original CDC guidelines:

IgM antibodies required to meet positive criteria were bands 22-25, 39, and 41.

IgG antibodies required 5 of the following: 18, 23, 28, 30, 39, 41, 45, 58, 66, and 93.

The reasoning for using fewer IgM bands is that theoretically IgM represents early infection, and so fewer antibodies will have developed. While IgG antibodies theoretically represent a longer term infection, and so a higher degree of antibodies will have formed. The problem is that all this is theory, and based upon the high number of dissenting physicians, does not seem to represent the norm. Much of it simply makes no sense either. Observe for instance that 31kd(OspA) is the most reactive and most studied protein of Bb. In fact a vaccine was created for Lyme disease based upon this one protein. However it was not even included as a required band. This is truly beyond belief! The same can be said for 34kd(OspB). Yet interestingly 66kd and 58kd are both included, which are not even unique to Bb! (Sorry for all the exclamations, but government involvement can sometimes be beyond lunacy.)

This criteria, it was later "learned" was not intended to diagnose Lyme disease, but meant for surveillance purposes. But why would this matter what your purpose was for creating such absurd guidelines to begin with? These guidelines only proved to demonstrate the ineptness of those involved since they later became adopted by medical boards, insurance companies, and even physicians in time. Today some changes have been made to include 31kd and 34kd in the reporting criteria. Again, ILADS "a positive 31 or 34 band is highly indicative of Borrelia burgdorferi exposure." [18]

But so much confusion and damage had been done due to the establishment of these original guidelines, that to this day many physicians are still adopting surveillance criteria in various ways for their own diagnostic interpretations. This is why it has repeatedly been said, and the CDC has made it clear, "Lyme is a clinical diagnosis."

So what practical value can be received from the western blot given it has so many flaws and limitations? Since so many of the assumptions that are accepted as being true in the administration of antibody tests for other diseases often do not apply to Lyme disease, there is very little diagnostic value when these tests do not coincide with clinical symptoms.

Such is the reason so much weight is placed on patient history and illness manifestations. Does one consider a patient to have Lyme disease who has no symptoms, yet has a positive test result more so than someone that has classic Lyme disease manifestions whose test is categorically negative? What is the answer? This will obviously need to be discussed between you and your doctor. However as a very practical guide, contrary to some authors, the IgM would seem to actually have more relevance than IgG in that IgM represents ongoing or current infection. Theoretically IgM antibodies should decline over time as the infection is resolved. But since this rarely occurs in Lyme disease, IgM antibodies may remain elevated. And since IgG antibodies can potentially decline over time, this does not fit the standard IgM/IgG antibody behavior either. Additionally, since many lipoproteins are variable and constantly changing, this will inevitably cause the constant formation of new (IgM) antibodies.

IgM should indicate new infection and should fade over time, while IgG levels should rise and indicate ongoing or past infection. Common sense, right? One Lyme-group post by two Lyme patients shared their frustration over this silly blind acceptance of test results that doesn't fit with reality. Due to privacy issues, they have been paraphrased.

"One doctor told me, the only time you show IgM antibodies is when you are first infected because it shows you have an active infection. This is only my opinion, but **HELLO**, if you still have Lyme disease and have Lyme symptoms, then it is still active no matter when you were infected!!!"

Another wrote: "Everyone is different. Some people test positive for IgM, but never IgG, while others test negative for IgM, but positive for IgG. Either way, we still have Lyme. I was sick for over 6 years when my test came up IgM positive. My physician interpreted this as me having a recent infection. But I knew that was a load of crap! There was no way what had been making me sick for all that time was a recent infection. I was told that after 4 weeks or so my IgM would convert to IgG. Months later I was still only testing IgM positive. . . . You just can't win with most doctors no matter what your test shows."

From LymeMD, a physician cited a patient who was seronegative, but made a clinical diagnosis. Her initial Western Blot showed only 41kd

IgM and IgG bands. However after 4 months on antibiotics here were her test results:

IgM - 18 3+, 23 2+, 30 2+, 31 3+, 34 2+, 39 2+, 41 3+, 45 1+, 58 2+, 66 1+, 93 2+ IgG - 41 2+ [19] (Remember, band 41 is a non-specific flagella protein band that is possessed by other bacteria other than Bb.) There are reports of clinically and culture diagnosed Lyme patients without elevated IgG antibodies. [20-22]

When Jesus and his disciples were out gathering food on the sabbath, they were criticized for allegedly violating the sabbath. His response was, "The law was created to serve man, not for man to serve the law." When doctors allow test results that don't conform to their preconceived ideas to overrule patients clear symptoms, and withhold treatment, they are forcing patients to serve their tests, rather than their tests serve the patient. A common expression among doctors is, "treat the patient, not the test."

Common sense approach to Western Blot: If you even have one of the following bands, and you have clear Lyme symptoms, that is an indication that your body is producing antibodies to that protein. You don't even have to have one positive band for your doctor to give you a clinical diagnosis. But reacting to any is only supportive to your clinical symptoms.

To repeat, the Bb bands 18KD, 23-25KD(OspC), 31KD(OspA), 34KD(OspB), 37KD, 39KD, 83KD and 93KD are specific for indicating Bb exposure whether they are to IgM or IgG. Using any other proteins would have less significant value. In order to clear up any confusion, here is the current CDC criteria used for surveillance purposes. This is NOT to be used as a diagnostic tool by your physician. Taken directly from the CDC website:

CDC Lyme Disease National Surveillance Case Definition is as follows:

1. *A person with erythema migrans; or*
2. *A person with at least one late manifestation and laboratory confirmation of infection*

Note: **It should be emphasized that is an epidemiologic case definition intended for surveillance purposes only.**

Laboratory confirmation of infection with B. burgdorferi is established when a laboratory isolates the spirochete from tissue or body fluid, detects diagnostic levels of IgM or IgG antibodies to the spirochete in serum or CSF, or detects a significant change in antibody levels in paired acute and convalescent serum samples. States may determine the criteria for laboratory confirmation and diagnostic levels of antibody. Syphilis and other known causes of biologic false positive serologic test results should be excluded, as appropriate, when laboratory confirmation has been based on serologic testing alone. CDC 52.60 Rev. 02-2006 LYME DISEASE CASE REPORT [23]

Remember, what you have just read is ONLY a surveillance case definition. That means that the CDC is not the one preventing or limiting your doctor's authority to determine according to his own diagnosis whether or not you have Lyme disease as he is not bound by any CDC criteria in order to make a clinical diagnosis.

However, each state and their medical boards may set diagnostic and/or treatment guidelines as they see fit. *"States may determine the criteria for laboratory confirmation and diagnostic levels of antibody"*. This then takes the battle yet into another arena. Many state's medical boards adopt guidelines similar to those established by the Infectious Disease Society of America (IDSA). (Yes that is the very organization mentioned earlier that has denied convincing evidence of the benefits of long-term antibiotic care for Lyme disease, as well as denying the reality of chronic Lyme disease.) These medical boards then seek to punish and even revoke the licenses of physicians that (according to their guidelines) improperly diagnose and/or treat Lyme disease. Physicians live in fear of these boards and often choose to not accept Lyme patients for this reason. Or perhaps they will withhold a diagnosis. Since each state has the right to establish its own guidelines, the situation will be different depending on where you live. Often Lyme patients are forced to travel to another state to receive a diagnosis and proper treatment. Interesting how driving over state lines can give you Lyme disease! It becomes a sad state of affairs when you are denied patient care for the most rapidly spreading infectious disease in the country.

Observation: Here is what appears to be happening. The CDC has often been criticized for their original establishment of ludicrous criteria for Lyme disease reporting. Many doctors had implemented those guidelines however for diagnostic purposes. Since the CDC knew that a potential Lyme patient would need to be tested using the CDC's recommended laboratory confirmation guidelines anyways to see if they met those criteria for reporting, this was an awfully suspicious action to begin with. When an outcry took place since those original guidelines were using ridiculously conservative criteria, and leaving many if not most Lyme patients without a diagnosis despite obvious Lyme symptoms, they rescinded (excuse me, "clarified") their position by saying the guidelines were not for diagnostic, but rather for reporting purposes, and that Lyme was a clinical diagnosis. In other words, the doctors were told, "Don't worry about using the criteria for patient diagnosis and treatment, the criteria is only for reporting. You may diagnose and treat as you see fit."

However on the other hand, the same US government that runs the CDC also provides funds for a non-government medical society (IDSA) which creates guidelines for diagnosis and treating Lyme patients, which in turn individual states end up adopting. The CDC knows this. In fact the CDC's own website lists and provides a link to this society's website for Lyme treatment. Rather than adopting ILADS guidelines which is a much more scientifically and intellectually honest medical society, the CDC is promoting the IDSA guidelines, and in doing so, accomplishes the same goal of leaving patients without a diagnosis or long-term care, because states end up adopting the CDC's recommened IDSA guidelines instead. The IDSA denies the very existence of chronic Lyme disease. And so states and their medical boards also adopt this idea. This way, the CDC is off the hook and cannot be blamed for bad criteria, while the IDSA can claim they have no authority over what guidelines are adopted by individual state medical boards. So in the absence of state legislatures listening to the voice of the people to determine their own laws and guidelines, the Federal government, through the CDC, is by proxy (IDSA) setting Lyme disease standards and guidelines of state medical boards by promoting and encouraging the acceptance of often unscientific and misleading conclusions regarding their research. Because they are heavily funded by government grants, they are given more credibility, even though the majority of intellectually honest researchers and doctors have refuted many of their misguided conclusions. This collusion between gov't and non-government organizations is much like fascism in old Nazi Germany wherein the government developed a relationship with organizations and corporations to do their dirty work. Make no mistake; this is by design, not by chance.

It is my personal belief that the CDC has had a multi-tier plan to deceive the public. It is quite literally beyond believability. The first is by attempting to keep the focus on ticks as being the source of infection, without even considering other obvious, as well as already proven vectors. For example, the very case definition for reporting, states, "Lyme disease is a systemic tick-borne disease . . . ." It does not say it is a disease caused by the bacterium Borrelia Burdgorferi! Why would it be more important to state the transmission vector of the disease in the reporting definition rather than even the bacteria itself? The bacterium is not even mentioned in the definition. Ticks do not cause Lyme disease. A bacterium called Borrelia Burgdorferi does. They are trying to drive home the emphasis on focusing on one particular vector in order to distract from the reality that this bacterial infection is already in millions of people who have not yet succumbed to its threat, nor have ever been bitten by a tick.

The CDC provides two maps. One shows the endemic areas where Borrelia-infected tick populations are most prevalent. The other shows where Lyme disease is mostly reported. They have a rather similar appearance. One could almost be laid over the other. In one report provided on the CDC website, Surveillance for Lyme Disease—United States, 1992-1998, "Lyme disease has a highly focal distribution within the United States . . . . This focal distribution of human cases correlates well with the distribution, density, and infection prevalence of I. scapularis [ticks] in the northeastern and north-central United States." [24]

By overlaying a tick-infestation map on top of a CDC Lyme disease reporting map, and seeing the similar pattern, you are deliberately being led to believe that Lyme disease only comes from ticks; and that if you live in another area of the country, you are unlikely to develop Lyme Disease. What you are not being told is that it is estimated even by the CDC itself that the actual cases of Lyme disease are much higher. Most scientists believe they are easily underreported by as much as 90% or more! Therefore, no one actually knows what the representative map would look like if all Lyme disease cases were reported, not just those meeting CDC criteria. What they hope you won't catch on to is that the reason they set the reporting criteria so high is because it is the tick-borne strains of Borrelia that are the most highly pathogenic. These strains are much more likely to exhibit a positive ELISA and WB test result over other strains found in other parts of the country. These other strains also induce Lyme disease, but usually do not affect as many physiological systems as do the northeastern and pacific tick-born strains, nor are they as likely to induce the same degree of antibody development, and hence as many Western Blot bands. As a result, less virulent strains are not going to present as many bands, hence will not meet their criteria. However the infections caused by these other strains are just as difficult to eradicate. Thus, the logical result is that many victims of Bb infection are deliberately being excluded from any formal statistics since they would not have been reported. One can therefore see how distorted and (I believe deliberately) deceiving the Lyme disease reporting map was intended to be.

If in fact it were possible to view a map which displayed all Lyme disease cases, including all those that met CDC reporting criteria, those clinically diagnosed with Lyme disease, as well as those that are sick with the illness who are never officially given a diagnosis by a doctor, the results would be staggering and would likely completely change the map results. Therefore my personal view is that the reason why the CDC maintains such unrealistic reporting standards is to deliberately create the illusion that Lyme disease only comes from ticks and is not as wide-spread as its reality. When one takes off his rose-colored glasses believing everything the government tells him is true, this can be the only logical explanation.

Additionally, the other criteria besides lab confirmation that they use for reporting Lyme disease is *erythema migrans* (the bull's eye rash*).* This will of course almost exclusively be observed in a tick bite since ticks seem to be significant carriers of the spirochete form. And even though we have already cited that spiders and mosquitoe-vectored infections have been observed to also induce the bull's eye rash, other vectors of infection that have been scientifically proven to exist as carriers of the spirochete and variant forms, by Dr. Mattman and others, are not mentioned.

What could possibly on this earth have caused any intelligent or rational person to set the standard for reporting so high as exclude as many as 90% of Lyme victims from the reporting? If they were genuinely interested in finding an accurate reporting figure, one way to escape this problem would simply be to lower the reporting criteria to more realistically reflect the reality of actual Lyme diagnoses. The other would be to develop tests which incorporate the less virulent strains into antibody tests. One test could utilize the less virulent strains, leaving out the more reactive strains, while still maintaining the common two or three strain approach currently being used by some labs. This would more realistically jive with what is actually taking place. Instead, they seem to be happy using one type of test that virtually guarantees that many if not most of those testing will test false according to their criteria.

A BETTER TEST?

There is one test that, although also measures antibody response, has a distinct advantage over other tests in that it does not measure the variable proteins. This test is called C6 LPE (Lyme Peptide ELISA) and was developed around 2000. Chapter 4 discussed the difference between the variable and invariable (or conserved) proteins of Bb. The C6 peptide is one immunodominant major protein that does not change, and is targeted by C-6 antibodies. This invariable or conserved protein is not only unique to Bb, but is also possessed by all known Borrelia strains.

This fact alone gives it a distinct advantage due to the fact that most western blot tests only use a few representative highly reactive strains found in the northeast, which may not accurately represent some of the less reactive strains endemic to other parts of the country. That means that no matter which strain is infecting you, and no matter what the variations of other proteins may be at any given time, your immune system is likely to respond in a more consistent manner, thus making the test more reliable. Variable proteins are more difficult to measure since they change over time. The problem with a weakened immune response would still be applicable, but at least you will have eliminated two prominent causes of inaccurate testing, and will be way ahead of the game.

Another advantage of measuring C6 antibodies is that they are theoretically created throughout the course of infection, so in theory might be used to monitor the progression of the disease. This may differ from western blot tests in that they include the variable proteins which are used to measure IgG antibody response. As has been cited, since variable proteins can change over time, the measuring of IgG antibody production as represented in the various bands seen on these tests, can become reduced and sometimes are not measurable at all, particularly in immune compromised individuals. What that means is that the variations of the proteins used in the western blot tests may not be a close enough match to the antibodies which have developed from the current strain infecting the patient. Either the bacteria in the test, or in the body have varied enough to not elicit a strong enough response to be measured positive. Hence it is sometimes assumed that there is no infection, when in fact the antibodies are simply not matching with the protein, or have not been challenged to be produced in sufficient quantity.

There is a limitation that has been observed however in these tests. Sometimes they have been used as a gauge to monitor the disease, assuming that the C-6 antibody production will drop as the infection improves. This may or may not occur, as we said, the rules that apply to other pathogens do not always apply in Lyme disease due to Bb's immune down-regulating ability. A study was done to observe the correlation between Lyme patients that had been treated with antibiotics, and their levels of C-6 antibodies post-treatment. It was expected that following successful treatment with antibiotics, a parallel drop in antibody levels would be observed. This in fact was not the case. The study concluded "no correlation was found between a decline of C-6 antibody titer of any magnitude and treatment or clinical outcome." [25] In fact what this study does demonstrate is that with the ongoing presence and persistence of C-6 antibodies, so-called "post-Lyme syndrome" is not consistent with these results. Even with so-called "successful treatment" and reduced symptoms, evidence of active infection persists, which is what many Lyme-literate medical doctors and their patients have been saying all along. Therefore, even with a more accurate test, patient symptoms and clinical observations are still tantamount to relying on serological testing.

One final test deserves mentioning briefly. PCR, polymerase chain reaction tests are designed to capture essentially DNA fragments from the spirochete. However, much like fishing in a pond, they only indicate a positive result if they catch a borrelia antigen in the serum or bodily fluids. If no antigens are found, a negative test can be the result. This test is actually far less accurate than Western Blot tests due to the fact that Borrelia has an affinity for tissues and joints. It hates the bloodstream since that is where it is vulnerable to both antibiotics and immune cells. Spirochetes use their cork-screw capacity to both hide inside cells, and to burrow thru blood vessels into tissue and joints where they can hide. So when PCR tests do not find Borrelia antigens in the blood, like a fisherman, they then conclude there are no fish in the pond just because they couldn't catch one.

But what if you don't receive a positive test result for your infection in spite of obvious clinical symptoms and positive response to antimicrobial treatments? Do you continue to test? Tests such as PCR actually require you to be off of anti-biotics for an extended time in order to give sufficient time for microbial infections to advance into a detectable range. Where does that leave the patient? He/she must deliberately become even sicker in order to receive what may in fact end up being another negative test result. Or perhaps the particular pathogen infecting the patient was not even the target of the test, leaving them with even more costs, and sicker than before. Add to that, doctors cannot legally prescribe long-term care in the absence of a definitive diagnosis, what then is the patient to do? For those with insurance, they will be denied further care since they received negative results. For those without insurance, they could go bankrupt before they find out what is wrong with them, on top of leaving them with no way to pay for a therapy having spent all their money on tests.

TREATING THE PATIENT

Lab testing is supposed to be used to help aid a doctor in confirming Lyme, not be the defining factor. It is just not possible. So in the absence of, or after the elimination of other possibilities, if your symptoms are suggestive of Lyme disease, then one of the most important things you can do that has actually become an important indicator of Borrelia-like infection, when lab tests are inconclusive, is the practical application of anti-lyme treatments, and observe the responses you have toward them. Doctors will often give a patient a test trial of abx just to see how they respond. If they seem to either improve, or temporarily get worse due to herxing, that may be indicative of an infection. But coinfections can exhibit similar symptoms. Therefore you don't necessarily know if the herx reaction is coming from Bb, or some other pathogen. But at least the administration of anti-lyme treatments and the subsequent herx reaction becomes a very important telling sign that will indicate an underlying pathogenic cause. In the words of LymeMD, "Treat the patient, not the lab result."

Lyme patients will often receive test after negative test, often spending thousands of dollars if they are uninsured, leaving little money for treatment. It is not the people receiving a positive test result that have the problems, since they know where they stand, and how to move forward. It is those that are borderline or false negative in light of clinical symptoms who don't know. The real question is, what do you do when you have Lyme disease, but no positive test to confirm it? How do you move forward? What do you treat, and how do you treat your illness if you don't know what you are battling?

Some practical advice. First, eliminate any other conditions such as coinfections, which should also include mycoplasma in addition to the traditional panels of Ehrlichia, Bartonella, Babesia. The problem with mycoplasma is that it is often even more difficult to receive a definite positive test result than Lyme. If you received negative Western Blot tests for both Lyme and coinfections, likely your doctor may put you on a course of antibiotics for a few weeks if you display clinical symptoms of Lyme. This will challenge your infection, and cause a mass killing of bacteria which will often then raise your antibody counts. Then you can retest. If you have been treating with antimicrobials for some time however, Bb will often not be found in the blood, synovial fluid, or urine as they often bind to nerve and joint tissue. Hence PCR tests would not be useful.

At this point, if you still have not received a positive test for anything, you are now on a road many have traveled before you. Your doctor will begin to look at many other factors that could be contributing to your Lyme-like symptoms. But the most reliable and practical way to point you in the right direction is the taking of antimicrobials that have specific action. If you improve on antibiotics or temporarily get worse, then you will know that a bacterial infection is a strong component to your symptoms. You will at least be able to partially eliminate both a fungal and viral component. Or if you take a substance that specifically targets a fungal infection with no results, that is of course very significant. Discovering what you *don't have* based upon how a specific antimicrobial is designed to work can eliminate other suspected possibilities. These will of course be discussed with your doctor.

If your symptoms have been consistent with Lyme, then your doctor may give you a clinical diagnosis. At this point, regardless of your lack of absolute certainty as to whether you actually have Lyme disease, if you have symptoms which are consistent with either Lyme or mycoplasma or Bartonella, and you respond positively to a particular antibiotic or antibacterial herbal product(s), then in the absence of anything more definitive, move in that direction while periodically retesting. Due to the fact that Lyme will likely require the addressing of multiple systems, you will necessarily need to deal with various healing modalities in order to reduce your overall toxin load, mineral deficiencies, neurotransmitter balancing, gut issues, probiotics, antioxidants, etc. This will enable you to maintain your overall condition while you focus on the battle of direct killing of your bacterial infection, whether it is Lyme or another related symptom-producing pathogen. Fortunately some of the treatments listed in this book address both Bb and mycoplasma, while others are very broad in their antimicrobial applications in that they address all categories of pathogens, such as monolaurin and some of the oxygen therapies for example.

ENDNOTES

1. *Recommendations for the Use of Lyme Disease Vaccine* Morbidity and Mortality Report Centerts For Disease Control and Prevention June 4, 1999 / Vol. 48 / No. RR-7 http://www.cdc.gov/mmwr/PDF/RR/RR4807.pdf Retrieved Feb. 3, 2013

2. *Problems that affect the reliability of the confirmatory Lyme disease test, the Western blot* From the LymeLight Newsletter of the Lyme Disease Foundation Archived webpage. Retrieved http://www.lyme.org/westernblot.html from June 13, 2010 at archive.org

3. *Two Texas Lyme Disease Bills Target Gap In Treatment* AMERICAN-STATESMAN by Chuck Lindell April 28, 2011 http://mylymediseasetreatment.com/lyme-disease-general/two-texas-lyme-disease-bills-target-gap-in-treatment/ Retrieved Feb. 3, 2013

4. *Basic Information About Lyme Disease* International Lyme and Associated Diseases Society website http://www.ilads.org/lyme_disease/about_lyme.html Retrieved Feb. 3, 2013

5. *The Clinical Assessment, Treatment, and Prevention of Lyme Disease, Human Granulocytic Anaplasmosis, and Babesiosis: Clinical Practice Guidelines by the Infectious Diseases Society of America* Gary P. Wormser, Raymond J. Dattwyler, Eugene D. Shapiro, John J. Halperin, Allen C. Steere, Mark S. Klempner, Peter J. Krause, Johan S. Bakken, Franc Strle, Gerold Stanek, Linda Bockenstedt, Durland Fish, J. Stephen Dumler, and Robert B. Nadelman IDSA Guidelines IDSA CID 2006:43 (1 November), Pp.1089-1134. http://www.uphs.upenn.edu/bugdrug/antibiotic_manual/idsalyme06.pdf Retrieved Feb. 3, 2013

6. *Chronic Lyme: An Evidence-based Review* by Steven Phillips MD 2007 Presentation from International Lyme and Associated Diseases Society website http://www.ilads.org/lyme_research/chronic_lyme.html Retrieved Feb. 3, 2013

7. *Astonishment as Medical Panel Rubber Stamps its own Controversial Guidelines* Dr. Robert Bransfield, MD, DLFAPA Article 27 April, 2010 09: ILADS website Archived on archive.org from Nov. 20, 2011 http://www.ilads.org/news/lyme_press_releases/72.html

8. *Research on microbial biofilms* (PA-03-047). NIH, National Heart, Lung, and Blood Institute. 2002-12-20. http://grants.nih.gov/grants/guide/pa-files/PA-03-047.html.

9. *Problems that affect the reliability of the confirmatory Lyme disease test, the Western blot* From the LymeLight Newsletter of the Lyme Disease Foundation Archived webpage. Retrieved http://www.lyme.org/westernblot.html from June 13, 2010 at archive.org

10. Schaller, J. (2005). *Amazing special darkfield images of tick diseases using fluorescent antibodies.* Retrieved July 26, 2005 from Personal Consult Website http://www.personalconsult.com/articles/bowenresearch.html Retrieved Feb. 3, 2013

11. Article from ILADS website: *Medical Society applauds Connecticut Lawmakers for passing a bill that protects physicians who treat Lyme disease* 22 June, 2009 http://www.ilads.org/news/lyme_press_releases/55.html

12. *Determination of members of a Borrelia afzelli-related group isolated from Ixodas nipponensis in Korea as Borrelia valaisiana.* Masuzawa, T., Fukui, T., Miyake, M., Oh, H.B., Cho, M.K., Chang, W.H., Imai, Y., & Yanagihara, Y. International Journal of Systematic Bacteriology, 1999 VOL(4), 1409-1415.

13. *Seronegative or False Negative Lyme Disease* research demonstrating false negatives in Lyme testing presented by Pacificfrontiermedical.com http://web.archive.org/web/20110517043138/http://www.pacificfrontiermedical.com/pdfs/38.pdf Retrieved Feb. 3, 2013

14. *Bartonella quintana lipopolysaccharide is a natural antagonist of Toll-like receptor 4.* Infect Immun. 2007 Oct;75(10):4831-7. Epub 2007 Jul 2.

15. *The Bartonella Plague Ignored: A Common Reason Lyme Treatment Fails* by Dr. James Schaller M.D.http://www.publichealthalert.org/Articles/jamesschaller/The%20Bartonella%20Plague%20Ignored.html

16. *Western Blots Made Easy* by Dr. James Schaller, M.D. Linda's Lyme disease journal Monday, August 18, 2008 http://lindaslymediseasejournal.blogspot.com/2008/08/western-blots-made-easy-by-dr-james.html

17. *Basic Information About Lyme Disease* International Lyme and Associated Diseases Society website http://www.ilads.org/lyme_disease/about_lyme.html Retrieved Feb. 3, 2013

18. Ibid.
19. *Seronegative Lyme* LymeMD blog Feb. 12, 2009 http://lymemd.blogspot. com/2009/02/seronegative-lyme.html Retrieved Feb. 3, 2013
20. *Seroprevalence of Borrelia IgG antibodies among young Swedish children in relation to reported tick bites, symptoms and previous treatment for Lyme borreliosis: a population-based survey.* Skogman BH, Ekerfelt C, Ludvigsson J, Forsberg P. Arch Dis Child. 2010 Dec;95(12):1013-6.
21. *Antibodies against whole sonicated Borrelia burgdorferi spirochetes, 41-kilodalton flagellin, and P39 protein in patients with PCR- or culture-proven late Lyme borreliosis.* Oksi J, Uksila J, Marjamäki M, Nikoskelainen J, Viljanen MK. J Clin Microbiology 1995 Sep; 33(9): 2260-4 (PDF):
22. *Video-microscopy and pictures of Borrelia burgdorferi and other spirochete like structures links collection* Eldøen et al. Tidsskr Nor Lægeforen 2001; 121: 2008-11 Quote from Norwegian study cited from http://lymerick.net/ videomicroscopy.htm Retreived Jan. 2013.
23. *LYME DISEASE CASE REPORT* CDC 52.60 Rev. 02-2006 http://www. cdc.gov/ncidod/dvbid/lyme/resources/LymeDiseaseCaseReportForm.pdf
24. *Morbidity and Mortality Weekly Report* April 28, 2000 / Vol. 49 / No. SS-3 CDC Surveillance Summaries pg. 8. http://www.cdc.gov/mmwr/PDF/ss/ ss4903.pdf
25. *Pre-treatment and post-treatment assessment of the C(6) test in patients with persistent symptoms and a history of Lyme borreliosis.* Fleming RV, Marques AR, Klempner MS, Schmid CH, Dally LG, Martin DS, Philipp MT. Eur J Clin Microbiol Infect Dis 2004 Aug;23(8):615-8. Epub 2004 Jul 8.

CHAPTER 8

Strains and How They Can Affect Test Results

As if testing for Bb were not confusing enough as it is, a case could be made that due to the shear number of Bb strains and the human variables involved, it's a wonder that some of these tests have any accuracy at all. Although there are over 300 Borrelia strains, not all are pathogenic in humans. But those that are have a multitude of potential variance factors that can affect the way any particular immune system reacts to them, as well as the way the disease is manifested in the body. That is why the term "Lyme disease" is truly more of a general term since it encompasses a wide range of strains as well as disease manifestations. The group *Borrelia Burgdorferi sensu lato*, covers those strains known to be pathogenic and cause lyme-like symptoms. They include 3 sub-specie groups called *Borrelia Burgdorferi sensu stricto* (strictly speaking), and two primarily European strains, *B. garinii* and *B. afzelli*. The Bb sensu stricto group includes mostly US strains. In this group there are over 40 strains. In addition there are *B. bissetti* strains (a California group), and *B. andersonii* strains.

The topic of Bb strains is very involved. In 1982 Willy Burgdorferi MD was the one given credit for discovering a particular bacteria that caused the illness and named it after himself. In those early days there were only a few strains that were thought to cause the disease. In time, it was learned that many more strains cause similar symptoms, and the way they manifest themselves in the body. It became evident that a small handful of strains were much more virulent than the others. Although not exclusive, strains Bb31, Bb297, Bb2591, and Bb N40 as well as others are commonly cited in research as being particularly virulent.

Due to the fact that not all strains are identical in their ability to evoke an immune response, and given that no two person's immune systems are going to respond to any given bacterial antigen in a uniform manner, to seek to apply one test, or even group of tests to encompass such a large scope is in itself part of the problem. And that is the reason why ultimately relying on test results which cannot be definitive in those that test negative or borderline positive is a wrong approach.

So perhaps there is no one name that can be given to an illness that has so many variables or faces. A person is not battling a name. He/she is battling their own particular strain of bacteria that are manifesting themselves thru many different pleomorphic forms, which are each going to possess their own immune inducing properties. And each form in turn is going to be expressing its own particular lipoproteins differently, which is also going to affect antibody responses differently at any given time. (This is why even your Igenex tests read "Because of the low sensitivity of this assay, for patients with negative results, we recommend testing by another method and/or repeating the serology in 4-6 weeks.") Add to that not only that Borrelia is going to attack the most vulnerable systems in the body first, but given that co-infections also affect overall antibody productions, they in turn will affect how the disease is manifested, and the degree to which testing will be accurate.

In the early years when one obvious vector or source of Lyme disease was first discovered to be from tick bites, an assumption was made, and it just kind of stuck in people's minds, that ticks were the only source of the disease. And in fact perhaps that made sense in the beginning. In those early days an explosion of research began examining the various species of ticks that were carriers, as well as the different varieties or strains of Borrelia that caused the disease. Soon what was called Lyme disease began to spread like wildfire across the northeastern states. And laboratories began to develop tests that could help doctors identify the disease based upon focusing on those few strains that were identified as producing similar symptoms.

Before this, symptoms similar to Lyme had been reported and were known to exist in ill patients, and in those in psychiatric wards in the US and Europe. It had out-seated syphilis as the Great Imitator of other diseases. But until now the causes were not obvious or definable. It was simply a disease that included a list of symptoms with an unidentified cause that was masquerading as other diseases.

It seems obvious therefore that Lyme disease in various forms had been around for a long time, even before the US outbreak in 1975. What made this particular outbreak in Lyme, Connecticut especially unique was that the symptoms were not subtle, and all those manifesting symptoms were very similar, in addition to being in the same geographical area and all relatively at the same time. However what was also notably different was that this illness was much more virulent or severe. One example was the bull's eye rash which is an indication of a very strong local immune response. The other is pronounced arthritic and neurological symptoms, which although present in other Lyme-like diseases before 1975, was considerably acute. Also the onset was usually sudden. So it's as though a new form of the disease had sprung up in a much more pathogenic form in the middle of Lyme, Connecticut with no apparent cause. Had ticks just all of the sudden become infected with some strange mutant and the intensity of this outbreak was so severe that it required a brand new name?

In time we of course learned of the research that was being done on ticks at the US government Plum Island biological warfare research facility across the bay from Lyme, Connecticut. There is obviously controversy as to this being the official source, as we will probably never be able to prove this. One thing is for certain, the strains of Borrelia that infect those ticks are a much more virulent form than is found in the rest of the country. And since then most of the research that sprang from this newly-found disease centered on those ticks that were discovered to be carriers.

Now we of course know that there are many more strains of Borrelia that cause similar symptoms than just the more virulent varieties found in the northeastern US, as they have been around causing disease in people for a long time. Some of these strains are known to exhibit symptoms associated with their name such as the "relapsing fever group", or "southern-tick associated rash illness" or "STARI". The latter was first suspected to come from Bb 1352 strain of Borrelia called *lonestari*, because a PCR test identified that particular strain as the causative agent of a person bitten by the Lonestar tick. Although some literature maintains that the cause of STARI is unknown due to the inability to culture B. lonestari from lesions of 31 patients with Lone Star tick bites, it was later confirmed by the first culture isolation of Borrelia lonestari from a lone star tick in 2004. [1] STARI is very similar and in some cases identical to Lyme disease in its symptoms. The bite of the Lone Star tick also exhibits a bull's eye rash like Lyme disease. The difference is the severity of symptoms. The similarities other than that can be almost identical, including the response to anti-biotic treatment. This became known as Master's Disease named after Dr. Edwin Masters who treated the first case in Missouri.

It is interesting that attempts at culturing a spirochete from this illness for many years was unsuccessful, leading some to conclude that the causative agent not only was not Borrelia Burgdorferi, but wasn't from a spirochete at all even though the symptoms were in many cases identical, right down to the bull's eye rash. [2] A different culture medium was necessary to grow spirochetes of this strain. Recall that the spirochete from Treponema Pallidum, the agent of syphilis has not yet been able to be cultured at all. Spirochetes, known to be pleomorphic, not only require highly specific cultures, but they love the culture of animal and human bodily fluids. Medical science is still resistant to accepting sometimes the obvious. It is a sad note that still virtually all research centers around ticks, when it has been widely demonstrated both thru cultures and flourescent antibody that ticks are not the only carriers of Borrelia species, nor are they the only vector of infection.

Lonestari strains do possess some crossreactive proteins, and the spirochete did in fact respond to 41kd antibody known to be common to Borrelia flagellin varieties. However, although it may show some positive WB bands, it does not generally show up positive on Lyme tests, this inspite of the fact the Bb 1352 is considered a Borrelia Burgdorferi sensu stricto strain. This demonstrates that in spite of what we are told, the strains used in even the best of tests do not accurately represent all known strains that cause Lyme disease or Borrelia-vectored illnesses. In spite of the massive research that has gone into the various strains of Bb over the past 30 years, this is only one illustration that shows how that even now we are still in the infancy stages of understanding the massive complexity of Lyme infections and their causes.

ENDNOTES

1. *First Culture Isolation of Borrelia lonestari, Putative Agent of Southern Tick-Associated Rash Illness* Andrea S. Varela, M. Page Luttrell, Elizabeth W. Howerth, Victor A. Moore, William R. Davidson, David E. Stallknecht and Susan E. Little J. Clin Microbiol. 2004 March; 42(3): 1163-1169.

2. *STARI or Master's Disease: More like Lyme than Lyme?* Blog article. July 19, 2009 http://spirochetesunwound.blogspot.com/2009/07/stari-or-masters-disease-more-like-lyme.html Retrieved Feb. 3, 2013

CHAPTER 9

Therapies

To those critics, it is interesting that very few of the non-drug therapies that are discussed in this book are being used by traditional medicine, or have been considered by conventional medicine to be "proven" treatments. Because they are not "proven" they are scoffed at, to which I reply, "go ahead and scoff while I heal." Living in a world of pure science without understanding the limitations of science leaves one vulnerable to seeing science as a religion rather than a tool which was meant to aid man, not impede him from understanding that not all of life is able to be viewed under a microscope. Is it necessary to be able to explain how an automobile engine works in order to drive a car? Can science explain why a "proven" medicine does not work for everyone that has the same condition for which it was designed? Of course not. If science is your religion, you will forever remain a skeptic until something is "proven" to be true. And that is a pretty sad way to live, but has become the modern paradigm of conventional medicine's model which has taken the wonder and possibilities out of life.

Of course the direction you choose is your responsibility, and your decision. However what many have discovered in time is the same thing that other Lyme patients before them have learned: antibiotics have been largely ineffective at dealing with chronic Lyme disease. Although certainly these drugs have improved the quality of life of many Lyme patients, rarely does one hear a story of a chronic Lyme disease patient that has been cured of the disease. Rather, the usual course of treatment involves years of continuous antibiotic use. And even then, the conditions of many of these patients continues to deteriorate since most of them, wanting to get off their meds, end up going thru a cycle of on and off antibiotics, remaining in limbo. This cycle virtually guarantees they will remain ill in the long term.

Even those that are regular and religious about their abx intake are only able to suppress the spirochete and cyst forms long enough to lower their symptoms. As soon as they stop however, often the entire cycle begins all over again. And remember, the taking of abx over time can actually entrench the disease making it even more permanent since they tend to drive Bb to create biofilms for protection, which can nearly completely solidify the disease in the body making it permanent.

Conventional medical science is very different from natural or alternative medicine in this regard: allopathic medicine generally seeks to match one drug with one disease, or one medicine with one microbe, or combination of medicines in order to address your illness. Sometimes specific lab tests are often necessary to identify the cause of your infection so the proper drug can be matched with the specific germ. This has become the standard motis operandi for dealing with infectious diseases. However in the absence of positive identification of an infectious agent, only short course medicine is given. This can translate into "refusal of future treatment." Since Borrelia infection is often difficult to serologically identify, and since there are no antibiotics that have been proven to eradicate Borrelia in all of its forms, this allopathic system is ill-equipped to adequately treat chronic Lyme disase.

However in natural medicine no such policy exists. You have free reign to use whatever medicines offer you benefit. Not only does it address the whole person, but the very natures of the medicines that are generally available also happen to affect a wide range of pathogens and conditions. For instance, not only does olive leaf extract possess strong antibacterial properties, it is also antifungal and antiviral, which would be far more advantageous than taking an antibiotic alone since antibiotics can make the conditions right for the development and spread of intestinal yeast growth. The antiviral properties would benefit any susceptible viral infections, as some viruses are also known to be coinfective with Lyme disease, for example Epstein Barr and Herpes simplex. It also possesses antiflammatory as well as antioxidant activity which will support the body as a whole. Additionally it does not have the grueling side affects of some antibiotics. And natural herbal products generally don't destroy the intestinal flora necessary to maintain a healthy gut, and hence the immune system since the vast majority of immune cells reside in the gut.

Therefore, since most of the therapies and non-drug substances listed in this book have broad spectrum applications against a number of infectious microbes, whether you have Borrelia Burgdorferi sensu stricto brand Lyme disease, a mycoplasma infection, Bartonella, Master's disease, or any number of other coinfections which can closely resemble Lyme disease, most of these are going to respond positively.

Substance abuse

Over the years so many substances have had claims made concerning their ability to cure Lyme disease that it is difficult to examine many of these therapies in a balanced and unbiased manner. Instead of looking for a "miracle medicine", it is far more realistic to realize that each herbal or non-drug substance is going to offer its own unique potential to address some aspect of your illness. And rather than spoon feed the sick by promoting a single product or two with the hopes that they will once and for all cure your condition, only to find yourself disappointed, I have chosen rather to share with you real world information that gives you a realistic perspective so decisions can be intelligently made. In fact, that is the entire premise of the philosophy that is being espoused. By finding primary and supportive treatments, rotating and continuously altering them, you will constantly challenge pleomorphic Borrelia in order to short-circuit its system so it can no longer be used as an evasion tool. Simultaneously it will become necessary to treat biofilms. Without this most important step, complete resolution may likely escape you.

Doing the same thing you've always done, you will keep getting the same results. If you keep using any one or two therapies against Borrelia, even if they are natural antimicrobials, unless you are one of the very lucky few, you might as well plan on having the disease for the rest of your life since your approach is likely not going to address the true nature of this bacterial infection. It would be great to be able to find one or two therapies that could be used against Lyme. Although treatments such as the salt/C protocol, the Marshall protocol, Teasel root,

Rife, Samento, or antibiotics have been used by some to find degress of success, the truth is that most people will not find complete healing from Lyme using a single or even two substance therapy approach. Even with those mentioned above, virtually everyone used more than one therapy in addition to them.

Depending on the state of your health and how far along you are in the healing process you have thus far come, there are some important things to consider before beginning any new therapy(s). Yes this may be a sort of disclaimer, but not in the legal sense. These are extremely important practical guidelines to follow. Remember, you are ultimately responsible for your own health, and any decisions you make ought to be made safely, intelligently, methodically, and in a well advised manner.

1. Do your homework. Don't just take someone's word that something is true. And don't follow someone else like the Pied Piper. Not only does that apply to something a friend has told you, or some internet blog, or some book you've read, but it also applies to your own healthcare practitioner. Make sure you understand what is being said, and that it makes sense to you.

2. Discuss what you are considering with your doctor. Remember to take the right information to the right doctor. If your doctor is not open to or is not knowledgeable about some of the therapies you are considering, see someone who is. Or at the very least discuss having him/her monitor what you are doing to work in conjunction with safe practices. Some physicians will only prescribe their own therapies. The problem is that Lyme disease is a rather unique illness. And if you are only going to do what has already been done that doesn't work, is that what you want to do?

3. Start out slowly. ALWAYS begin slowly with any new therapy you are considering. Homeostasis, the natural chemical balance your body maintains to keep you functioning at your optimum is thrown off when you introduce something new whether it is a drug, or some natural substance. It needs time to adjust. Also, you need time to listen to your body for the way it may react to something new before you increase the therapy, or add another

substance. If you begin to react negatively, it is better to be caught early so you can adjust, or stop if necessary.

4. Only begin taking one new supplement or substance at a time. You need to monitor what is taking place. If you are taking several things at once, you won't know which one is affecting you, or what their combined action is if you begin too aggressively.

5. Keep a log of what you are doing. Keep it simple and brief. But record what you are taking, how much, and any reactions you are noticing from it. Not only will this help you to remember what you are doing, but what is working or isn't. It also gives your doctor a way to monitor what is happening.

Chronic Lyme disease is one of those kinds of illnesses that doesn't really have a standard protocol per se. Other than being put on antibiotics in the early stages of Lyme and giving a patient a series of tests, once the stage of Lyme has advanced too far for abx to be curative, it becomes far too complicated to create some standardized one-size fits all strategy that works for everyone. That is why so much monitoring is done by physicians, and also why it can quickly drain you financially even if you have health insurance. And health insurance generally is not going to cover alternative therapies which are really most people's real only hope of getting well in my opinion.

Having said that, there are important things to consider no matter what approach is taken to get well not necessarily in this order:

1. Any underlying health conditions you already have may need to be taken into consideration before beginning some new therapy. For instance diabetes, allergies to foods or drugs, blood pressure problems, liver functions, mineral deficiencies, pregnancy, etc. These can be affected negatively when you begin to consider taking some new supplements or develop a therapy or protocol you would like to consider trying. These absolutely need to be discussed with your doctor.

2. The state of your intestinal health will rank as perhaps one of the most important considerations. You need to aggressively and consistently take probiotics since some of these therapies

act as powerful antimicrobials which can also weaken or kill off the good bacteria. This absolutely cannot be emphasized enough. If you have never had candidiasis which is perhaps the most common condition associated with long term antibiotic therapies, it can be almost as serious a condition as Lyme disease, and almost as difficult to eradicate. Many people who develop Lyme disease also develop this condition. Although I have described a therapy that can eliminate the condition, there is no sense going thru it in the first place when it can easily be prevented. Let taking probiotics become a part of your life from now on which may rank even more importantly than taking your daily vitamins when you are doing therapies for Lyme disease.

3. Listening to your body. This may sound obvious. But you are your own doctor in the sense that you must pay attention to what is happening inside yourself and closely monitor any changes that may seem out of the ordinary. Then back off if necessary.

4. Be consistent and aggressive. By this I mean be determined you are going to get well. If something doesn't work, try something else. There are so many options to try that the possibilities are nearly endless. However part of the therapy process also involves rest and taking a break to allow your body time to recover between herxes. Generally however, if you are having massive herxes, that means you may be too aggressive. If you push yourself too hard not only will you feel horrible and get discouraged, but it could be dangerous. On the other hand, herxheimer reactions can be your friend in that sometimes it is the only way you know for sure that a therapy may be working. Over time, the period following your herx you will generally find your symptoms becoming less severe. These are the rewards from your consistency.

5. The growth and reproductive cycle that Bb may be going thru at any time may affect the response of a particular therapy. As new colonies of Bb go thru a growth and incubation cycle, they regularly "hatch" new spirochetes from their cyst form. When this happens, those new spirochetes are highly susceptible to antimicrobials. You may be doing your protocols for several weeks with no significant reactions only to suddenly find yourself

having what you think is a setback when your symptoms seem to return with a vengeance.

Although this may seem discouraging at first, actually this is a good sign to be alert for. It means that your consistency paid off. On the other hand, sometimes it is a good idea to deliberately give yourself some time off. I mean completely stop all antimicrobials for perhaps even several weeks. (Take this time to load up on the immune boosters and probiotics.) You never know what the cycle of growth may be in. Some of the therapies are more prone to kill spirochetes, while others are more effective against the cyst or CWD form. Consistently taking a particular therapy for a prolonged period of time would force the bacteria to remain dormant in that form and actually slow down the killing process. Sometimes it is advantageous to allow them time to feel the coast is clear, and emerge or morph into another form that will once again allow them to be susceptible to being killed. Then begin a new therapy with a vengeance.

6. Keep the bacteria off guard. This goes along with number 5. Keep rotating or altering the therapies. This has already been discussed in what I believe is the most important key to successfully battling Lyme disease. Do not let them have enough time to adjust to your therapies. In fact, it may be said that the longer you keep doing the same therapy on a continuous basis, the longer you will prolong the disease. Use a multi-faceted approach to your therapies in order to address all forms of the bacteria. Keep rotating, adjusting and altering the treatments. You must exploit their weakness.

7. On the other hand, if you have found a therapy that you are receiving a lot of herxes from that are not letting up, you may have found one that Bb is particularly vulnerable to, or at least that particular form that is expressing itself. Stay on that therapy until you find that its effects are subsiding. Then switch to another. By this I don't mean you don't take time to rest between herxes. But you need to learn to adjust your therapies so that you don't have massive herxes that completely wipe you out. Sometimes this will happen of course especially in the beginning

of a new therapy when you have no history as yet as to how it will affect you, or what dosage you need. But a slow and steady pace will allow you to have a more normal life while you are getting better.

8. Never do only one therapy at a time. This may sound like a contradiction to number 4 under the advisements section, but it's not. When you first begin any new therapy, yes, only use one substance at a time to see what affect it is having you, and to see if it is benefiting you, as well as any safety precautions in case you experience some allergic or other negative affects from them. But once that has been established, incorporate that as a conjunctive therapy as part of a multi-dimensional attack protocol. Some therapies may not be compatible. In fact, some may actually be dangerous when combined indiscriminately. (Although I have personally not experienced any problems with the mixing of substances, in some people this may not be the case.) These are the things that should be discussed with your doctor. However as has already been discussed, allowing defensive lipoprotein expressions to take place gives the microbe a distinct advantage. We want to have the upper hand.

9. You must make the decision to fundamentally change your diet. This is an absolute must. Eating simple sugars and simple carbohydrates must be eliminated from your diet. This also means fruit juices and sodas. This one point could exponentially improve the speed of your recovery, yet is the one area that is most often ignored. Most patients tend to rely upon their antibiotics/antimicrobials to do the work and assume they will get well. After all, that is the way most other bacterial infections are resolved. If you won't do this important step, then you might as well plan on having Lyme disease the rest of your life—pure and simple. Look into the "hunter/gatherers" diet. Also there are now good books on Lyme diet available.

10. Incorporate Rife or electromagnetics if possible into your over-all plan of attack. As has already been discussed, Rife has the potential to do what no other known therapy can do. It can penetrate where drugs and natural products taken internally have a difficult time reaching, and as such can have a huge advantage over these products. Borrelia and other pathogens can hide even

inside bone cavities, and deep inside joints so deeply, without aggressive therapy, it is not known whether these could ever be reached using standard abx or herbal products; whereas Rife holds the potential to penetrate even bone, or connective tissue.

Note—Rife doesn't work for everyone. Some receive great benefit, while others find no benefit at all, despite trying various machines and multiple frequencies. But it is certainly to your advantage to be able to add this therapy to your arsenal. One of the better arguments for the use of Rife is that it may also hold the potential to kill pathogens in biofilms, something few therapies can do, although its use in this manner has yet to be thoroughly explored.

Finding a practitioner or someone who owns a Rife machine would be a good starting point rather than lay out the expense, only to later find it does not work for you. Try several kinds. But as a precaution, you need to stop taking oral antimicrobials for a month or so before trying the machines. This is because Rife appears to target primarily spirochetes. If you have been taking abx or antimicrobials for any length of time before beginning to Rife, you may find very diminished results, since the spiros have been driven into other pleomorphic forms which may not be susceptible to rifing, or at least to the frequencies or machine you are using.

Consistency is very important in your Lyme therapies, whichever ones you decide to choose. You must decide within yourself what your goal is when developing any treatment protocol. If you only wish to feel better, but do not go beyond that goal, then you will likely be sentencing yourself to a lifetime of chronic illness that you will never get over. Many of the therapies listed herein, or that your doctor prescribes will accomplish that goal quite easily. But if your goal is to completely eradicate Lyme once and for all, then your outlook will be different, and so will your approach. You will be looking beyond merely feeling better, because at that stage, you are only in the beginning phase of eliminating the disease. Remember what we said about your paradigm or the structure from which you develop your outlook. If your paradigm is one of complete victory over Lyme, then you need to look beyond merely feeling better. Because there will be times when you feel very well, like maybe you are close to having completely kicked the illness. However in time, if you stop your therapies, or even reduce them at this point, relapsing is the norm. For myself, instead of stopping, I decided that it was time to develop a new strategy or change my therapies, or combination of therapies to go even deeper. I realized that I had completed another layer of the onion, and it was now time to move even deeper. Each time I have done this, I have been rewarded with herxes. Take notice that your paradigm should be just the opposite of how many Lyme sufferers typically design or approach their plan of attack. Rather than easing up on your therapies once are feeling better, you need to drive them on even deeper. Continue on the offensive. Kick your opponent when he is down. In this way you are not allowing yourself to be deceived or allowing the enemy to gain the upper hand. In fact, it may be a good idea to continue your therapies for at least 4-6 months beyond the point when you feel completely well. Remember, the reduction of planktonic bacteria, or therapies that inhibit quorum sensing capabilities can lead you to believe you are well. Be aware of this and ever mindful.

The following is a partial list of therapies/natural medicines or supplements I have taken over the years for Lyme disease. These do no include every product that has been tried. But most of these have been used either as having a direct killing affect, or playing a supportive role for the body specifically as it relates Lyme disease. There is no particular order or sequence. Many others have been tried but did not justify mentioning since they seemed to show little benefit. You may be surprised at the sheer number of different kinds of products I have used and wonder why, if natural and non-drug based therapies are so effective, it took so long to get well. Actually, not all of the therapies I have taken over the years did much by way of directly affecting my Lyme disease. As I say, I learned what worked, and what didn't. However as I will share later, as effective or beneficial as any one product was, the approach I took ensured that I would remain ill. It is the same approach generally offered by conventional medicine. Once I broke away from it, my healing began to accelerate exponentially.

Herbs or extracts: Carnivora (Venus flytrap extract), Samento (Toa-free Cat's claw), Cat's claw, Grapefruit seed extract, Garlic, Olive leaf extract, Swedish bitters, bitter melon, Artemisisin, Teasel Root, celery seed extract, Spiro X (Siberian milkweed, Tarragon leaves, Litchi seeds, Changii Root, Fringtree bark, Raphari seeds, Wahoo bark, poppy seeds, mandrake root, yellow sophora fruit, Buckhorn Bark), Cayenne pepper, Bioperine, Uva Ursi, Bloodroot, goldenseal, clove, moringa, chlorella, Sutherlandia Frutescans, Haritaki, Kalmegh, Monolaurin, curcumin.

Oils: Krill, Coconut, Niaouli, Moringa, Eucalyptus, Lemon, Lime, Orange, White Thyme, Cinnamon Bark, Rosemary, Sage, Oregano, Clove, Squalene, Tea tree, Manuka.

Drugs: Minocycline, Tinidazole, Cephalexin, Klaritromisin, Doxy, Amoxicillin, Cipro, Flagyl, Naltrexone.

Misc: ACZ nanozeolite, ACS 200 silver, 8 other brands of silver products, Oxy E, Destroxin, humic acid, fulvic acid, Gallium Nitrate, Cesium Chloride, Potassium Iodide, sodium chlorite (aka MMS), calcium hypochlorite (aka MMS2), Ursolic Acid, Ellagic Acid, Ace Immune, various aloe extracts, MPS-Gold, Boron, Hydrogen peroxide therapy, Manuka honey, Ezorb (Calcium aspartate anhydrous), Willard water, Glyoxilide, serrapeptase, Lumbrokinase, nattokinase, sodium bisulfate.

Therapies: Colloidal silver IV's, H2O2 IV's, Lipsomal encapsulated vit C, resveratrol, glutathione, "SALT/C". Rife, Ledum homeopathic, Budwig diet.

Mexican clinic—shark placenta injections.

The Townsend Letter Colostrum Therapy

Electromagnetic pulsing—Rob Allen's High Power Magnetic Pulser, PEMF.

DC electrifier—Sends an electric current deeply thru the tissues to potentially destroy or inhibit bacteria and viruses.

Pap Imi electromagnetic pulser—known as the worlds most powerful therapeutic pulsing device creates cellular electroporesis, increases the transmembrane potential of cells, and induces calcium ions into chronically diseased cells. Some studies have indicated the electromagnetic fields have the potential to kill some microorganisms.

Molecular enhancer/Multi-wave oscillator with violet ray tube.

Radionics—Advanced Biophoton Analyzer.

William Hitt Center—Tijuana Mexico. Series of ionic silver and Vit C IV's.

I want to state this again since it bears repeating. The entire point of this book is to reveal a new way to view Bb. The conventional medicine model has taught us to utilize a one or two substance approach to killing off this bacterial infection. As a result, that model has mostly been a dismal failure because it does not take into consideration the biochemistry of Bb. By taking not only a multi-substance approach, but also constantly altering the therapies, in addition to including antibiofilm strategies, you are allowing for the potential to exponentially speed your recovery from Lyme disease at a rate far exceeding anything you may have tried in the past, as well as going deeper than using even a 2 or 3 medicine approach. This cannot be overemphasized.

However one caveat or warning to this approach is that it should NOT be used aggressively when your bacterial load is high, or when first using these therapies. The approach you are going to learn is so powerful that it can potentially force massive herxes and wipe you out for potentially weeks. This material was written with the chronic patient in mind since the chronic condition is by its very nature very resistant to most therapies due to often years of employing the old conventional medicine paradigm. No matter whether you have been taking antibiotics, or using a non-drug approach, you may still have been relying upon a method that employs the repetitive use of substances which actually encourages Bb to change and guarantees its survival. Don't get caught in this trap.

In hindsight, my choices and approach to these therapies was admittedly wrong. That was the reason why so many different ones were tried, and why it took so long to find healing. Twelve years ago no one had yet blazed a trail, and many natural and herbal therapies were being tried hit and miss without a logical game plan or plan of attack. It was like trying to fight an enemy by shooting in the dark. Near the conclusion, logical sense will be made of the seemingly endless list of potential therapies that now exist for Lyme. There are simply too many excellent treatments for Lyme disease that even the poor-boy do-it-yourselfer will have a multitude of strategies to develop which will aid him/her by lighting the trail.

I suppose over the years I've probably tried more treatments than anyone I personally know. Each contributed to varying degrees to my overall success in finding healing. However I have also learned what is ineffective and what is worth keeping. But one thing is important for me to report. I say this as my own personal experience and not to downgrade or belittle. Sadly probably 15% of my success and 85% of the cost I would attribute to the allopathic medical profession; while 85% of my success and 15% of my costs over the years were due to my diligence in finding natural or alternative therapies which worked. They are these I wish to report to you as to how they have helped me personally. In hindsight, what I learned was that I was using these natural therapies the same way conventional medicine does. I kept doing the same thing over and over, except I used a different therapy. It was when I made one fundamental change did I see dramatic results.

However keep in mind, that while these benefited me, I make no claims as to how they benefit anyone who may choose to try them as well. These are being shared for your own consideration. As a legal disclaimer, later I will list a number of therapies which are known for their antimicrobial effectiveness in a number of applications. However that does not necessarily mean they will be effective for your personal condition. That is the nature of results-oriented medicine. What works for you, may not work for everyone the same. However, it should also be pointed out that neither can drug-based or evidence-based medicine tell you that you will find either partial or total healing from their use. That is the lie of conventional medicine. When it comes to evidence-based medicine, even it is ultimately subject to the real test of whether or not the patient gets results. And if that is your goal, then it is up to you to find your own healing.

CHAPTER 10

The Best Medicine

Today there is a wealth of information available to Lyme sufferers that didn't exist even a few years ago. However, whether you gain your knowledge from books, the internet, or a healthcare practitioner, the greater portion of this information deals with the chronic phase where most of us get trapped. In chronic Lyme the infection has spread beyond merely the dreaded spirochete. Borrelia has transformed itself into every form imaginable. The pandemonium and havoc this wreaks on the systems of the body involve lymphatics and detoxification impairment, nervous system, hormonal, cellular energy, brain and emotional, allergies, digestive, etc. They promote biofilms, heavy metal and neuro-toxicity, co-infections, chronic pain, impaired and down-regulated immunity, mouth, teeth and nasal problems, never-ending inflammation, etc. All of these systems and adverse conditions inter-relate as Lyme disease is no longer merely a bacterial infection, but needs to be viewed as a whole body problem. I don't know of a single person with chronic Lyme disease who has ever gotten well that didn't address most of these areas since chronic Lyme affects to some degree the breakdown and collapse of nearly every system in the body. Lyme may pull the proverbial leg out from under a person. However once this happens, it isn't a matter of just fixing the leg anymore.

What happens over time is that most Lyme patients become mired down in this phase of Lyme, like getting lost in a vast forest. And many stay there going from therapy to therapy doing just enough to see if "something works", then moving on to something else, but never really improving, or doing so at a snail's pace.

I would like to interject something at this point. I will tell you what I believe to be the single most important medicine that you must take, and never stop taking as long as you have Lyme disease. It is not something you can receive from your MD, or from a practitioner of natural health or integrated medicine. Their offices don't carry this particular product.

I have never seen it in a health food store, although I have been to many. I thought for sure it would be found doing a Google search on the internet. But still could not find this.

I will tell you what this medicine is and where to find it. The name of the medicine is called the Iron Will and can only be found inside you. Without the absolute determination and resolve that you are a conqueror, and not a victim you will remain in this chronic phase indefinitely, because it is the most difficult phase to get thru. I promise you this. There are many terrible diseases in this world. Many we have been told are incurable. However, some have laughed in the face of that word, defied it, and won. If you accept "incurable" then you will be its victim, *of that it is certain*. Those whom I have known that have defeated Lyme disease all have one thing in common: they possessed an absolute resolve to get well, and never accepted the condition they were in. They always believed they would get better. If you do not possess this absolute Iron Will and conqueror's spirit, get it. Look within you. See that others have beaten this, but only a few. And it wasn't necessarily the doctor they were seeing, or the drug they were taking, or the medicine that got them well. They found it within. It is this Iron Will that allows all other medicines to work. I'm not talking about the placebo affect here. I am speaking about the drive necessary to keep using the tools you have at your disposal. If you stop using the best tools in the world, then none of them will work, no matter how much they cost.

During your journey it will be necessary to address all of the systems of the body that are affected by Lyme. But once you have begun to address them one by one, and find youself improving, then you move onto the next phase of chronic Lyme where you must address some of the more subtle aspects of the illness. This involves the deeply entrenched forms of Borrelia, any remaining co-infections, and the variant or CWD forms which have been resistant to most of the therapies you have used up until this point. And of course biofilms. In fact it may very well be that it was the very therapies that killed off the spirochetes that lead to the deeper infection. What kills spirochetes has the ironic unintended consequences of entrenching the disease on a deeper level. In fact oftentimes the symptoms of Lyme at this stage have become so reduced, many mistakenly believe themselves to be cured when they compare their symptoms now to what they were at the height of their early acute phase. However there are still layers of the onion yet to be revealed.

What must be done at this point is to utilize therapies which have the potential to deal with these deeper layers and highly resistant forms in order affect the next level of infection. Unless this next level is addressed, you will remain in a chronic "sub-clinical" condition staying just well enough to have your life back, but never achieving complete healing. This is where many of us who have been using Lyme therapies have found ourselves. I say this not as a healthcare practitioner obviously, but purely as an observation in myself and others I have known who also have had Lyme disease for a long time—the longer a person goes thru various therapies, the longer it seems to take for them to get well. What is meant by that is that by taking a slow methodical non-aggressive approach to therapy, wishing to see how well you respond, then trying another medicine, then another, then another, the illness is actually prolonged and allows more generations of bacteria whose immunity has been challenged to overcome the previous therapy, to further develop if not more resistance, then at least more entrenchment.

Certain forms of Bb tend to be more intracellular in nature, such as L-forms. Another one of the many reasons why Lyme disease takes such a long time to completely recover from is because most antimicrobials simply are not taken up by infected cells. Noni extract has been used to aid in the expelling of intracellular infections over time. Apoptosis or programmed cell suicide normally signals phagocytes to devour intracellulary infected cells. But in certain forms Borrelia infections, this process becomes impaired. So sometimes the only true means to eventually dissipate and reduce the infection is shear time that it takes for infected human cells to die off, and relinquish their intracellular infectious agents over time. This process is one that is not easily sped up, and is one prime reason why Lyme disease takes such a long time to resolve. However, if you are very passively treating your infection, and not attempting to maintain aggressive therapy, then as generations of intracellular infected cells die off with their host bacterial forms, rather than immune cells scavenging them along with the removal of dying cells, the now expelled host bacteria are free to move on to a fresh new home to continue the process of infection in perpetuity. Whereas if you were maintaining a continuous antimicrobial presence, they would be killed as they exit their host.

Your level of commitment, your determination, and your aggressive approach to therapy will determine whether you remain in the chronic phase of Lyme disease, or whether you move inward and onward to deeper levels of healing that can only be attained when you choose with your will to remain actively involved in the healing process.

Note: At this point a word deserves to be mentioned about a popular therapy that is offering hope to many, called the Marshall Protocol. This is one therapy that in fact moves counter to the aforementioned approach. In brief, this therapy is based on research that identified L-form (CWD) bacteria as producers of a by-product of Vitamin D called 1,25 dihydroxyvitamin-D which suppresses the immune system. This enables L-forms to persist in the body by inhibiting immune response. The therapy works by reducing Vitamin D levels to normal, and thus enables immunity to regain a foothold. Many have used this therapy with good results.

However I do not spend time explaining this therapy for several reasons. First, it is extremely difficult to follow and almost completely disrupts your life (as if Lyme sufferers have a normal life to begin with). Hence you end up modifying the protocol and reduce its effectiveness. Second, it is not a quick fix. It can take up to two years or more, and still does not address biofilms, which in my opinion is the primary reason why Lyme becomes chronic. Many have beaten Lyme disease without using the protocol. Also, intracellular infections have been addressed by other means such as PC Noni as described by Dr. Klinghardt. [1] So it is not the only means of defeating L-form bacteria. I don't know of anyone that has become cured of Lyme using this protocol, although many have testified of significant improvement. However for those interested the site is listed for your consideration at marshallprotocol.com.

ENDNOTES

1. Lyme disease: A Look Beyond Antibiotics Dietrich K.Klinghardt, MD, PhD   pg.27   www.klinghardtacademy.com/images/stories/Lyme_Disease/ Lyme_protocol_Jan06.pdf

CHAPTER 11

Healing Substances

"Plant medicines are intelligent, human medications are usually quite dumb."

Dietrich K.Klinghardt, MD, PhD

Although I have designed this book with the end goal being to give to the reader practical ideas and therapies that have worked for me and others, these therapies will not serve you if they are not implemented within a framework of the true nature of Lyme disease. By that I mean, if you are of the philosophy that simply taking antibiotics for a few weeks or even months will cure you of the disease, then that is the paradigm or framework from which you will view not only the therapies you try, but the length of time you decide to take them. That is based upon a false idea that this bacterium is just like most others. Gaining a proper understanding as to what makes Borrelia different will change the therapeutic approach you take. It will also help you to understand why it is important to remain on those therapies considerably longer than one would for a typical staph infection for example. This is why it is important to understand the biochemistry of Borrelia, and why we have spent so much time helping you gain a rudimentary understanding.

In order for a patient to be in charge of his own health, he must decide for himself what approach to take. If you are hoping for and are fortunate enough to receive a definitive test result for any type of infection, it is obviously just a matter then of deciding on the course of action. However if not, considering a results-oriented approach would be your only other alternative by incorporating integrative alternative healthcare practitioners and natural remedies in cooperation with your MD or DO.

Antimicrobial substances, whether drug-based anti-biotics, herbal supplements, or other non-drug substances, are always preferred as a secondary choice over our own innate and primary defenses. However in the case of Lyme disease, history has shown that our own immune systems are not usually sufficient to overcome the infection alone. But whenever possible, it would be advised to seek out therapies that would support your own immune system rather than complete reliance on a medicine.

For example, Advanced Cell Training developed by Gary Blier would be a good first option, as the primary focus of this modality is to naturally restore your immune system's response specifically as it relates to Lyme disease. Another is one called Lymestop, which is a technique developed by Dr. Tony Smith DC of Coeur d' Alene, Idaho. His therapy works on the principle of balancing trigger points in the body that allows the person's own immune system to heal the Lyme. He has had remarkable success helping Lyme patients and neutralizing allergies very rapidly. Dr. Smith's therapies are some of the most remarkable and fast acting I have ever seen. They will support the Lyme patient by directing and enhancing the immune system towards self-healing and normalization. Dr. Smith has also developed his own highly effective therapies which seem to work much faster than NAET described in the beginning of this book. These will aid by allowing the body to turn off allergic conditions which Lyme patients commonly develop due to a perpetual hyper immune condition as well as chronic antibiotic use. However the therapy does not have the ability to address biofilms, since the immune system alone often does not seem to have the capacity to resolve this aspect of the disease.

One of the observations I have personally made having been exposed to and worked with many good Lyme therapies over the years, is that many are very subjective to each patient. Not only that, but there seems to be a point that each patient reaches where a particular modality can only take them so far, and will help no further, and is time to move on to the next level. There are a number of reasons for this other than just the obvious individual bacteriocidal effects any particular medicine is directly having at the level of the microbe.

For instance any underlying hormonal and endocrine imbalances are going to have a dramatic affect on your degree of improvement. And the effectiveness of any particular therapy you are doing could be related to how it affects for example your mood, glands, metabolism, nervous system, etc. I can recall how that one of the effects of a particular therapy I was on was a feeling of profound nervousness. I recall at times actually having feelings of paralyzing fear running thru my body. I didn't understand it at the time, but later after it had subsided, I realized it was the affects of the toxic die-off from using the therapy. So when it happened again, I could handle it since I knew what was causing it. And eventually it went away altogether. That in turn led to some emotional healing, which in turn allowed me to move still deeper to the next level and further therapies.

The amount of personal emotional issues a person has can have a dramatic effect on the immune system. As a general rule, think about who you are as a person, and any emotional issues you have in dealing with not only your own self-image, but how you deal with others. Now picture your own immune system as a mirror of your own emotional condition, and you will get a good idea of the state of your own immunity. Your immune system will often, if not usually behave towards pathogens the same way your underlying emotional reactions are in your own personality. That is because who you are, or who I am as a person is in every cell of the body. That is why oftentimes emotional traumas can precede declines in health. The two are intricately connected.

But when our efforts at balancing our immune system and healing our emotions have taken us as far as we can, that is when it is time to take the next step by receiving the God-given healing modalities that were designed for that very purpose. Lyme disease is such a powerful illness. And that is why even the healthiest, most emotionally balanced and happy people can succumb to it. Don't be misled by some well-intentioned person who doesn't understand the seriousness and complexities of Lyme disease. That is ok to be naïve in the beginning. But then it is time to mature, and see reality for what it is, and deal with it head on with all of the weapons at your disposal as possible.

How to View the Following Information

In a perfect world, we as Lyme sufferers would love to be able to take one pill, or one therapy that we knew if we followed the instructions consistently would cure us. (Of course if we lived in a perfect world, we would not have Lyme disease in the first place.) We would love to know that that product or medicine had been tried on other Lyme patients, that it was safe, that we would only have the take so much and for so long, and we would be well. In the beginning as we learn we may have Lyme disease, that is what we hope and pray our doctors will give us. We soon learn that is not the case with this disease.

Some may wonder why so many different therapies are being examined. After all, haven't some Lyme patients gotten well using simple therapies such as salt/C or teasel root? For those fortunate enough to have what I consider more simple infections, simple therapies may work. Now certainly no Lyme infection is a "simple" infection. However to the degree that both biofilms have developed, and the co-infectious agents that occupy those films along with the higher resistance they invoke, they become much more complex and difficult to eradicate. So as effective as these therapies may be in some people, in others they may only represent a partial answer. The following therapies represent a huge arsenal from which even the most resistant infections can be dealt with.

I remember when I first learned I had Lyme disease. Because of all that I had previously gone thru with my health issues; because of the years I had spent learning about medicine, both natural and energy, and the tremendous success I ultimately found, I figured it would be a walk in the park for me to find a cure for Lyme. As I began reading and hearing of people having the disease for 10, 15, and even 20 years or more, I sort of thought in the back of my mind, "What is wrong with these people? Why don't they get serious about getting well? How could someone have a disease this long, be on anti-biotics for that many years, and still be suffering from their disease?" I thought to myself, "I am not going to let that happen to me. I'll find a way to a cure. I'm not going to be like those people."

Well over the years, and as time passed, even with access to the best therapies available and following the advice of those that had been having success in their own lives, still, the hope of ever finding healing seemed like an illusion. In time I came to realize that even with all that I knew, and with all that I had at my disposal living in a country where we have access in one way or another to virtually any product, medicine, herb, device, therapy, or gadget, (even if we had to go outside what is considered the "approved legal medical establishment"), this was not going to be the stroll in the park I thought it was.

The following list of information is not a list of proven Lyme disease cures. The fact is, there is no such thing as a "proven cure" for chronic Lyme disease, at least not one that gives consistent results to those that follow it. Even the best doctors in the world who have at their disposal every possible medication available can only hope to completely heal a small percentage of their patients, since even those few that have found complete cessation of their symptoms using antibiotics often relapse, demonstrating they were not completely cured to begin with. This is more the rule than the exception. Too many variables exist in this disease. Even those drugs or medicines, or natural products that seem to help one person, may not be found to benefit another. And even if one were to find something is effective for them, that one thing by itself is not likely going to be the sole answer. It will take a combination of therapies addressing various aspects of the illness, and each one will do something very specific. And even then, it may only work or be beneficial for a given time. Then once it has done all it can to take you to one level of healing, it will be necessary to move on to something else that will address healing at another level. If you ask any person who has found healing from their own Lyme disease, I promise you that is likely the story you will hear. Lyme disease therapies are like taking courses in school in that the taking of any one course does not a graduate make. As a requirement for graduation you will have to take some courses along the way that may not seem related to your goals, or don't seem to benefit you. But they are part of the process necessary that will ultimately lead you fulfilling your obligation to graduate.

What follows are substances or therapies that have either been used by Lyme sufferers who have attested to their benefit in some fashion or degree, or because of either studies that have been done or even anecdotally showing potential, are included for your consideration. Some may have demonstrated success or benefit as an antibiotic or antimicrobial in a similar kind of infection, and has either been used for Lyme disease by some, or holds potential. And any particular substance may address one level of where you may find yourself now or the current life cycle of the microbe. Some, because of their properties may only benefit you once you've reached another level, even though you find it doesn't seem to be very effective at doing anything at your current level.

The listed items are of course not FDA approved for Lyme disease since only drugs require FDA approval. However having said that, as we are already aware, FDA approved antibiotics have often been inadequate, even sometimes poor choices for chronic Lyme disease. [1] Except in extremely rare cases, (there is always an exception to every rule) these drugs have only shown limited and temporary benefit in chronic Lyme disease. One must change his/her way of thinking with this illness since almost everything about Lyme disease does not fit a mould and is unlike any other illnesses in that regard.

Someone may ask, "Then are these 'proven' therapies?" Although all hold potential due to what is known of their benefit to those that have already tried them, some are yet to be used by the masses for Lyme disease specifically. And even if someone ultimately found healing using a certain therapy or group of therapies, it doesn't guarantee it will be a "proven therapy" *for you.* That is a journey that must be taken by each individual.

I have been a gold prospector for many years. There is wise advice given to those that want to know where they can go to find gold. "You search for gold where it has already been known to have been found in the past." That is where you begin your search. But that does not guarantee you will find it there. In that case you must set out to search for it where there is at least a preponderance of evidence showing potential. Ultimately, "Gold is where you find it." Good prospecting.

SUPPLEMENTS:

Ursolic Acid chemically is from the family of terpenes found in plants such as basil, apples, oregano, thyme, cranberries, rosemary, and others. One product on the market is being sold as a sage extract. UA has been discovered to have the capability of inhibiting cancer cells. It was used primarily first in the cosmetic industry, but has been the subject of research demonstrating powerful anti-inflammatory, anti-tumor, as well as antibacterial and antifungal properties. It is relatively well tolerated and non-toxic both externally and internally. It has also been the focus of study for the protective properties it has against chemically induced liver injury. This product should be near the top of the list for Lyme patients. Its bacteriocidal and anti-inflammatory benefits were experienced as being very potent. [2, 3]

In addition to its immune modulating and antimicrobial activities, Ursolic acid could also be taken as a conjunctive treatment to help protect the liver when taking essential oils internally. Can be purchased as a supplement.

Olive leaf extract—Hydroxytyrosol is a plant phytochemical whose antioxidant and free-radical scavenging capacity is one of the most powerful known. It is found as a by-product of processing olives and is a constituent of olive leaves. This may be the primary polyphenol found in Olive Leaf Extract known for its antimicrobial properties. Research has demonstrated effectiveness against various strains of mycoplamsa, a co-infection of Lyme disease. A plethora of studies have been done on this substance, as well as having been used by Lyme sufferers for years indicating it may one of the most important natural weapons in a Lyme therapy arsenal. [4, 5] The extract of olive leaf which contains hydroxytyrosol has many known antibacterial, anti-viral and antifungal agents. This should be one of your primary herbal medicines against Borrelia.

I personally found this to be very effective. Although hydroxytyrosol is probably the most effective constituent of Olive Leaf Extract, it may be purchased in concentrated form in Olivinol as one source.

Liposomal Enapsulated Vitamin C—Probably the most dynamic advance in delivery system since IV vitamin C. Developed from nano-technology, liposomes are micro-sized spheres encapsulated in a lipid base that allows them to be absorbed intracellularly, not just in the blood stream. The lipid coating protects the liposome from being destroyed during the digestion process. Due to its nano size and due to the fact that human cell walls are composed of the same phospholipid coatings as the liposome, they are capable of being absorbed thru the cell membrane.

Most vitamin C is around 19% absorbable in the body. So to receive 190 mg, you need to take 1000 mg, whereas liposomal vitamin C is 93% absorbed, making it significantly more bioavailable to the cells where it is needed most. Dr. Thomas Levy MD, an expert in Vitamin C administration for incurable diseases, and author of the book, *Curing the Incurables*, testifies that liposomal vitamin C is more clinically effective than IV administered vitamin C!

For the better part of two years, I actually ignored my own medical observations, since they were in complete conflict with what I felt just had to be true. Also, until the past nine months or so, I had not bothered to educate myself extensively on the body of liposome science that has been accumulating for the past 45 years or so. In a nutshell, I found that liposome encapsulated vitamin C, taken orally, was roughly 10 times more effective clinically in resolving infectious diseases than the IV-C. Having given thousands of IV-Cs and taken hundreds myself, this was difficult to comprehend, even though the clinical observation was quite straightforward. I subsequently realized that the liposome gave the ultimate bioavailability: intracellular delivery, including the mitochondria, endoplasmic reticulum, and even the nucleus. Furthermore, it was delivered in a non-energy-consuming fashion. IV vitamin C requires an expenditure of energy to eventually reach the intracellular compartment, but liposome encapsulated vitamin C does not. If possible, you do not want to consume energy to get energy-carrying substances inside the cell. It defeats the basic purpose. But let me clear, if it is possible, give a patient both IV-C and oral liposome encapsulated vitamin C. However, if only one is available, the best application is with liposomes orally. [6]

The effectiveness of this form of Vitamin C is staggering. And the conjunctive use as a Lyme treatment, particularly for the salt/c protocol would potentially exponentially increase its effectivness. However, there are other products that are also available thru liposomal encapsulation, for instance resveratrol and glutathione. Additionally, it is now possible to actually make your own liposomal supplements using an inexpensive ultrasonic cleaner purchased from Harbor Freight. This holds endless possibilities to be able to make your own more absorbable form of not only Vitamin C, but other products as well. [7-9] I now make my own liposomal vitamin C at home. Imagine being able to take a form of vitamin C so absorbable and powerful that it may be 10 times more effective than even IV vitamin C!

Even if one takes a good Vitamin C product, it is not likely to functionally hold the same potency activities as liposomes. This product could completely replace your current C supplement, and end up costing you less with more effectiveness.

To make your own liposomal vitamin C, you need to purchase an ultrasonic cleaner from Harbor Freight. It is item # 95563. (You can buy a smaller one, but the volume will be so small, you will end up making a very small amount per batch.) You will also need Non-GMO soy lecithin granules. Buy a good quality pharmaceutical grade ascorbic acid vitamin C powder. Have two small containers at hand and spring water. In one add ¾ cup of water to 1 ½ tablespoons of ascorbic acid powder. Let dissolve. In the other, add 1 ½ cups of water to 4 ½ tablespoons of lecithin powder. Let this set for a few hours to dissolve. (Note: It will not dissolve completely, but turn into a slime. Using warm water will speed up the process.)

Then add both containers to a blender, and blend on high speed for at least 3-5 minutes. This will often be sufficient for a good general quality liposome. But the smaller the liposomes the more absorbable they are. So, take this mixed solution from the blender, and pour into your ultrasonic cleaner. Activate for 6 minutes. This will result in a good quality liposomal C. There are ready-made liposomal C products that can be purchased on the internet. But this method is by far a less expensive alternative. More details will be discussed under the salt/c therapy.

SSKI—Stands for saturated solution Potassium Iodide. This product holds phenomenal potential for a number of conditions. It is most known for its potential to reduce radiation absorption by the thyroid gland in case of nuclear disasters. However it has been used as a natural disinfectant for cuts, to purify water before drinking, to cure some bladder infections, to reduce and eliminate fibrous conditions such as ovarian cysts in women and keloids or thick scar tissue. It is known for its powerful antibacterial, antifungal, and antiviral properties including a wide range of bacterial infections and herpes simplex infections; can eliminate hemorrhoids quickly. One LLMD has commented "The most critical element in the Lyme patient is iodine." [10]

Over time Potassium Iodide can turn yellow which is the result of oxidation. SSKI is easily oxidized, so would be best not taken if you are using MMS, ozone, or hydrogen peroxide therapy. If taking high doses internally over extended period of time, monitoring of thyroid should be done by your doctor. It should be taken with a full glass of water or juice. As it passes thru the bloodstream it would actively kill all vulnerable pathogens. Work up to 3-6 drops per day in water taking periodic breaks. Very high dosages of fewer than 9 drops per day may be used for short periods. But again, thyroid should be monitored, or product discontinued periodically. Is available for purchase without a prescription. [11]

Cesium Chloride—Has been a powerful mineral salt used in the treatment of cancer and tumors. There have been several theories as to how it works. One is that is raises PH levels in cancer cells which allows the cell to undergo programmed cell-death, thus shortening the life of the cell. The other theory is that cancer cells actively uptake the cesium faster than they can release it. This causes an excessive build-up inside the cell thus killing the cell. For several years I have been researching the relationships between intracellular infections and cancer. This had been a significant area of research of Dr. William Koch, the developer of

Glyoxilide, the most effective cancer cure of its kind in his day. Cancer can begin as an intracellular infection by a virus, bacteria or sometimes a fungus. These cancers are precipitated by damage to the mechanisms within the cell that allow for cellular respiration to take place needed for the subsequent burning of glucose for fuel. As a result, infected cells become highly acidic due to lactic acid accumulation. When this occurs, cellular energy becomes reduced, and apoptosis (programmed cell death) is not able to be initiated. Thus, these cells grow unchecked and can form tumors.

Borrelia Burdorferi can also be an intracellular infection which also holds the possibility of inhibiting cellular respiration. Although Bb does not likely spark cancer, the therapy holds the potential however to either shut down infected cells since they would likely also have lost their oxidative capabilities and lost the capacity for apoptosis, or the cesium uptake in the infected/damaged cells would kill the cell. However it works, the end result would be a mass expelling and release of spirochetes as infected cells die off and spill into the bloodstream resulting in a large herx. By the time this theory occurred to me, I had already killed off most of the spirochetes long ago from therapies I had already been finding success in. So by the time I tried it, I found little effects from it. However, the seller of the product from Essense-of-Life.com has shared with me that users of Cesium Choride for Lyme disease have experienced massive herxing, and should be taken slowly and cautiously. This may be one of the few Lyme therapies that holds the potential to address intracellular infections. Caution: Cesium chloride should always be supplemented with potassium as it seems to deplete or replace it in the body's cells. This ideally needs to be monitored by a doctor.

Gallium Nitrate—This substance is rather unique, and may have a significant affect on some biofilms. GN as a drug was originally used to reduce hypercalcemia (too much calcium in the blood) that resulted from chemotherapy. Later it was learned it possessed the ability to dissolve kidney stones which are made up of calcium and other minerals coating what have been termed "Nanobacteria", indicating a possible link between these "microbes" and the formation of mineral deposits. (Some controversy surrounds exactly what "nanobacteria" really are.) George Eby, a scientist and researcher began researching other far more interesting properties of GN too many to cite here. It was given to horses both orally and topically and, in many cases, completely eliminated arthritic conditions very quickly. Testimonies from human use also found dramatic and sometimes complete cessation of chronic pain within days of use. In many cases these rheumatoid arthritic conditions were completely healed with no return of arthritic conditions. The effects were not caused by some temporary analgesic properties. It is theorized that biofilm-related infection may quickly be resolved in some kinds of infections. Rheumatoid arthritis is believed by many doctors to be caused by pathogen infection in the joints.

Studies have demonstrated that GN possesses powerful antimicrobial properties. Gallium maltolate, a newer more absorbable form of gallium has been developed by Titan Pharmaceuticals. It possesses similar properties as GN, but will only be available by prescription. GN is however currently available from internet sources. A description of Gallium maltolate is provided from Titan:

> *Gallium maltolate is our novel oral agent for the potential treatment of chronic bacterial infections, bone disease, and cancer. Gallium deprives bacteria of iron required for growth and renders resistant bacteria in biofilms susceptible to treatment. Gallium acts upon bone by enhancing the formation of osteoblasts and inhibiting osteoclasts, thereby increasing bone deposition and reducing bone turnover. Additionally, gallium also inhibits ribonucleotide reductase, a key enzyme essential for DNA replication in cancer cells.*

> *In preclinical studies with an animal model for persistent infection due to bacterial biofilms, oral dosing of gallium maltolate was effective in eradicating infection in a dose dependent manner. Based on these results, we believe that gallium maltolate may have potential in the treatment of chronic bacterial biofilm-based infections, including lung infections associated with cystic fibrosis or urinary tract infections.* [12]

It is believed that gallium functions by replacing iron within susceptible bacteria which require it. It is molecularly similar to iron, and is taken up by the bacteria which normally utilize the iron into their biochemistry. However, enzyme and delivery systems which require iron are not able to utilize the gallium in the same manner as the iron. Thus the bacteria die from the inability to process normal cellular functions. Hence the gallium acts with antibacterial and anti-biofilm activity. It also possesses powerful anti-inflammatory properties.

Borrelia Burgdorferi however does not appear to be directly or significantly affected biochemically by gallium due to its requiring little iron. However, since gallium also functions by affecting calcium that is associated with biofilm formation, it may contribute to the weakening of Bb induced biofilms. Also, co-infective pathogens (which may be iron-susceptible) which are known to associate in biofilms with other microbial species may be affected, hence the reason for citing GN as a potentially valuable tool in reducing bacterial biofilms. Babesia is one such common co-infection associated with Lyme disease which may respond to gallium nitrate since it utilizes a significant amount of iron.

My use of gallium nitrate resulted in a significant reduction in pain at old injury sites. It was used for several months to receive optimum benefit. Gallium nitrate may aid in dissolving calcium deposits associated with biofilms. Although gallium nitrate acts as an antibiotic against iron-dependant bactera, Bb seems little affected by gallium when taken alone. However, since its biofilm is vulnerable, as with other anti-biofilm substances, it needs to be taken in conjunction with (followed by) antibacterial agents which Bb is susceptible to. This makes gallium nitrate a potentially prime anti-biofilm product. If choosing to take an antibiotic with gallium nitrate, minocycline may be an ideal medicine since tetracycline antibiotics in general (of which minocycline is a member) are the only ones known to also kill nanobacteria. These tiny microorganisms are also strongly implicated in calcium deposits, chronic inflammatory disease, heart and other tissue calcifications, kidney stones, and are known to develop biofilms. They are a potential co-inhabitant of Bb biofilms. Bb has been shown to also be vulnerable to minocycline.

Some people who do in fact have bacterial infections which are susceptible to GN seem to resolve very quickly. Others may require longer therapy to give time for the GN to dissolve calcium deposits.

Biofilms seem to have a strong propensity to populate around old injuries. This is due to several factors that have been touched on already—acid formation and low oxygen within injured cells makes intracellular infection a preferred refuge for both anaerobic and microaerophilic pathogens. And subsequent inactivation of apoptosis enables the infection zone to be less vulnerable to immune cells.

Gallium nitrate should ideally be administered by a physician due to the mineral leaching affect it can have, and the monitoring that may be required as a long term therapy. However you are unlikely to find a physician who is willing to use GN in an off-label manner. It is very important that minerals, particularly potassium, be supplemented in the diet, as they will be leached out of tissues and could cause serious spasms if not maintained. They should not be taken concurrently.

Although considered a drug by FDA definition, technically GN is a mineral salt which must be taken in a liquid form due to dilution necessities. It is sold as 14% solution, but must be highly diluted down to 1% solution. This is done by combining 13 parts water to one part 14% solution. This will yield 1% GN. *Then, when taken internally, it must additionally be reduced* at the rate of about ⅛-¼ cup of this 1% solution added to a full glass of water. Those interested in GN for its therapeutic potential should thoroughly research before use in order to understand the specific manner in which it should be diluted and is being used by others. [13] GN is technically more involved as specialized precautions need to be observed when taking gallium nitrate internally. Again, potassium supplementation is vital with GN.

GN is a strong biofilm effector. Nanobacteria have been implicated as contributing to degenerative biofilms. And although little information is available as to the relationship between Lyme disease and nanobacteria infections, they may play a contributive role in immune compromised individuals. Regardless of the controversy some have engaged in regarding whether nanobacteria are living organisms or not, the fact is that Nanobacteria, whatever they are develop biofilms. And gallium nitrate is highly effective at dissolving biofilms. Calcium formations occur in both nanobacteria and likely contribute to the formation of Bb biofilms. But it is interesting that nanobacteria are vulnerable to tetracycline antibiotics. Minocycline, a member of the tetracycline family, is often used as a longer term drug against not only Bb infections, but also mycoplasma. And of course is effective to various degrees against nanobacteria. That Bb, mycoplasma and nanobacteria all develop biofilms, all have been implicated in degenerative disease, and all require long-term therapy to be resolved, makes GN and Minocycline a good potential combination treatment option for long term biofilm and Lyme/mycoplasma/nanobacteria infections. There are probably no natural alternatives to this combination as their activities are unique in the way they affect the biochemistry of both biofilms and infectious bacteria.

Zeolite—This has become a popular supplement due to its ability to trap and remove toxins from the body. Zeolites are highly porous minerals mined from ancient volcanic sources. Molecularly they have a property termed "sieves" which acts much like a screen mesh which can capture positively charged molecules. Zeolites possess a negative ion charge (anions), whereas most toxins and free-radicals tend to be positively charged (cations). These sieves or pores act much like a cage that captures toxins that possess a vulnerable electrical charge. Some of these toxins include heavy metals such as mercury, lead, arsenic, etc., but also chemical toxins and microbial toxins. Some micronized zeolites have been processed such that they have the ability to cross the blood-brain barrier, making them an ideal therapy for Lyme disease. Not only are spirochetes known to live in the brain, but their neurotoxins released are perhaps one of the most hideous and horrific symptoms experienced by Lyme victims. The brain fog, depression, emotional rage, and neuronal disruption have been reduced by those testifying of zeolites activity. Systemically zeolites can reduce the overall toxin load acting as a free-radical scavenger. Free radicals are simply molecules which possess an electrical ionic charge that tears electrons from their orbit from molecules making up the cells and tissues, thus damaging or destroying them. So zeolites could be termed a kind of super free radical scavenger since they are known to capture those free radicals which possess a positive ionic charge.

One of the interesting aspects of biofilm formation is the reliance upon autoinducers for quorum sensing—the communication system used by bacteria that allows them to make cooperative decisions that affects their virulence. One of the auto-inducers of Bb has been identified as a by-product of its metabolism, hence contributes to toxicity in the body. Zeolites would then hold the potential of actually inhibiting biofilm formation by reducing the positively-charged free-floating autoinducers in the body thus inhibiting the propagation of bacterial colonies.

Additionally, by zeolite's trapping viral components before they can fully assemble, they are known to possess viral-inhibiting activities to a number of strains. It also raises blood ph levels to more normal levels, has liver protective qualities, and is a natural chelator.

Not only this, but due to zeolite's anionic property, it actually promotes a calming state within the body. If you've ever come inside from a hot day and turned on the air conditioner and found yourself suddenly wanting to fall asleep, you've experienced the affects of negative ions. They are relaxing. Scientific studies also have demonstrated this to be true. Many taking zeolites often experience a lifting of depression, clarity of thinking, and an overall feeling of balance.

There are now quite a number of good zeolite products on the market. Some are more effective than others. So do your homework. As I said, the micronized and nano sized zeolites will tend to cross the blood brain barrier better. A few brands are, ACZ Nano, Natural Cellular Defense, Liquid Zeolite, and Destroxin. This latter brand, although a powdered form which is not as well absorbed into the blood, has the added benefit of being enhanced with Vitamin B-12 and works very well to stabilize emotional mood. Taking small spread out doses works much better than large doses since zeolite will only "process" available toxins or free radicals that are present at any given time. This should become a permanent part of any Lyme sufferers overall therapy program, right up there with the taking of probiotics. [14]

To any Lyme sufferer in an overloaded condition, experiencing a herxheimer reaction, or just having a relapse and need to feel better fast, Destroxin may be one of the best supplements to bridge you over due to its B-12/zeolite combination. It is best to keep this product on hand.

*Cilantro extract, chlorophyll based greens such as chlorella, spirulina, blue-green algae, barley and wheat grass are other products that have toxin-absorbing properties.

Before moving on to this next substance, it is important to point out that although some people might wish to jump forward to just begin the "therapies", to others it helps to understand the reasoning behind a therapy, otherwise they simply will not make the important connection and see the relevance. So here it is.

Most of us Lyme sufferers follow the same chain of thinking as those that suffer from other kinds of infections. We think that because we have a bacterial infection, it stands to reason that in order to overcome the infection, we need to find those herbs and substances which are known to stimulate the immune cells to attack and destroy the infection as any other bacterial or viral infection. On the surface this appears to make perfect sense. We then consider taking supplements that focus on enhancing immunity as a means to fight the infection. Certainly this is part of the solution.

But we know that even those that have the healthiest immune systems seldom overcome this illness by natural immunity alone, no matter what immune-enhancing measures they take. What we also know is that Bb always seems to elude eradication and actually proliferates regardless of the measures that are taken. In fact, to our frustration, attempting to make our immune systems stronger alone can actually stimulate Bb to act even more defensively.

Borrelia Burdorferi is a master of taking advantage of the weakness of its victim. What your immune response will be is already anticipated. The responses are encoded in Bb's plasmids. So it knows what your immune system's efforts will be—step up the attack! It knows this because that is what the predictable immune response has been in the past.

Do you remember the Star Trek nemesis—The Borg? They were called the "collective" because they conquered their enemies and incorporated everything their enemies knew into their collective consciousness, hence its defenses. And so they could anticipate and prepare to respond to further attacks based upon the actions and memories made in the past of those they already conquered. In this way they had the upper hand and could win virtually every battle with every enemy. They possessed all the thoughts and defensive actions already made by those whom they battled and conquered in the past, and could thus be prepared for any offensive and defensive measure from its enemies.

What I have just described is *exactly* what Bb has the potential of doing. Plasmids display genetic-like capabilities wherein they have incorporated into their memory information that has recorded what the immune responses have been from previous hosts their bacterial ancestors have infected. They then call upon that information and send signals for lipoproteins to form structures that can resist and confuse the body's immune cells. It already knows that it can subvert natural immunity because of what it has learned in the past. The immune response is predictable. It already knows that the immune system will in fact escalate its offensives just as it has always done. Plasmids encode information for the bacterium to respond in a manner that will not only be defensive, but offensive. What have some have termed "neuro-toxins" are nothing more than proteins that are so poisonous to cells, that they interrupt communication between cells. Because immune cells are not able to communicate properly, they continue the assault, and act to perpetuate the problem. Bb is a master of disguise and a master of confusion.

In a manner of speaking, it is the very act of escalation and "strengthening of the immune system" that can contribute to the entrenchment of the disease. Read that again. The real problem is not due to a "weakened immune system", but that the tactics employed by the enemy are subverting or sabotaging the efforts of the immune system by disrupting its communication. The result is frustration and hyper stimulation. Immunity is forced to act in the only manner it knows how—to throw more firepower at it. This is not the long term solution.

In order to take back control of the disease, it is necessary to step back and observe that this is happening. This hyper-immune response leads to non-productive hyper-inflammation, which further damages tissues. In Lyme disease inflammation appears to be the immune system's universal response to nearly every offensive and defensive maneuver enacted by this bacterium. Thus, that response only perpetuates more inflammation by eliciting more activating plasmids to further find new ways to attack or defend itself. And the cycle repeats.

Thus a different strategy would be required that stops the cycle of perpetuation and escalation we already know doesn't work. Although natural immunity, even in the healthiest of persons, isn't likely to eradicate Lyme disease, the down-ward spiral which causes the health of the person to dramatically decline can be stopped and reversed while antibiotics and/or antimicrobials focus on direct killing. Enter galactomannans.

Galactomannans—Aloe vera is perhaps one of the most studied plants on earth. It is far more than a folk medicine as hundreds of scientific studies have been done on its properties. The most important agents found in Aloe are its polysaccharides, or group chains of sugars. Aloe's primary saccharides are galactose and mannose which combine to form galactomannan. The benefits of these chains of sugars are dependant upon the length or size of the polysaccharide molecules linked together. These sugars are not broken down by stomach acids, hence become bioavailable to cells. In order to make these available as a supplement, the polysaccharides need to go thru a special process to become highly concentrated from the aloe. Their potency and hence their healing potential is dependant upon both the size of the molecule, the length of the chains, and the concentration levels. The levels necessary for immune modification for certain illnesses cannot be obtained in sufficient quantity by simply taking any aloe vera product from a health food store. The galactomannans are highly processed and extracted making them much more potent and effective.

Galactomannans are generally divided into small, medium, long, and very long chain polysaccharides. Each of these classes has been studied and found to possess its own unique properties and functions not found in the other classes. For instance, according to Dr. Ivan Danhof, an expert in Aloe Vera research and author of the book *Remarkable Aloe*, small chain GM's have the ability to reduce blood sugar in both type 1 and type 2 diabetics, as well as are inhibitors of leukotrienes which are produced in response to an injury and infection for healing purposes. Thus it induces a strong anti-inflammatory effect. Medium chain GM's have potent antioxidant capacities. Long chains have very powerful antibacterial, antiviral, and antifungal capacities, as well as immune stimulating signaling. The very long chains seem to hold special benefits which would address specific immune activities affecting chronic Lyme disease. They stimulate lymphocytes to produce antibodies, increase natural killer cells, and enhance the release of chemotactic factor. (These are special molecules used by the immune system to direct white blood cells to specific areas of infection and injury.) And these are only a few examples.

The new science of glycobiology has helped us to understand how galactomannans have the potential to perform these functions. Scientists have discovered that there are certain proteins on every cell wall in the body called glycoproteins (glyco short for sugar). These proteins are imbedded in the cell wall with a chain of saccharides attached to it much like an antennae protruding from the protein. These glycoproteins are the means that cells use to communicate with one another. They act much like a two-way radio that can both broadcast and receive communication. Thus the functions of these saccharides and polysaccharides are specific. However when these saccharides are absent or lacking this communication system breaks down, or may cease to function. Cell to cell communication therefore is the foundation upon which all immune activities are able to operate, whether by innate or adaptive immune cells. One can have a "strong" immune system, but if cells can't communicate properly with other immune cells, it will be ineffective and may actually overreact, thus further enhancing ineffective inflammation. In order to understand the complexity involved for immunity to function properly, and to realize the importance these communication molecules hold, consider how the process works:

Adaptive immunity is first communicated to by what is called *innate immunity*. The innate system may be considered a sort of general first response to microbes, and identifies them. These cells then present antigens or threats to the adaptive immune system. Adaptive immunity is more complex and can recognize pathogens by developing receptors based upon specific antibody coupling. Memory B and T cells retain both specific and variable receptors which recall pathogen exposure and are able to prepare for future attacks. Thus they are able to adapt or modify themselves depending on the infection.

The process goes something like this: Innate immunity begins with exposure to a germ through the use of special antigen-presenting cells called dendritic cells. Germs or pieces of protein molecules are captured by these cells and display them on their surface by what are called *major histocompatibility complex* (MHC) proteins. This newly formed complex which contains the pathogen molecules becomes presented to an aid to T-cells called *helper T-cells* or the *CD4+ adhesion molecule*. The presentation of the displayed pathogen protein with the MHC becomes the ligand molecule (interface or signaling molecule) which is presented to CD4. Here is where the crucial part comes. As long as an interaction takes place with the ligand presented CD4 and the T-cell, the ligand will deliver its message, an agonist, and enter into the T-cell for response mechanisms to become activated to neutralize or kill the pathogen. When this occurs, the T-cell becomes a killer T-cell and stimulates other functions such as chemokine responses, bacteriocidal cells such as phagocytes, macrophages, anti-body production, etc., and will destroy infected human cells to accomplish this if necessary. But the activation process can only occur when the CD4 molecule presents the ligand to the T-cell, and the receptor is not being blocked by an antagonist (receptor blocker).

However, sometimes an interaction between the CD4 and T-cell does not take place. Specific signal-generating properties responsible for this would appear to be missing or in short supply. Additionally, viruses have been known to block ligand communication signaling. [15] However any number of specific ligands called *antagonists* can act by blocking the T-cell receptor, preventing the coupling of the helper T-cell with the T-cell. When these antagonists are present, the activation process cannot occur, even though the T-cell itself is able to identify the pathogen peptide molecule being carried by the MHC proteins. From a purely biochemical standpoint, the activation process can only occur when the CD4 molecule presents the ligand to the T-cell, and the receptor is not being blocked by an antagonist.

One can see therefore just from this tiny overview how important cell to cell communication is particularly as it relates to immune cells. It is far more complex than this, but you get the idea.

During this entire process, glycoproteins on the surfaces of these cells would have been necessary for every aspect of communication. Any breakdown or miscommunication along the way could have inhibited the subsequent chain reactions from occuring. Thus it is not difficult to understand how vitally important the role these polysaccharide chains play. This is especially important in Lyme disease where these "antagonists", or ligands which compete with receptors on cell surfaces are likely Borrelia waste by-products or toxins, and lipoproteins acting as antagonists interfering with cell to cell communication. By increasing galactomannans, you have the capacity to directly compete with Borellia's toxic interference with the immune system by saturating your cells with vital communication molecules to give your immunity the upper hand. So it is not necessarily a general "strenghthening" that is needed, so much as restored and enhanced communication. That is why sugars designed specifically to enhance communication ultimately leads to a more effective immune response.

Another advantage of galactomannan is its potential against bacterial adhesions which are involved in biofilm formation. Mannose is a component of this polysaccharide which has been known for its ability to aid in the treatment of urinary tract infections. Cranberry supplements are often recommended for this condition. This is due to its mannose content. Laurance Johnston, Ph.D in an article *Urinary Tract Infections* writes:

> *The cell wall of the UTI-causing E. coli has tiny finger-like projections that contain complex molecules called lectins on their surfaces. These lectins are cellular glue that binds the bacteria to the bladder wall so they cannot be readily rinsed out by urination. However, because D-mannose molecules will glom on to these lectins and fill up all of the bacterial anchoring sites, the bacteria can no longer attach to the bladder wall and are, therefore, flushed away.* [16]

The results of taking galactomannose in supplement form as testified by those taking the product is nothing short of amazing. Space won't permit me to tell all the incredible benefits and stories. I began taking the product very late in my recovery process, and wish I had learned of it sooner. Its benefits I would classify as in the top 3 products for all Lyme patients. That along with ursolic acid accelerated my recovery exponentially beyond anything I had previously experienced. The over-all anti-inflammatory effects surpassed any product I had ever taken, even the gallium nitrate.

There are several products which fit into the category of galactomannans. It is important however to be certain to acquire an aloe product that contains the entire spectrum of polysaccharides, not one that only contains one or two of these sugars. These are only 4 of them. AV Ace Immune, WLA-132, MPS Gold, and Digestacure, although I am sure there are others. The developer of MPS Gold seems to demonstrate some evidence that this product is superior to the others. I have used both the AV Ace Immune and the MPS Gold. Very little of this product is necessary for the benefits you receive. Note: The taking of galactomannans with ursolic acid seems to have an extremely potent immune-enhancing and anti-inflammoty effect that also possesses a very effective anti-microbial component.

Manuka honey—Most of the antibacterial activity of common clover honeys and other plant sources is due to its hydrogen peroxide content in small amounts, as well as a recently discovered antibacterial agent known as defensin-1. However the unique Manuka honey has antibacterial benefits far superior to other forms of honey. That is because it is harvested from bees that acquire the honey from a certain plant called the manuka bush (Leptospermum scoparium), or tea tree which is native to New Zealand (not to be confused with Melaleuca alternifolia, tea tree of Australia). The unique properties of this honey come from a compound that has been isolated called *methyglyoxal*, which possesses powerful antibacterial activity. Its notable properties of being genotoxic (toxic to genes and chromosomes) in some studies, as noted by some cellular biologists, is perhaps what gives it the notoriety of killing even the highly resistant forms of bacteria such as MRSA, as well as E. coli, and H. pylori. This property would explain why even these highly antibiotic-resistant bacteria are vulnerable since it has the potential to disrupt bacterial genes that would normally adapt and resist antimicrobial activities of plant chemicals. One study demonstrated the intracellular effects of methygloxal from manuka honey in Staphylococcus areus, and found that it prevented normal cell division from taking place. [17]

Although methyglyoxal has been considered by some to be toxic due to this genotoxic activity, methyglyoxal is well known for its anticancer activities and therapies. Due to the fact that honeys are known to possess some 800 constituents, there are likely some other unknown components that combine with the methylglyoxal that makes bacteria vulnerable, but human cells unaffected. (One study demonstrated that the oil of this Manuka tea tree possessed antioxidant activity which might support this idea. [18] I have not been able to find any reports of toxicity from consuming this honey, or any other negative reports. They are basically non-existent as far as I can tell.) [19]

Manuka honey has been given a rating system which helps to somewhat standardize its antibacterial activity. Not all manuka honeys possess these properties. Only the "active" honey is considered antibacterial. The rating is called the UMF rating system (and an older one with a different name). Most Manuka honey containers will say "Active 12+" or "Active 16+" etc. The higher the number the higher the methylglyoxal content.

Manuka honey is also beneficial in addressing biofilms.

> *Honeymark scientists studied six different strains of bacteria, five of which came from injuries. The bacteria were grown in a laboratory to form biofilms, which are notoriously difficult to treat when they appear as hospital infections. Biofilms prevent healing in wounds and may lead to chronic ulcers. The laboratory grown samples were treated with Manuka Honey, then unattached bacteria were washed off and the remaining slime layer was studied after different time periods. In every sample, the biofilm was disrupted making it more susceptible to the treatment . . .* [20]

I add Manuka honey to my "oil tea" which will be explained later. It is primarily an adjunctive addition to other therapies. By adding to your therapy, you gain the benefits of methyglyoxal and its potential to inhibit bacterial replication and biofilm development which has been demonstrated in multiple scientific studies. However Manuka honey can also be eaten whole as any other honey to receive the benefits mentioned as this form has far more antibacterial benefits that ordinary clover honey.

Humic acid/fulvic acid—These are the terms used to describe several acids which are the by-product of the microbial degradation of plant matter. They have been used in agriculture as a powerful natural fertilizer/enhancer for a long time. But the health benefits from human consumption only recently have become popular. Humic acids have unique molecular properties which are very diverse and complex that enables them to perform many different functions, not all of which are understood. They act as catalysts and enzymes which can break down inorganic matter and possess a molecular structure and ion charge that enables them to act as chelators of heavy metals and toxins. They have been observed to remove salt acids from cell walls allowing them to become more permeable; possess antimicrobial properties, yet can enhance the growth of intestinal flora; act as signal enhancers of biological activities involved in cell communication and cell nutrition, provide important minerals and electrolytes; increase absorption from the intestinal tract and help to form a protective film that can block microbial toxins; have a strong ability to alkalize the blood; due to its negative ion charge and high flavonoid content it possesses strong antioxidant capacity, and the list goes on. [21, 22]

One of the unique qualities of humic acid is its ability to selectively coat receptor-binding proteins of viruses. [23] These are the proteins which allow them to attach to human cells. They are then marked for immune cells to attack and remove them. Many people who suffer from Lyme disease have some form of viral co-infection which not only exacerbates the condition, but enables the toxins of viruses to actually stimulate and enhance the virulence of certain pathogenic bacteria, as it is known that many pathogenic germs possess toxins which are poisonous to one another. Thus by reducing the viral activity you potentially weaken the virulence of the bacterial infection as well. This may also hold potential for the weakening of mycoplasma infections as one Lyme researcher has stated that mycoplasma is the single most common co-infection of Lyme disease. [24] Mycoplasmas possess qualities of both bacteria and viruses. In fact it may be that some who believe they have Lyme disease actually have a mycoplasma infection.

Humic and fulvic acids also possess their own antibacterial activities which involve influencing the metabolism of their proteins and carbohydrates. As well, by molecularly bonding with their toxins they can reduce the bacteria's quorum-sensing ability much the same as was described in the section on zeolite. [25]

There are a number of sources of supplemental humic and fulvic acids. They both have their own specific function, but also have similarities. They can be taken along with zeolite to enhance its chelating qualities. Sometimes they can be purchased together in one product. Rather than interfering with other therapies, humic acid's catalytic qualities may actually enhance other products absorption into cells.

Salt/C—This one has become a solid standard protocol used by many Lyme patients with good success. It is also being used by some doctors either as a primary alternative treatment, or in addition to other treatments. Marc Fett wrote a book on this protocol and has apparently been symptom free. There are several versions of the therapy, and each needs to be adjusted to each person since tolerance levels will vary from person to person.

I am including my version here as I believe it may be more tolerable. But there is no exact formula per se. The idea here is that the salt has not only a direct anti-microbial affect, but studies have demonstrated that elevated salt levels increase the human leukocyte elastase. [26, 27] This is an enzyme that breaks down elastin, which together with collagen forms connective tissue. However neutrophils use elastase to break down the proteins of bacterial walls. Elastase has been proven to be effective at killing Bb. [28]

There are a number of studies showing its antibacterial and antiviral affects. Due to its fiber and protein-breakdown properties and enzyme activities, elevated elastase levels would also seem to be ideal for combating biofilms.

The vitamin C on the other hand is used to help as a detoxifier, antioxidant, as well as to activate immune cells. However it needs to be taken in relatively high doses. In some people, high dose vitamin C can cause gastrointestinal problems. Only so much vitamin C can be absorbed into the blood stream before it begins to back up in the bowels causing diarrhea. So your bowel tolerance level needs to be determined. In many people it can be as low as a few grams per day, in others 10 or more is tolerable. Keeping your vitamin C intake just below this tolerance level will allow you to take your maximum absorption level. However, as a word of warning, depression is one of the main symptoms of Lyme disease. And Vitamin C in high doses can actually inhibit neurotransmitter levels in the brain, thus actually making you feel worse as it begins to build up in the blood stream. Because of these two problems it is suggested that vitamin C in ascorbic acid form be replaced with liposomal vitamin C. This form is highly absorbable. It is 3-5 times more absorbable than any other form, is extremely unlikely to cause diarrhea, and due to its intracellular absorption, it doesn't seem to interfere quite as much with neurotransmitter activities because it is not "building up" like the less absorbable form. Another added bonus is that due to liposomal C being much more highly absorbable, it is more cost effective since you can take less.

The form of salt used in the original formula was taken in tablet form. This form of salt may cause stomach problems in some people as it required some time to dissolve. A better form is to use sea salt. One of the best sea salts available due to its trace mineral content is Himalayan sea salt. This is a much more balanced form of salt with other naturally occurring dissolved minerals. But most sea salts would work.

Here is the protocol: Approximately 1.5 grams of salt per 20 lbs of body weight. (Some formulas say to use as high as 1 gram for every 10 pounds of body weight.) Six grams of salt converts to approximately 1 teaspoon. So a 160 lb person for example would use 2 teaspoons. This is taken throughout the day. The vitamin C is taken throughout the day in divided doses as well just below your bowel tolerance level. If you are taking the liposomal C, you will use a lower dosage. What I have personally found to be easiest to do is to use a two liter bottle filled with spring water, add the salt, and carry it with you throughout the day with the vitamin C. So for instance, depending on your weight, the kind of vitamin C you are taking, and your maximum dosage, your protocol might look something like this:

Two teaspoons sea salt dissolved in 2 liters of water. Drink this in divided doses during the day approximately every 1-2 hours. With each dose also take 1-2 grams of vitamin C. By evening you will have taken 10-12 grams of C and the entire bottle of water. The therapy is not taken at night. But begin again in the morning.

This is only an example. You need to adjust to your own requirements. Also, as a general guideline, you may take about 1/3 the same amount of vitamin C if taking the liposomal C. However having said that, the liposomal C allows you to take higher doses, so you may not even achieve a bowel tolerance level with this product. I personally experimented with this product just to see what my bowel tolerance level was compared to regular ascorbic acid capsules. I took around 10 grams of liposomal C per day. Based upon approximate equivalent absorption amounts that would convert to perhaps 40+ grams of ascorbic acid capsules per day with no bowel problems! (Normally my bowel tolerance level would be around 12 grams.)

Start the therapy slowly as you would any other therapy until you reach maximum levels. Then do the therapy for approximately a month, giving yourself a rest for about a week. You may reduce the dosage of the vitamin C during that time. But do not completely stop the vitamin C. Just significantly reduce the dosage. Then repeat until symptoms are gone.

*Reminder—You are responsible for your own health. Do your own research and your own homework before beginning any therapies listed. Consult a health care practitioner before beginning any therapies you may have reservations about.

As a word of caution, those with high blood pressure need to be monitoring this as higher salt intake may aggravate your condition. If so, see your doctor or eliminate this therapy as an option. Another word on this therapy is that it takes time, especially those with deep seated biofilms. We have been told that sticking with this therapy will pay off if it is done consistently and for long enough time to slowly see a dissolution of symptoms. Six months to a year or more would not be uncommon. This therapy would not be compatible with MMS (activated sodium chlorite) due to vitamin C's antioxidant capacity to inhibit the oxidation of chlorine dioxide.) However it may be rotated. As long as you wait approximately 4 hours after taking the vitamin C. Good luck.

*Since the original salt/C therapy was introduced, others have added their own variations and additional supplements to increase its effectiveness. The original idea was simple and straightforward. Some have added GSE, or other antimicrobial supplements to the mix. Given what we now know of biofilm formation, the need for chelating, as well as deeper absorption properties that can enhance its effectiveness and yet even more potent immune stimulating medicines, I personally developed my own version. In addition to the salt/C, I took 3 gm niacinamide spread out throughout the day, (niacinamide is discussed in the next section) which may have even more immune enhancing abilities than vitamin C. However to reduce the potential for liver accumulation, it may be best to take smaller doses more frequently throughout the day. 2 gm per day total may be a better dosage, divided into 200 mg taken every two hours. 3 gm per day divided into 500 mg doses after continuous use for 3 months did seem to be my limit since at this level and length of dosage I began to experience a slight pain in my right side, which I interpreted as aggravation in the liver. Upon ceasing its use, it went away. Note: This is another reason why it is best to be under the supervision of a healthcare practitioner. Even though natural medicine is infinitely safer than conventional drugs, even they can be so potent as to necessitate caution and oversight by a medical professional.

Then I added 1 teaspoon Haritaki, 1 teaspoon Xylitol, ⅓ teaspoon sodium borate to the 2 liter mix, along with taking MSM (in capsule form) to enhance absorption. But these additions should be added slowly and in smaller amounts to allow time for the body to adjust. Haritaki and xylitol possess potential anti-biofilm properties. (A very noticeable improvement of symptoms and reduction of inflammation was experienced upon adding the xylitol.) The sodium borate significantly adds alkalinity to the solution, is highly anti-inflammatory, but is also a powerful chelator. Sodium borate, aka Borax, is a mined natural mineral, and this amount is generally well-tolerated, but should not be used for prolonged periods to reduce the possibility of accumulating in the body producing potential toxicity issues. Note: For those interested in adding sodium borate, begin using smaller amounts such as1/8 teaspoon per 2 liters of water. Then slowly build up. Do not exceed ½ level teaspoon in 24 hours as this amount is very high dosage. This should be periodically used, and not become a permanent part of the protocol. Listen to your body. Also, the Haritaki doesn't mix well in water. You may wish to put in a blender and mix a little before adding to the salt solution, or take in capsule form.

To enhance the therapy even more, add 1 teaspoon of non-GMO lecithin granules. Put all in a blender and mix.

If someone wanted to begin with a therapy, this salt/C/niacinamide/ Haritaki/xylitol/ solution may be one of the few that contains all the components to address the major aspects of Lyme disease. However, as we have said before, never continually use only one therapy. Rotate them in order to continually challenge Bb.

Niacinamide—If ever there was a substance with medicinal properties ideally suited for Lyme disease, it may be niacinamide. Although commonly known as vitamin B3, niacinamide holds potentials beyond what most people are aware of. And after learning of the research and uses of niacinamide, I was quite frankly shocked as to why I had never heard of this before.

Niacin is of course the precursor to niacinamide (also called nicotinamide), but is converted in the body to niacinamide. Niacin is known for its ability to affect cholesterol levels, and is also the form that produces an uncomfortable "flushing" as a supplement, which although is temporary, can be quite intolerable. Niacinamide however does not possess these same properties, nor is it considered as toxic in high doses.

However although well tolerated, the safety zone for niacinamide seems to be in the mega dose range not exceeding 3 gm per day, as there is a potential of it becoming toxic to the liver in higher doses, though this seems to be rare. But niacin/niacinamide has been found to have remarkable benefits beyond its role as an essential B vitamin.

With the cooperative efforts of several major researchers and in part sponsored by the NIH (National Institutes of Health), recent research has shown that high-dose niacinamide was used to dramatically increase the activity of white blood cells called neutrophils to enhance its ability to kill both Staphylococcus aureus, as well as the notoriously resistant super bug, MRSA (methicillin-resistant Staphylococcus aureus). In fact it was shown to enhance this ability by up to an astounding 1000 times. Phenomenal research such as this is often played down ironically and most often by medical professionals who warn us not to draw conclusions from such studies. However obviously neutrophils are not selective to staph bacteria, and based on historical usage and other reports, is likely to benefit most infections that rely upon white blood cells as a first line of defense. [29]

Niacinamide has also been shown to "directly disrupt key Candida reproductive enzymes leading to weaker strains of Candida, an inability to form infectious biofilms, and gross aberrations in the DNA of Candida." [30] It is also being used in the skin care arena where it is commonly being used to replace antibiotics such as Clindamycin.

High-dose niacinamide has become known to have powerful antiinflammory benefits, and has been used by many sufferers to find healing or relief. William Kaufman, M.D., Ph.D. has been a long time user of high dose niacinamide in his practice. In a 1998 article *SOME NOTES ON NIACINAMIDE THERAPY FOR ARTHRITIS*, he says:

> *It measurably improves joint mobility, muscle strength, decreases fatigability. It increases maximal muscle working capacity, reduces or completely eliminates arthritic joint pain. Niacinamide heals broken strands of DNA and improves many kinds of CNS functioning.* [31]

He wrote a paper in the *Journal of the American Geriatrics Society* in 1955 wherein he noted that many cases of arthritis were completely healed. Although these were not univsersal, most received significant improvement, and it did demonstrate clinical evidence of the effectiveness of high dose niacinamide. He noted that more frequent doses of around 250 mg are some 40-50% more effective than 500 mg spread out less frequently. This is taken up to a maximum 3000 mg per day. At this level it was well tolerable. Some arthritic conditions were more resistant and took up to 3 months to see significant improvement. Some showed little improvement. [32]

In a laboratory test, it essentially cured Alzheimer's disease in rats after 4 months of administration. [33]

It also exhibits powerful anti-anxiety properties that have a calming effect similar to benzodiazepines and other anti-anxiety drugs. [34]

Dr. Abram Hoffer MD has treated 5000 schizophrenic patients using niacin, as well as patients with severe chronic depression. [35] Although he used the niacin form, niacinamide appears to have the same benefits. Niacin and niacinamide have been used by many as a natural replacement/alternative for anti-depressant medication. Orthomolecular Medicine News Service, October 7, 2005, reported high dose niacin is being used by doctors to treat a number of psychiatric disorders, including depression. [36]

Although niacin is known to cause flushing, and is known to affect cholesterol levels in the body, and whereas niacinamide does not have these properties; the use of both niacinamide or niacin alike appear to posses the above advantages. Therefore niacinamide would be the better choice since it can be taken in high doses without the problem and temporary discomfort of flushing.

As one can see, niacinamide may address many of the problems associated with Lyme disease, including influencing pathogens either directly or indirectly; supercharges neutrophils thus significantly enhancing immunity; anxiety and depression both of which are well known neurological symptoms; treats arthritis, also a major symptom of Lyme.

One safety caution. Again, when taking high dosages of different substances, especially at the same time, remember to additionally take liver protecting supplements much as you would with the essential oils. These would include curcumin, ursolic acid, milk thistle, and Haritaki. Given the incredible healing benefits of medicines such as niacinamide, these would help reduce any potential complications from taking such high dosages over time. Even though they have been demonstrated very safe in clinical applications, what is not known is how the adding of other substances that you will also be using during your course of therapies against Lyme disease will place added stress on the liver. It is thus always safer to err on the side of caution.

HERBS

The area of herbal medicine has become more and more popular as much has been learned of their anti-microbial properties. They have been the only natural medicines given to us by God which have been used for thousands of years in many cultures. And even today they continue to be researched in the field of orthomolecular medicine. Some have resisted the idea that herbs can have any significant role in fighting infections, let alone used to fight Lyme disease. As you study more and more the therapies of LLMD's, you are finding in many cases the total abandonment of antibiotic drugs in favor of the (in many cases) much more effective herbal products. In most cases, abx are designed to have a specific way they fight bacteria. Most attack the cell wall; others slow the replication process by inhibiting transcription of proteins. However Borrelia very effectively has learned to evade these mechanisms by reverting to a form, or by expressing enzymes or lipoprotein variations that renders them weakened at least, or completely ineffective at most. While most abx work most effectively on spirochete forms, they almost always force them into a form which is no longer vulnerable. Once stopped, they may revert back to the spirochete, and the whole process starts again.

Of course perhaps the single most significant problem with abx are detrimental side effects they have with long term use. Usually short courses are tolerable. But this is one disease that is going to absolutely require long term use of not just one, but usually several antimicrobials over the course of the disease, whether you choose the natural route or conventional antibiotics. We already know of their effectiveness when caught early in the disease. In fact abx have proven to be an excellent first line of defense once caught very early on in the infection. Other than that, once chronic Lyme disease has developed, keep this one thing in mind as it is very important to know: except for very rare cases, almost no one is cured of Lyme disease by taking abx, as a high percentage of patients tend to relapse. This doesn't mean there haven't been those isolated cases when no symptoms recurred. But you will find that those that eventually find healing from Lyme are far and away those that have taken the natural approach. You may choose your own route, and follow your own belief systems when it comes to Lyme disease. But unless you are one of those rare cases, you will be spending most of your time and money repeating the same cycle as those that have gone before you—going on and off abx for 2, 5, 10, 15 + years. You will virtually guarantee to remain a Lyme disease victim for the rest of your life. I am sorry to tell you this, but that is the truth. I say this not because I am an authority, but because it doesn't take a rocket scientist to observe this is true. And unless some new drug is discovered to change that, your odds based upon pure observation and the history of those having taken abx as their primary medicine of choice, are slim that you will find permanent healing from Lyme disease.

Personally, I have found herbal and non-drug therapies to be far superior in their effectiveness against Lyme. That is my own personal experience, as well as the experience of those whom I have known that have found the most consistent success. Others may have had a different experience, but then of course it depends on what therapies you are comparing to drugs. I have used for various periods of time about 8 different antibiotics for Lyme. Most of them simply stopped working, or didn't work at all. I always had to go back on my herbal and non-drug therapies in order for my condition to improve.

Having said that, one of the advantages of herbs is that not only do they not have the adverse side effects as do drugs, but they actually have the side benefits. Depending on the herbs, some of these include antioxidant capabilities, liver protective properties, cell communication enhancing activities, less stress on natural intestinal flora, anti-fungal and anti-viral actions in addition to the anti-bacterial properties. Also, many herbal products have more than one action against bacteria, making them less likely to develop resistance. And finally, most actually work with the body, rather than create poisonous stressors as do abx. These become a significantly better choice especially for long term use. You get the point. You choose your own weapon.

Cumanda/Samento/Burbur—This protocol was graciously put up on the internet by Dr. Lee Cowden MD. For those not familiar with Dr. Cowden, he is a strong advocate for natural and integrative medicines, and is well-known for his alternative medical approaches to all kinds of illnesses. I had the pleasure of receiving treatment from Dr. Cowden many years ago while still suffering from "environmental illness", allergies and candidiasis, and found his intuition and discernment unparalleled. Using kinesiology he was able to share things about my condition that were later confirmed by testing, and at the time I thought "How could he possibly know that?"

The protocol speaks for itself and I will not add anything to it. I have personally used both Samento and Cumanda, but not in the manner listed in Dr. Cowden's protocol. [37]

Samento is a Peruvian herb also called Cat's Claw. There are two kinds of Cat's Claw—one with, and the other without tetracyclic oxindole alkaloids (TOA), also called TOA-free. The TOA is said to inhibit the affects of pentacyclic oxindole alkaloids, which are believed to be the antibacterial and immune enhancing properties of the herb. Samento is therefore considered to be TOA-free Cat's Claw, the form used for Lyme disease. There is one author who has cited that the other works better. However I personally tried both forms in the early stages of Lyme disease. The ordinary Cat's Claw had no affect on my condition. But taking of the TOA-free Samento induced significant herx reactions. You may try both forms if you have any doubts as to which may be effective for you. Samento was one of the first herbal products I used for Lyme disease. At the time I was using it I did not yet know what I do now about Lyme disease—that you cannot use single product therapies against Lyme, since it actually encourages it to morph into another form or alter lipoprotein expression, thus actually increasing its resistance as well as prolonging the disease. As previously shared, and as cited in Dr. Cowden's protocol, use it in conjunction with another therapy or rotate it.

Cumanda comes from the bark of a tree (campsiandra angustifolia) found in the Peruvian and Brazilian rainforests. It is an extract and distributed in the USA by Nutramedix. This herb is unique in that it is said to have antimicrobial activity in all four major categories, anti-bacterial, anti-viral, anti-fungal, and anti-parasitic, with the added benefit of being anti-inflammory and analgesic, making it ideal as Lyme treatment therapy. One internet site cited studies at a university in Equador that demonstrated Cumanda to have nearly the same anti-inflammatory properties as the drug Feldane, and had no toxic side effects. It has been used extensively by Lyme patients as part of Dr. Cowdan's protocol with great success, particularly in the earlier stages of Lyme, and will produce herxes. I personally had used Cumanda, but had already been so far along in my progress that I experienced very few noticeable benefits. The one noticeable affect I experienced was as an anti-depressant, probably due to its analgesic properties. Cumanda may be more ideal in its use against the spirochete form. Most of the remaining infection at the time for me were the CWD form and biofilms based upon low level of response I had been receiving from those specific therapies which are known to affect spirochetes. However the degrees of response as in any patient are subjective. [38]

Burbur—Another South American herb. Burbur is an extract from the leaves of a perennial plant called Desmodium molliculum, or Manayupa depending the citing. Its chemical composition is made up of saponins which are metabolites which have soap-like properties. They also possess steroid properties and other anti-inflammatory qualities as well. However its use in Lyme disease is primarily for its cleansing properties. It is added as a detoxifier both in the digestive tract as well as for the blood to aid in the reduction of herx reactions in response to the anti-spirochetal affects of the Samento and Cumanda.

These are only three of the primary herbs used in his beginning protocol. Not all have been listed here. Dr. Cowden's company he works with is Nutramedix. They have developed these and other special extracts and herbal products designed specifically for Lyme disease and its co-infections. Their formulations are somewhat unique. So purchasing similar products may not yield the same results as has been testified by some users. This protocol for Lyme patients has undergone changes or evolved due to the addition of new products and the way they are administered. The protocol is designed to address the major problems faced by the Lyme patient with the understanding that most Lymies not only have co-infections, but toxicity from several sources other than just Borrelia. The products are taken in a particular fashion where they are rotated, or staggered for two primary reasons: to reduce the speed at which Borrelia can develop resistance or morph into a resistant form, as well as interfere with its natural cycle of replication, but also to reduce the likelihood of developing allergies to the substances. Lyme sufferers are very susceptible to allergies due to their weakened immune state and the likelihood of them developing intestinal hyperpermeability.

Here is the basic protocol and a list of the products used:

1. Taken 3 times per day mixed in water:
   Burbur—10 drops, Amantilla—10 drops, Pinella—10 drops.

2. Take twice per day before breakfast and supper mixed in water:
   Parsely Detox—10 drops, Trace Minerals—15 drops, Cumanda—1 drop to start gradually moving up to 30 drops, Carvivora—4 capsules.

3. Mixed in water twice daily after meals:
   Adrenal support—20 drops, Burbur—10 drops.
   Magnesium Malate 2-6 capsules twice daily.

On day 18 of protocol take the following at bedtime mixed in water:

Samento—20 drops, Parsely Detox—10 drops, Amantilla—15 drops, Trace Minerals—15 drops.—Each third night take Algas 10 drops mixed with the above.

After 2 months of taking the above therapy after having increased the Cumanda to 30 drops, replace it with Quina, alternating between

Quina and Cumanda every two weeks for four months. Take Quina for 12 ½ days, waiting for 36 hours, then Cumanda for 12 ½ days, waiting 36 hours, etc. This may need to be taken for up to 6 months depending on the patient.

This is based upon an average body weight of between 120 and 170 lbs.

This is the core of the therapy; although more detailed supplementation for other problems are mentioned. Credit is given to Dr. Cowden for sharing the therapy to those who can't see him in person. More specific and detailed information can be found online. [39]

Included are additional herbal products also recommended for consideration:

Takuna, Quina, Mora, Lakato, Enula, Banderol, Barberry.

Kalmegh—(Andrographis Paniculata)—This is a small annual shrub found in northern India and southern Asia. As an Ayurvedic herb, it had been used long before antibiotics to treat infections. It has also been called Maha-tita, meaning "king of bitters", also Hempedu Bumi meaning "bile of the earth" because of its strong bitter taste. The main constituent of the plant that gives it both its bitter taste as well as its medicinal properties is an extract of the leaves called Andrographolide. This plant and extract has been researched for its potential use in drug applications, and found to have potent qualities as an antibiotic, anti-inflammatory, anti-fungal, antihepatitic (hepatitis c), anti-snake venom, and others. It is also known as an immune stimulant as it has been shown to significantly raise CD4 lymphocytes levels in HIV patients, as well as interleukin and tumor necrosis factor in cancer studies. [40] Its traditional use also included a treatment for parasites. It has been cited anecdotally that treatment of parasites and spirochetes may have similar actions. Also, andrographis has been used as a treatment for treponema pallidum, the spirochete that causes syphilis. [41]

In a paper by Subhuti Dharmananda, Ph.D., Director, Institute for Traditional Medicine, Portland, Oregon, *Lyme Disease Treatment with Chinese Herbs*, Dr. Dharmananda cited in the Modern Study and

Application of Materia Medica, information regarding laboratory testing of herbs that inhibited or killed leptospira. Leptospirosis is another spirochetal disease. Andrographis was one of the herbs listed that demonstrated antispirochetal activities. [42] Stephen Buhner, herbalist and author of *Healing Lyme*, describes andrographis as both an anti-lyme treatment as well as an anti-inflammory. Many have used the product with Lyme and experienced herxing as well as improvement over time.

This is a strong herb. Some human studies indicate it is well tolerated with few adverse reactions, while others showed it may cause gastric upset, headache and fatique. However in some with certain infections they may be experiencing a herx response. While in others it may involve intolerance to the herb. There is no known toxicity. [43]

There are no known human studies on Lyme disease with this herb. However due to its known antispirochetal activity, immune enhancing properties, antitoxin activity, and anti-inflammatory actions, as well as the anecdotal evidence by those taking the herb, this may be a powerful addition to your Lyme therapies.

Typical dosage of andrographis has been between 400 and 1000mg 3 times per day. It is also available in a liquid extract which is more bioavailable. These are only general guidelines and should be monitored by your healthcare provider. This herb should be especially taken slowly do to its strong antimicrobial actions, as well as its affects on many physiological functions.

Moringa Oleifera—Aka the Miracle Plant, is a small tree that is native to the northern India Himalayas, but has become cultivated in Asian and now in Africa for its tremendous health benefits. In fact it may contain more nutrition and health benefits than any other plant known—a virtual tree of life. The seed pods, leaves, and roots are edible. The leaves are reported to have 4 times the vitamin A as carrots, 7 times the vitamin C of oranges, 3 times the potassium of bananas, 4 times the calcium of milk, twice the protein of yogurt, and 18 amino acids including the 8 essential amino acids. The plant is said to actually thrive in drought conditions, making it an ideal crop for growing in poor third world countries where no other crops will grow. But even more amazing are the therapeutic benefits it is reported to have affected.

Scientific studies have reported Moringa possesses over 90 nutrients, some 45 antioxidant and 36 anti-inflammatory properties. It appears to reduce cholesterol and triglycerides, helps balance sugar levels, boosts immunity, strengthens cells, increases metabolism, protects the liver and kidneys, and the list goes on. Moringa has been used by AIDS patients to prevent the normal wasting condition that is usually experienced. But this appears to be doing far more than merely providing nutrition. The amount of research and information on Moringa is vast. So it is not one of your typical folk remedies.

For more than 50 years moringa has been known to possess anti-microbial properties, making it the perfect food for chronically ill patients with infectious conditions. A number of derivatives of benzyl isothiocyanate were identified has having anti-bacterial activities against a number of species of microbes. Also thiocarbamate has been found to have anti-tumor and antiviral properties. One study demonstrated fresh leaf juice from the moringa plant to have 1 ½ times the antibacterial activity of tetracycline against 10 gram positive and negative germs under controlled conditions. Moringa oil is also edible and resists rancidity longer than many other botanical oils and may contain antimicrobial properties as well.

Moringa leaf powder can be purchased inexpensively and can be added to any therapy not only for overall nutritional support, but for its immune stimulating and antimicrobial properties. I add it to smoothies and antimicrobial tea mixes. But a word of caution: although it is a highly absorbable plant, only take up to about a tablespoon maximum at a time (less than this in the beginning until you see how well your body responds) as it will stimulate the bowels at higher levels. Additional amounts may be taken spread out during the day. I recall when I first learned of Moringa and purchased some, there was very little information provided as to dosages. So being in a large bag in a powdered form, and knowing it was an edible plant, I treated it as I would a protein powder and shoveled in several large tablespoons. I'm here to testify that I and my toilet seat had a family reunion for the next 24 hours! So take it slow and easy. [44-48]

Sanicle—There are several species of Sanicle. Most studied is sanicula europaea, a perennial herb which grows in Europe, also known as Poolroot or Self-Heal. Its American cousin (of a different gene family) sanicula marilandica, is called Black Snakeroot (not to be confused with Black Cohosh, also called snakeroot.) Both in its European and American use it has been termed "cure all" and "self heal" due to its ability to address virtually any problem in the body. The American sanicle has been used traditionally by N. American Indians to treat sore throat, fever, and skin and streptococcal infections. The European version has been reported to have been used for chronic cough, ulcers, dysentery, hemorrhoids, and to draw out snakebite poisons. It has been used as a blood thinner, yet has also been traditionally used to help stop or slow internal bleeding due to its astringent properties. However it seems to stand out most as a healer of wounds, both internal and external, even long-standing old injuries. The testimonials of those using this product have been nothing short of amazing.

One of Sanicle's constituents is called *allantoin* which has the ability to speed the healing of tissue. This is because allantoin possesses keratolytic activity, meaning it can break down dead and dying tissue.[49] One research study done comparing sanicle with TFG-Beta3 (transforming growth factor) observed that sanicle had antibiotic activity, but particularly observed was its "wound debridement" capacity. [50] This means that it possesses an ability to remove dead cells. This supports its use in herbal medicine as an internal blood cleanser as it relates to wound infections and toxicity issues, also its alleged tumor resolving ability.

Additionally, a triterpene saponin glycoside called *saniculoside N* was discovered in the europaea specie to have anti-HIV activity. [51] Studies have shown Sanicle possesses anti-viral substances in other applications. [52, 53]

It is interesting how that so much of what has been known of the traditional use of herbs becomes verified or explained in modern research. For example, Sanicle also contains rosmarinic acid, which is known to possess anti-bacterial, and anti-fungal, anti-oxidant, as well as anti-inflammatory properties. Rosmarinic acid has been demonstrated to break up neuritic amyloid plaques in the brains of Alzheimer patients. [54] These plaques are made up of specific amyloid proteins produced by the body, but which accumulate in sticky plaques in Alzheimer patients and has been thought to be the cause of the illness. However it has recently been learned that these proteins actually possess antibacterial activities which some believe are attempts by the body itself to destroy certain pathogens, and may rewrite how these proteins are viewed. Derek Lowe PhD in organic chemistry writes:

> *It's been known for a long time that there's a big inflammation component to the disease—perhaps the problem (or at least the trigger) is an underlying infection that sets off the innate immune system in the brain. Larger than normal amounts of beta-amyloid are produced in response, but it starts to precipitate out.* [55]

According to Dr. Lida Mattman, Alzheimer's disease has been strongly associated with Borrelia-infected patients. [56] Given what is known of Bb to associate in biofilms, it is possible that Borrlia or other pathogens somehow contribute to this plaque formation. And if rosmarinic acid is known to break up plaques, as well as allantoins ability to break down proteins associated with dead cells, perhaps Sanicle might be considered for its potential to affect biofilm activities, as well for its anti-bacterial properties. Cell-wall deficient forms have been known to cloak themselves in human cellular debri as a means to mimic human cells and evade immune cells. Also, human cell components are said to become incorporated into biofilms for this same reason. If Sanicle has been traditionally used to help remove dying and dead cells thru its own natural chemical mechanisms, this may be an ideal herb for affecting or inhibiting two of the most difficult to affect forms of Borrelia, biofilms and CWD forms.

Perhaps the longstanding traditional claims of using this product are not unfounded.

From Altmed.com:

> *The American herbal practitioner, Jethro Kloss, in his monumental work "Back to Eden," aptly describes Sanicle in this manner: "This is one of the herbs that could be called a cure-all,*

because it possesses powerful cleansing and healing virtues both internally and externally."

Sanicle's great strength includes its uncanny ability to seek out and find anything which needs correcting and works on that area first which needs it most. It also deserves distinction as a "thinking herb." In other words, if you've got it, Sanicle will find it and fix it, whether it be in the reproductive organs, brain, nervous system, lungs, throat, urinary system or elsewhere.

Sanicle is a bulldozer and builder. There may be temporary discomfort when Sanicle contacts an unwanted obstruction, but it is your reassurance that Sanicle has scored a direct hit. Skin disorders, tumors (also brain tumors), and all manner of morbid material are resolved by Sanicle. [57]

As an extract Sanicle's dosage is 40 drops 3 times per day internally. However it can additionally be applied externally, particularly on areas of old injury or scars. As an adjunct, rosmarinic acid extract is also available in supplement form which may further enhance the affects of Sanicle.

GSE—Grapefruit seed extract is actually a synthetic product that is the result of processing grapefruit seeds using a multi-stage process. The end active anti-microbial ingredient is *diphenol hydroxybenzene*. This substance has very powerful activities against all classes of pathogens, viruses, bacteria, fungi, and parasites. It is said to function by affecting the cytoplasmic membrane of pathogenic cells which prevents them from uptaking necessary amino acids for formation and development. It also causes leakage of the membrane, as well as affects normal cellular respiration of the germs.

This product is one of the most popular natural antibiotics and anti-fungals used.

Note—There has recently been controversy over this product claiming that GSE is not an organic product, and that the claims of it being antimicrobial are false. When one reads thru the literature, it appears that it is an attempt to discredit the product by citing that there is a contaminant in the product that is actually the source of the anti-microbial property, not the pure GSE itself. The fact is that the process that GSE goes thru results in a change in the chemical properties called *quarternary ammonium compounds*, of which diphenol hydroxybenzene is the primary constituent. So what they are calling a "contaminant" is not some added substance. It is the end product of the synthesis process.

GSE has also been used internally for acute and chronic inflammations, and for secondary infection control in AIDS patients. It is well tolerated and non-toxic even at much higher doses than is recommended. However it may cause some upset at very high doses. This was one of the very first products I used in my battle against Lyme disease. It will produce herxes. Laboratory research has demonstrated that GSE has a powerful killing affect against Bb spirochetes and cyst forms. [58]

This is one of the best all around products against Lyme, and is one of the antimicrobials that possesses both anti-bacterial as well as anti-fungal properties making it ideal to be rotated given it reduces fungal overgrowth associated with long-term anti-bacterial use. I personally used this at very high dosages, sometimes pulsing it for several days at a time at 10 triple strength capsules per day with no negative side effects. For Lyme disease, I would personally use this in combination with other herbs to attack Borrelia and other co-infections from various angles. It seems to have few interaction problems with other herbal products. Always dilute the liquid form, and drink plenty of water with the product.

Terminalia Chebula—This is a tree that grows in Asia that goes by several names, Black or Chebulic Myrobalan, Hirada, Kadukkai, and others. In Ayur-Vedic medicine it is called *Haritaki*. Indian stores in the USA call it "Harde Whole". It bears a nut-like fruit which contains the healing properties.

This is one of the most powerful and most used herbs in Ayer-Vedic medicine. Its reputed benefits are nearly endless as it is considered a "panacea". It is said to inhibit malignant tumors, aids in digestion, stimulates the liver, relieves nervous irritability, cures chronic coughs by inhibiting mucous, acts as a laxative, heals hemorrhoids, is adaptogenic (balances immune responses). It is used for sore throats, gum and tooth problems, as an anti-diarrhetic, anti-histamine, anti-oxidant, all sorts of skin disorders, heartburn and other gastrointestinal disorders (GERD). [59]

In clinical research it has been shown to have anti-bacterial and anti-viral activity with HIV, and cytomegalovirus inhibiting properties.[60] It is known to work against tumors, acceleration in the healing of wounds, anti-candida and candida biofilm inhibition. [61]

There are numerous properties found in terminalia chebula that have bacteria inhibiting substances: gallic acid, chebulinic acid, tannic acid, oxalic acid, and ellagic acid. There is solid research that demonstrates these properties of TC have effective anti-biofilm activities. In fact, I have seen more studies on its biofilm activities than any other substances. [62-70]

However of the compounds cited, two specific acids in TC were found to have "profound inhibitory" activities against certain bacteria. They were oxalic acid and ellagic acid. Organic acids such as oxalic acid have the affect of penetrating the walls of susceptible bacteria, altering ph levels, and disrupting metabolic activities. They are natural chelators of metals and calcium.[71]

Of particular interest are ellagitannans. The biofilm properties of this substance have been well studied. Ellagic and tannic acid is found in many plants. They do not appear to have direct killing capabilities in most bacteria, but they do possess anti-quorum sensing properties in that they inhibit auto-inducers, particularly in the gram-negative bacterial group, of which Borrelia belongs. Quorum sensing auto-inducers are necessary for the growth of biofilms.

Some of the interest in using TC for biofilms was based upon novel research done by a young girl, Madhavi Gavini, whose grandfather was of Indian decent and a practitioner of Ayurvedic medicine. Her friend's aunt had developed cystic fibrosis. A particular bacterium called *Pseudomonas aeruginosa* is known to develop biofilms in this disease, and is deadly. Madhavi experimented with a number of traditional herbs to see which ones would inhibit this biofilm. RNA are the molecules necessary for the development of proteins which become the building blocks of bacteria cellular structures and membranes. It was discovered that TC was able to inhibit RNA in the bacteria which enabled them to form biofilms.

Whether or not this same inhibition is functional in Borrelia is yet to be studied. However given TC's broad spectrum activities against all kinds of bacterial species, and its wide range of chemical constituents that perform multiple functions in the human body, and given the multiple compounds found in TC that are known to inhibit biofilms, this would be worthy of consideration.[72] It should be noted of importance however that biofilm inhibition must be accompanied by anti-bacterials. While the goal should be to slow, stop and eventually destroy biofilms, unless the killing of bacteria developing those films is simultaneously addressed, they may continue to form as fast or faster than they are being inhibited. This may be one reason why some never find complete healing from Lyme. Insufficient or non-aggressive enough treatment may be to blame. Terminalia Chebula possesses both anti-biofilm and anti-bacterial properties.

As a note: Greg Lee, acupuncturist at the Two Frogs Healing center in Frederick, Maryland has been having good success by incorporating TC in the Lyme protocols when combining with other herbs with his Lyme patients. So there are already those finding success using this product.

Terminalia Chebula is available both as a whole nut that can be ground into a powder, or purchased already in powdered form. A general dosage would be 3-6 gm. per day. This will need to be adjusted for your own use. Additionally, a product is available which is contains extracted ellagic acid from TC and has added bioperine to enhance absorption. It is called Ellagic Defense.[73] This would appear to be an ideal adjunct to taking the powder and may increase its biofilm inhibiting potential.

Carnivora—This herbal extract comes from a plant called *Dionaea Muscipula*, otherwise known as "Venus flytrap". It is a highly processed phytonutrient created by a Dr. Helmut Keller M.D. Carnivora is perhaps one of the most versatile of all herbal products known, and can effectively and powerfully treat infectious diseases of all sorts. Numerous compounds that possess highly specific immune-modulating activities have been identified in Carnivora. From the Carnivora website:

Droserone—Free radical scavenger—Hydroplumbagin, Immune Modulation / Stimulation Quercetin—Anti-oxidant, free radical scavenger, protectant

Formic Acid—Natural bactericidal

Myricetin—Bioflavonoid. Identical properties as Quercetin

Gallic Acid—Antioxidant, Immune stimulative

Arginine—Supports NK function. Improves immune responses to foreign entities, crucial for tissue repair

Asparagine—Explusion of harmful ammonia, increased resistance to fatigue and increase of endurance

Threonine—Aids in function of intestinal / digestive tracts. Assists in metabolism and assimilation of nutrients; Prevention of fat build-up in the liver

Glutamine—Helps maintain white blood cell population and T-cell production, supports intestinal health. Nature's brain food to improve mental capacities, decrease fatigue, controls craving for sugar

Alanine—Strengthens immune system by producing antibodies, important source of energy for muscle tissue, brain and central nervous system

Cysteine—Facilitates the production of glutathione, which enable white blood cells (lymphocytes such as T cells, B cells and NK cells) to reproduce to make antibodies to destroy foreign substances in the body

Serine—Component of production of immune antibodies. Antibodies bind with antigens which are toxins, etc. destroying them and removing them from the body

Histidine—Found abundantly in hemoglobin. This amino acid is used as a potent free-radical scavenger to normalize systemic functions in the body

Proteases—Known for their ability to enhance immunity, proteases are considered an important line of defense and intestinal toxicity are among the most common symptoms of protease deficiency

Lipopolysaccharides—Contribute to stimulation of the immune system. Contains properties that are highly potent against harmful cellular entities

Phytohormones—Plant-derived building blocks that your body can use to rapidly create any hormone that your body needs. These substances, also called phytosterols, are vital to a healthy balanced endocrine or hormonal system. [74]

But here is what makes Carnivora so unique. Dr. Keller had become fascinated with the Venus flytrap's ability to capture flies and other insects, then to digest them very similarly to the way food is digested in the stomach. However the compounds used in this digestion process did not harm the plant itself. He discovered that the juices only digest specific undifferentiated cells of its prey, the same kind found in the human body that leads to illness, as well as pathogenic microbes. From this he developed an extract from the plant that is used in multiple disease conditions.

In Dr. Keller's early work he worked with cancer patients, and had phenomenal success using his extract, even in some cases where the patients were sent home to die, many were restored. It became a powerful cancer treatment. Later it was learned that one of the chemical ingredients of Venus flytrap kills the AIDS virus, which was confirmed by a Beta-2 Microglobulin test which measures the proteins produced by HIV.[75] Bacterial infections are also addressed as it has been used in Mycoplamsa as well as Borrelia-born illnesses.

One particular case study was done of a young 14 year old girl that had been given multiple diagnoses for a condition that was causing pain in most of her joints and chest, severe headaches, fatigue, night sweats, "pain" in her brain, insomnia, frequent urination, inability to concentrate, as well as others. She had gone from an "A" student to unable to retain information. This had apparently been going on for quite a number of years having become rather acute by the age of 11. By the time she had received a diagnosis of Lyme disease she was no longer even able to focus her eyes and had become totally bedridden by the age of 14. She also had a positive test for Babesia. Her doctor said it was the worst case of Lyme disease he had ever seen.

She was started on Carnivora capsules, then the extract, as well as a lymph drainage tonic, along with some sea extracts. Within months her fatique went away, she began to be able to think clearly, and slowly her joint pain subsided. In time, she has been able to become fully active again attending ballet classes where she dances 2-4 hours per night. Eventually all of her symptoms disappeared completely and has had a full recovery.[76]

This demonstrates a rather unique case, as it is not common to have a complete recovery especially in such a short period of time. Perhaps in part it was due to her age and physical condition. It may also be that she had never been put on any antibiotics from the start, and began the Carnivora as her first antimicrobial therapy. We know that antibiotics not only drive Borrelia into evasive forms, but into forms which are not responsive to antibiotics. As a result it may be that Carnivora was able to effectively kill the microbe without driving it into other forms because of either its ability to arrest Borrelia before it could morph, or because it possessed the ability to affect cyst and CWD forms which no doubt likely had already become a factor in her illness. Whatever happened, it illustrates the potential of Carnivora as a powerful tool against infectious disease. It appears to work with the body by enhancing human immune properties that matches its own.

I had used Carnivora early on in my Lyme disease. I found it to be effective and experienced herxheimer reactions from its use. However I had stopped it after only 2 months due to financial circumstances preventing me from continuing at the time. As a result I began looking for less expensive treatment options. I was also using it as a stand-alone therapy which even in the case of this young girl was not used. However in hindsight had I been able to remain on the product, there is no telling how much quicker I could have advanced. The manufacturer of Carnivora has vastly increased its production, and it is now available at about half the cost as previously. So it is much more reasonable to apply this therapy than in the past. From the literature and testimonials it appears that the extract would be the preferred method of choice, as it would seem to get deeper due to its refinement. This is one of those products that might be ideal as a beginning treatment option before any other therapies have been used. But even so, it certainly is at the top of the list as effective Lyme disease treatments since it has been used by the Lyme community for years as an extremely effective substance that appears to be effective in a number of pathogenic conditions.

Goldenseal—(Aka, jaundice root, eye root, turmeric root, yellow root, Indian turmeric, as well as a host of other names, is a member of the Buttercup family, and should not be confused with turmeric or its active ingredient curcumin extract which is a member of the Ginger family.) This herb has its traditional origins as a medicine used by early Native American Indians. It is a small perennial plant that has multiple uses. It has been used as a digestive aid due to its bitterness, thus stimulating digestion. It was said to be used by the Cherokee as a cancer cure. In the American Materia Medica it was described as having liver protective properties, used for disorders of the stomach, gallstones, constipation, moved along mucous, swelling, and a laxative. However it is most well known today as having powerful antimicrobial and anti-inflammatory properties, although very few scientific studies have been done on the whole herb to demonstrate this. Most have centered on its isolated berberine, hydrastine, and canadine properties. These are called *alkaloids* which are known for their anti-inflammatory and antiseptic effects.

Goldenseal is a very common herb used in the US, but may not be ideal when used at higher dosages exceeding 500 mg, or for long-term use since there are toxicity issues. The good news is that it appears to be goldenseal's berberine content that may be the primary source of its therapeutic effects. And although the herbs Oregon grape and barberry also contain berberine, today berberine can be purchased as a supplement in extract form, and does not possess the toxicity issues as goldenseal.

The benefits offered by berberine are quite extensive and go way beyond the scope of this book. This is an extremely well researched substance. However we will mention a few as it is truly a wonder-supplement. In animal and/or human studies, it has been shown to increase immunoglobulins,[77] thus supporting and stimulating the immune system in fighting infection; inhibit tumors and cancer;[78,79] it induces apoptosis (programmed cell death of unhealthy cells);[80] lowers LDL cholesterol and triglycerides;[81] acts has a natural anti-depressant[82]; has been recognized for its potent anti-fungal, antibacterial, and antiviral applications[83-85]; is anti-inflammatory.[86]

It has been shown to inhibit bacteria from adhering to urinary bladder, much the same as cranberry. Since biofilms are the means by which bacteria are able to do this, berberine may have some anti-biofilm properties in additional to being antibacterial.[87]

In the chapter on Biofilms, we noted research that specifically alluded to berberine's ability to block the adherence of certain bacteria to human cells, but particularly fibronectin, which we also learned is a target for the binding of the Bb's RevA outer surface lipoprotein. But berberine can also inhibit fibronectin expression, thus aiding in the reduction of the excessive production of fibrin which is known to be associated with fibromyalgia-like and other chronic inflammatory conditions. Therefore, fibrinolytic and proteolytic enzymes followed by berberine may be a highly effective protocol particularly in the final stages for healing of deep seated biofilm-based infections, since the deeper tissues where the fibrin and fibronectin originally developed would now be exposed once the films have been razed or reduced.

Curcumin—Used in AyurVedic medicine, is the main constituent of the spice turmeric. It is what gives the spice the yellow-orange color and is a fat-soluble substance. Hence is not particularly well absorbed, and is often found in herbal preparations being combined with piperine (a pepper used to increase bioavailability). It is an antioxidant that protects cells against oxidative and chemical damage. It possesses anti-inflammatory properties that affect multiple avenues. It has been used for gastrointestinal problems and colon cancer, and recent research has shown it to be a powerful healer and inhibitor of liver cirrhosis, even reversing damage already done.[88] It has also been traditionally used as an antiarthritic to reduce joint pain, and has been compared in effectiveness to prescription drugs in some studies. Several studies have demonstrated that it exhibits protective qualities against neurodegenerative disease such as Multiple Sclerosis.[89] Curcumin also possesses anti-bacterial properties as is demonstrated in numerous research studies.[90]

Each one of curcumin's beneficial properties would directly affect Lyme disease. Pain and inflammation need to be reduced in both neuroborreliosis as well as Lyme arthritis. Medicines such as ibuprofen and Naproxen Sodium are notorious for causing sometimes life-threatening internal bleeding, and liver toxicity. While acetaminophen, though possessing analgesic or pain-reducing benefits, does little for inflammation, but is also a very dangerous drug that can also be poisonous to the liver. Curcumin would be an ideal substitute as it not only reduces inflammation, but actually helps to heal liver damage, as well as possesses anti-bacterial properties.

Especially noteworthy is one particular study which tested the anti-bacterial properties of the essential oil of turmeric. Essential oils are specific chemical properties of plants which allow them to resist microbial invasions. It was demonstrated against an entire group of bacteria to have the comparable antibiotic effectiveness as the drug *chloramphenicol*.[91] This particular antibiotic has very potent activity against a wide spectrum of bacteria, and has been used in the past among other things in the treatment of Lyme disease by inhibiting protein synthesis. However it is rarely used because of its severe side effects. However essential oils can be taken in a number of ways, even internally when combined with carrier oils such as coconut and moringa oils that are a safer alternative with comparable benefits.

I have personally used curcumin as an adjunct to other antimicrobial herbal therapies. I have also found it to effectively reduce inflammation and pain. However it may take some time for its anti-inflammatory benefits to begin to work. It has not shown any demonstrable toxicity issues even at high dosages. Curcumin is not easily absorbed. Bromelain is an enzyme of the pineapple which has been shown to enhance absorption of turmeric.

The dosage used for any particular application may differ widely from person to person since it is not a well absorbed herb. If enhanced with bromelain or bioperine, lower dosages would be required. A good starting dose would be 600-800mg twice per day. However some research has shown that doses as high as 2-3 grams twice per day may be necessary.

Sparganium and Zedoaria—These are both traditional Chinese medicines, today often used together due to their synergistic functions.

Sparganium, also called *san leng* (in TCM), is a rhizome or root stalk of a bitter grass-like plant that grows in wetlands. Its English name is Scirpus and is a member of the sedge family. Used in powder form, teas, or extracts, it has been used in Chinese medicine to promote the flow of chi. Accumulations and stagnations in various parts of the body as well as deep in the joints are said to be cleared, as the medicinal herb tends to move directly into these areas to free up, soften binds and dissolve blockages. These include lumps, masses and tumors as scirpus has been demonstrated in some animal studies to inhibit cancer growth.

Zedoaria, also called Zedoary Root or White Turmeric, is a rhizome from the plant family Zingiberaceae, and is also used in Eastern medicine. A pungent plant, like Sparganium, it promotes chi by moving blood in areas of stagnation. Traditionally it has been used to soften hardnesses, remove old lumps, and dissipate concretions. Particularly stubborn growths that fail to resolve on their own such as areas around old injuries, mineral deposits and excessive tissue growth are said to be addressed. These would seem to include any deposits or accumulations in the body that are not part of the necessary healing process or differentiated cells. In this manner it appears to have properties similar to Carnivora and Sanicle.

Sparganium and Zedoaria are often used together since they have similar functions. Subhuti Dharmananda Ph. D. of the Institute for Traditional Medicine describes their actions and how they have been traditionally been applied.

"Solid masses, including uterine fibroids, thyroid adenomas, and sclerodermic patches of tight skin, liver fibrosis, enlarged spleen, post-surgical adhesions, and other manifestations of blood statis are frequently treated with formulas that include the herbs sparganium and zedoaris." [92]

Greg Lee LAc. and Chinese Herbalist in Frederick Maryland uses these herbs as part of an over-all anti-Lyme therapy for their ability to aid in penetrating biofilms and cysts.[93] This pair has been included here since, based upon its function, it may have ideal properties for moving deeply into joints and areas of sequestered infection or biofilm structures, and draw other herbs into them as well for the dissolution of unhealed and unresolved fibrous deposits.

These herbs are sometimes combined along with frankinsence and myrrh into a formula which together work to perform similar functions. Frankinsence and myrrh are considered bitter herbs. "In modern Chinese Materia Medica, these two resins are classified as herbs for vitalizing circulation of blood and are utilized for treating traumatic injury, painful swellings, masses, and other disorders related to stasis syndromes." [94]

As a precaution, nerve damage *may* be aggravated by this formulation. Remember that Bb OspA is a close molecular match to myelin sheath covering nerves, and that Bb and spirochetal infections have been implicated in multiple sclerosis (MS). Therefore biofilms may be developing along nerve pathways in an attempt to mimic myelin and hide from immune cells. This formulation *may possibly* therefore aggravate this condition if nerve damage has resulted from biofilm infection. Aching or agitation may result. If this occurs, it is suggested to reduce the dose or stop taking the herbs, and see an Ayurvedic or

Chinese herbal practitioner for advice on how to best use this powerful herbal decoction.

Note: I had added this formula to my Lyme therapies and found that this agitation was due to the pair attacking the biofilms along nerves. In time they resolved as the biofilms eventually significantly were reduced.

Teasel Root—Teasel is rather unique as a Lyme disease remedy as it has been touted by an affable and humorous herbalist who affectionately calls herself LadyBarbara. She recalls her experience with what she says is 8 separate infections of Lyme disease over a 15 year period. Although that simply doesn't match any known experiences of Lyme sufferers, she makes the point that using teasel root completely eliminated her illness, and is now symptom-free.

Teasel is a family member of a group of tall flowering plants called Dipsacus, of which some 15 species are known. It has a tall flower head at the top, but the root is used for medicinal purposes. The various varieties grow in Europe, Asia and Africa. In traditional Chinese medicine it is used "to fix what is broken". This variety is called Dapsacus asperoides or japonica. However the specie that is suppose to be the most effective for Lyme is *Dapsacus sylvestris*, which is native to the US.

What makes this remedy different is that it doesn't appear to work in the same way as classical herbal remedies or drugs, where "more is better". Although some herbalists do prescribe it at higher dosages, LadyBarbara suggests no more than 9 drops per day total, and less if possible. That is all that is necessary. And although some experience herx reactions from it, as part of the therapy, taking it at these lower dosages would be far below the level that should cause uncomfortable herxes. Perhaps this is part of what makes this therapy unique. Virtually all Lyme therapies act by killing off masses of bacteria so viciously, that a back up in the lymph system may cause an energetic block that may affect the further progress of the teasel root. Although this is my own theory, LadyB she says that she believes teasel root works "with your body", to allow the immune system to do the killing, perhaps not necessarily the herb itself. This may have merit, as many taking the herb also find success. However LadyB even admits that it may not affect everyone the same way, just like any other kind of therapy.

What makes this herbal remedy particularly noteworthy is that based upon her testimony, she has been completely symptom-free for 9 years. This may be one of those therapies that a few find particularly successful, while others may only find limited success. It needs to be taken by itself in water or sublingually, away from food or other medicines. In this way, it seems to be similar acting as homeopathy, but not entirely, as homeopathy is generally potency dependent. LadyBarbara says, "What we've seen with Teasel over the years is that it appears to 'coax the beasts out of hiding' so that your own immune system (ideally) or something ELSE (if your immune system is just too compromised to do it) can kill them." [95] However she does admit to taking Grapefruit seed extract in addition to the teasel root. This no doubt in her was an effective combination.

She suggests starting out slowing and working up by adding a drop per day until the lowest effective dose is reached, then remain there.[96] Teasel sylvestris is available from several small vendors on the internet including myherbs.net.

Garlic—Garlic has been one of the most widely recognized herbs which also possesses strong medicinal properties. It is a mild blood thinner in that it reduces blood platelet aggregation and reduces fats in the bloodstream. So it has blood-pressure lowering abilities. It has been used for its anti-cancer, anti-inflammatory, and anti-oxidant activities. Allicin in garlic is reported to raise CD4-T cell count to enhance immunity.

But garlic is perhaps at the top of the list as a true antimicrobial for its powerful anti-bacterial, anti-viral, antifungal, and even anti-protozoal properties. There are several sulphur-containing compounds found in garlic which, to varying degrees, have germicidal properties. These are alliin, ajoene, diallylsulfide, dithiin, and S-allylcysteine. Sulphur has powerful anti-germ capabilities, and became the basis of sulphonamide antibiotic drugs. *Photoalexins* are also a group of properties found in garlic which also contain compounds known to "puncture the cell wall, delay maturation, disrupt metabolism or prevent reproduction of the pathogen in question." [97]

However allicin is by far the most potent of these antibacterial agents. At least in vitro. Early on allicin was researched due to its potential as a powerful natural anti-biotic. The problem is that allicin is very readily broken down in the body to other constituents, and is nearly undetectable in the bloodstream, even in massive doses. For this reason pharmaceutical companies abandoned allicin research since it was highly unstable.[98] Therefore much of the hype surrounding allicin's anti-germicidal capacity could not necessarily be converted to practical effectiveness.

Allicin is produced by the crushing of the garlic bulb. Contained in the garlic clove are two separate compartments, one containing alliin, and other an enzyme called *allinase*. Alliin does not possess antimicrobial activity itself. But once the two compartments are opened and released, they combine to form allicin. Taking garlic capsules does not show nearly the benefit as one would expect since it is not known whether any allicin remains after processing. Allicin begins to break down after forming. And any allicin that remains available however once consumed very quickly begins to react with proteins in the immediate environment, thus neutralizing it and reducing its potency. Some of the activity that produces the benefits is still active, but is very short lived and soon is dissipated. Also, stomach acids neutralize the alliin, thus preventing it from combining with allinase to form allicin. It is for these reasons that the germicidal benefits of garlic are only a small fraction of its potential.

There are other constituents of garlic however that are also known to possess antimicrobial activites. Ajoene is an associated molecule with allicin that appears to inhibit specific enzyme systems of certain infectious organisms, as well as the synthesis of phosphatidylcholine which has shown to be deadly to certain parasites.[99]

Garlic is an herb of many constituents and properties which together is greater than the sum of its parts. Isolating single compounds or phytochemicals have not been able to explain the benefits seen in its use against a wide range of pathogenic infections. And certainly the lack of allicin detection in the bloodstream after large intake leaves questions as to how garlic has earned its place as an important natural antibiotic. Some nutraceutical companies have been researching and developing stabilized forms of allicin which appear to have superior activity to garlic extracts and whole garlic capsules.

For instance Allimax Nutraceuticals US has developed a stabilized allicin extract that shows real promise against what is believed to be the spirochete and cystic forms. One 2006 unpublished study was done showing a 90-100% reversal of Lyme symptoms using their Allisure AC-23.[100]

Another allicin product is called Alligin. It is made by a special patented water soluable process that is combined with ginger to preserve the allicin. The allicin is pre-formed and stabilized prior to being put into capsules. So it does not rely on the combining of alliin and allinase in the body which yields little to no allicin at all.

Allicin has been shown to have a wide spectrum of activity even against drug resistant forms of bacteria.[101] This should be included as one of the standard products when creating antimicrobial formulations or cocktails for addressing Lyme and its co-infections as it affects not only many different bacteria, but also various pleomorphic forms.

A word of caution. The dosages of many of the substances that are discussed are deliberately left up to the patient and his/her healthcare provider to determine. This is for several reasons. Since most non-drug substances are not tested and standardized for their effective dosages as are drugs, ideal "effective dosages" may be unknown. Also, since the rule of thumb for most treatments is to start out slowly, then gradually build up until benefits are noticed, this will be different for every person. And since many of the remedies are being combined with other substances, the synergistic affect will be greater when taking a smaller dose than if it was being taken alone. Therefore it is best to heed the warning given earlier. That is, to always begin taking a new supplement by itself first, and gradually increase the dosage over time until you will see how your body reacts. This is especially important during acute stages of Lyme, since many substances can be so potent, that a dangerously reactive herx can be an unintended consequence. Remember too, never continuously do a particular therapy. That is part of the conventional model which we already know has proven time and again to be a failing system, especially when it comes to Lyme disease. Constantly rotate and vary your treatments in order to impede the morphing process. This will give you the upper hand and short-circuit the very process that gives Bb its advantage.

ENDNOTES

1.   *Growth, cysts and kinetics of Borrelia garinii (Spirochaetales: Spirochaetacea) in culture media.* Oliveira Ad, Fonseca AH, Costa CM, Mantovani E, Yoshinari NH. Mem Inst Oswaldo Cruz, 2005 105(5), 717-19

2.   *Pharmacology of oleanolic acid and ursolic acid.* J Ethnopharmacol. Liu J. 1995 Dec 1;49(2):57-68.

3.   *Antibacterial effects of Ursolic acid against cariogenic bacteria* H. Suzuki, M. Konishi, M. Kimura, and T. Ikemi, Nihon University, Matsudo, Japan Seq #124 - Clinical Microbiology of the Oral Cavity I Thursday, March 22, 2007 Ernest N. Morial Convention Center Exhibit Hall I2-J http://iadr.confex.com/iadr/2007orleans/techprogram/abstract_90701.htm

4.   Hydroxytyrosol http://en.wikipedia.org/wiki/Hydroxytyrosol

5.   *Antimycoplasmal Activity of Hydroxytyrosol* Pio Maria Furneri, Anna Piperno, Antonella Sajia, and Giuseppe Bisignano. Antimicrobial Agents and Chemotherapy, December 2004, p. 4892-4894, Vol. 48, No. 12

6.   *Liposomal Encapsulation Technology* http://www.racehorseherbal.com/Infections/LET/let.html

7.   *Liposomal VITAMIN C A NanoLiposomal Single Nutrient* http://www.nanoliposomals.com/Liposomal_VITAMIN__C.html

8.   *Liposome Science Liposome-encapsulated vitamin C delivers up to 800% more vitamin C into your body* http://www.livonlabs.com/

9.   *Homemade Liposomal C* http://www.pdazzler.com/archives/62

10. Dr. Klinghardt's Treatment of Lyme Disease Posted by: Dr. Mercola August 04 2009 Excerpted From the Writings of Dietrich Klinghardt, MD, Ph.D., edited by Eve Greenberg, LPC, CN, Explore Staff Reporter and Director of the Klinghardt Academy of Neurobiology http://web.archive.org/web/20120427104329/http://lymediseaseresource.com/wordpress/important-new-insights-from-dr-klinghardt-on-lyme-disease-and-its-treatment/

11. *Iodide—One Mineral Can Help A Myriad Of Conditions From Atherosclerosis To "COPD" to Zits* by Dr. Jonathan V. Wright, MD http://tahomaclinicblog.com/iodide/ Retrieved Feb. 3, 2013

12. Titan Pharmaceuticals excerpt from website. http://www.wikinvest.com/ stock/Titan_Pharmaceuticals_(TTNP)/Gallium_Maltolate Retrieved Feb. 4. 2013

13. Science News - Gallium: *A New Antibacterial Agent?* Science Daily March 16 2007 http://www.sciencedaily.com/releases/2007/03/070315210325. htm Retrieved Feb. 4, 2013

14. *All Natural Zeolite* All Natural Prevention http://www.allnaturalprevention. com/pages/zeolite-faq.htm Retrieved Feb. 4, 2013

15. *Viral evasion of natural killer cells* Orange JS, Fassett MS, Koopman LA, Boyson JE, Strominger JL. Nature Immunology 2002 3, 1006 - 1012

16. *Urinary Tract Infections* Laurence Johnston PhD Article http://www.sci-therapies.info/UTI.htm Retreived Feb. 4, 2013

17. *The intracellular effects of manuka honey on Staphylococcus aureus.* Henriques AF, Jenkins RE, Burton NF, Cooper RA. Eur J Clin Microbiol Infect Dis. 2010 Jan;29(1):45-50.

18. *Pharmacological and antimicrobial studies on different tea-tree oils (Melaleuca alternifolia, Leptospermum scoparium or Manuka and Kunzea ericoides or Kanuka), originating in Australia and New Zealand.* Lis-Balchin M, Hart SL, Deans SG. Phytother Res. 2000 Dec;14(8):623-9.

19. *Is Manuka Honey Safe?* Nov 16, 2008 Stephen Allen Christensen http:// www.suite101.com/content/is-manuka-honey-safe-a78850 Retrieved Feb. 4, 2013

20. *Manuka Honey Heals* Health News July 22, 2007 http://www.prleap.com/ pr/86675/ Retrieved Feb. 4, 2013.

21. *Fulvic Ionic Minerals* Description from Website http://www.optimallyorganic.com/Fulvic.htm Retrieved Feb. 4, 2013

22. *Nano Ra Energ Humic Acid* Healingwithin.com https://mall.ppcserver. net/mm5/merchant.mvc?Screen=PROD&Store_Code=healing&Product_ Code=597V&Category_Code=026 Retrieved Feb. 4, 2013.

23. *Vital HF™ Recharges the Body* Source PRWEB Article by: Nina Anderson SAFE GOODS PUBLISHING http://defazios.tripod.com/ healthproducts/id24.html Retrieved Feb. 4, 2013.

24. *Mycoplasma—Often Overlooked In Chronic Lyme Disease* Public Health Alert, v. 4, no. 7, 2009 by Scott Forsgren http://www. immed.org/infectious%20disease%20reports/InfectDiseaseReport06.11.0 9update/PHA_Nicolson_0709_v4.07.pdf Retrieved Feb. 4, 2013.

25. *More on Humic Acid* Article from website. http://www.terepia.com/ HumicAcid2.htm

26. *pH dependence of salt activation of human leukocyte elastase.* Oshima G, Akashi K, Yamada M. Arch Biochem Biophys. 1984 Aug 15;233(1):212-8.

27. *Liberation of human leukocyte elastase by hypertonic saline baths in psoriasis.* Wiedow O, Streit V, Christophers E, Ständer M. Hautarzt. 1989 Aug;40(8):518-22.

28. *Elastase Is the Only Human Neutrophil Granule Protein That Alone Is Responsible for In Vitro Killing of Borrelia burgdorferi* Rodolfo Garcia, Laura Gusmani, Rossella Murgia, Corrado Guarnaccia, Marina Cinco, and Giandomenico Rottini. Infect Immun, April 1998, p. 1408-1412, Vol. 66

29. *Vitamin B3 May Offer New Tool in Fight Against Staph Infections, 'Superbugs'* ScienceDaily (Aug. 27, 2012) http://www.sciencedaily.com/releases/2012/08/120827122258.htm

30. *Niacinamide Helps Combat Candida Albicans* Article by Byron Richards citing *Modulation of histone H3 lysine 56 acetylation as an antifungal therapeutic strategy* Hugo Wurtele, Sarah Tsao, Guylaine Lépine, Alaka Mullick, Jessy Tremblay, Paul Drogaris, Eun-Hye Lee, Pierre Thibault, Alain Verreault, Martine Raymond Nature Medicine 2010 July http://www.wellnessresources.com/studies/entry/niacinamide_helps_combat_candida_albicans Retrieved Feb. 4, 2013.

31. *Some Notes On Niacinamide Therapy for Arthritis* William Kaufman, M.D., Ph.D. Article from Doctoryourself.com http://www.doctoryourself.com/kaufman3.html Retrieved Feb. 4, 2013.

32. Ibid.

33. Nicotinamide Restores Cognition in Alzheimer's Disease Transgenic Mice via a Mechanism Involving Sirtuin Inhibition and Selective Reduction of Thr231-Phosphotau Kim N. Green, Joan S. Steffan, Hilda Martinez-Coria, Xuemin Sun, Steven S. Schreiber, Leslie Michels Thompson, and Frank M. LaFerla Journal of Neuronscience 5 November 2008 28(45) 11500-11510

34. *Niacinamide's Potent role in Alleviating Anxiety with its Benzodiazepine-like Properties: A Case Report* Posted on: 10/28/2008 22:24 Orthomolecular Health http://www.helpyourselfcommunity.org/features/niacinamide%E2%80%99s-potent-role-alleviating-anxiety-its-benzodiazepine-properties-case-report Retrieved Feb. 4, 2013.

35. Abram Hoffer, MD, PhD (1917-2009) *interview by Andrew W. Saul* From the Townsend Letter November 2009 http://www.townsendletter.com/Nov2009/hoffer1109.html

36. *Mental Health Treatment That Works* Orthomolecular Medicine News Service, October 7, 2005 http://orthomolecular.org/resources/omns/v01n11.shtml Retrieved Feb. 4, 2013.

37. *Protocol for Lyme Borreliosis* From Wm. Lee Cowden, MD http://www.lyme-disease-research-database.com/lymeprotocolfile5_files/SAMENTO-PROCOTOL-FOR-LYME-BORRELIOSOS___Wm.-Lee-Cowden-MD.pdf Retrieved Feb. 4, 2013.

38. Post from Samento user http://www.prohealth.com/me-cfs/blog/boarddetail.cfm?id=807568 Retrieved Feb. 4, 2013.

39. Dr. Cowden's Lyme Protocol http://www.encognitive.com/files/Dr.%20Cowden's%20Lyme%20Protocol.pdf Retrieved Feb. 4, 2013.

40. *Andrographis paniculata* http://en.wikipedia.org/wiki/Andrographis_paniculata Retrieved Feb. 4, 2013.

41. *Lyme Disease and Andrographis* Written by sshowalter, FoundHealth. http://www.foundhealth.com/lyme-disease/lyme-disease-and-andrographis Retrieved Feb. 4, 2013.

42. *LYME DISEASE: Treatment with Chinese Herbs* by Subhuti Dharmananda, Ph.D., Director, Institute for Traditional Medicine, Portland, Oregon http://www.itmonline.org/arts/lyme.htm Retrieved Feb. 4,

43. Andrographis [Andrographis paniculata] herbal supplement benefits and side effects, research studies, cold, immunity - updated on June 19, 2011 ZHION.COM http://www.zhion.com/herb/Andrographis.html Retrieved Feb. 4, 2013.

44. *Antibacterial Activity of Leaf Juice and Extracts of Moringa oleifera Lam. against Some Human Pathogenic Bacteria.* M. Mashiar Rahman, *M. Mominul, Islam Shiekh, Shamima Akhtar Sharmin, M. Soriful Islam, M. Atikur Rahman, M. Mizanur Rahman, and M. F. Alam* CMU. J. Nat. Sci. (2009) Vol. 8(2) c Vol. 8(2)

45. *Niaziminin, a thiocarbamate from the leaves of Moringa oleifera, holds a strict structural requirement for inhibition of tumor-promoter-induced Epstein-Barr virus activation.* Murakami A, Kitazono Y, Jiwajinda S, Koshimizu K, Ohigashi H. Planta Med. 1998 May;64(4):319-23.

46. *Moringa Health Benefits* Moringa Malunggay website http://www. edlagman.com/moringa/moringa-health-benefits.htm
47. *Moringa Tree of Life* Internationalresearch 2009-05-14 10:43 http:// internationalresearch.webnode.com/news/moringa-disease-treatment-and-prevention/ Also, *Moringa oleifera: A Review of the Medical Evidence for Its Nutritional, Therapeutic, and Prophylactic Properties.* Part 1. Jed W. Fahey, Sc.D. Johns Hopkins School of Medicine, Department of Pharmacology and Molecular Sciences, Lewis B. and Dorothy http://www.edlagman. com/moringa/John_Hopkins.pdf Retrieved Feb. 4, 2013.
48. *The Moringa-Tree, a wonderful present of the nature* http://www.alternative-technology.de/Reforestation/moringa_tree.doc Retrieved Feb. 4, 2013
49. *Allantoin* http://en.wikipedia.org/wiki/Allantoin Retrieved Feb. 4, 2013.
50. *The Effect of Transforming Growth Factor Beta (TGF-Beta3) and Sanicle on Wound Healing* C.B. Beggs, M.C.T. Denyer, A. Lemmerz, F. Sefat, C. Wright, and M. Youseffi Proceedings of The World Congress on Engineering 2010, pp572-577 http://www.iaeng.org/publication/ WCE2010/WCE2010_pp572-577.pdf
51. *Saniculoside N from Sanicula europaea* L Arda N, Gören N, Kuru A, Pengsuparp T, Pezzuto JM, Qiu SX, Cordell GA. J. Nat. Prod., 1997, *60* (11), pp 1170-1173.
52. *Antiviral activity of Sanicula europaea L. extracts on multiplication of human parainfluenza virus type 2.* Karagöz A, Arda N, Gören N, Nagata K, Kuru A. Phytother Res. 1999 Aug;13(5):436-8. http://www.ncbi.nlm.nih.gov/ pubmed/10441789
53. *Antiviral effect of Sanicula europaea L. leaves extract on influenza virus-infected cells.* Turan K, Nagata K, Kuru A. Biochem Biophys Res Commun. 1996 Aug 5;225(1):22-6.
54. *Alzheimer's Disease: a 21st Century Epidemic* by Lara Pizzorno, MDiv, MA, LMT http://www.lmreview.com/articles/view/alzheimers-disease-a-21st-century-epidemic/#fn-71-
55. *Beta-Amyloid: An Antibiotic?* By Derek Lowe In The Pipeline March 16, 2010 http://pipeline.corante.com/archives/2010/03/16/betaamyloid_an_ antibiotic.php Retrieved Feb. 10, 2013
56. *Stealth Pathogens* 2005 Presentation in Chicago by Lida Mattman PhD Autoimmunity Research Foundation's Chicago Conference http://www. youtube.com/watch?v=WozrCFW0mRM Retreived Feb. 10, 2013

57. *American sanicle: a cure-all* Altmeds.com http://www.altmeds.com/american-sanicle/articles/american-sanicle-a-cureall Retreived Feb. 10, 2013

58. *Grapefruit seed extract is a powerful in vitro agent against motile and cystic forms of Borrelia burgdorferi sensu lato.* Brorson O, Brorson SH. Infection. 2007 Jun;35(3):206-8.

59. *Terminalia Chebula Holistic Herbal Detox Ayurvedic Herb* http://www.holistic-herbalist.com/terminalia-chebula.html Retreived Feb. 10, 2013

60. *Cytomegalovirus infection and its possible treatment with herbal medicines* Shiraki K, Yukawa T, Kurokawa M, Kageyama S. Nippon Rinsho. 1998 Jan;56(1):156-60. http://www.ncbi.nlm.nih.gov/pubmed/9465682

61. *In vitro activity of gallic acid against Candida albicans biofilms.* Wang C, Cheng H, Guan Y, Wang Y, Yun Y: Zhongguo Zhong Yao Za Zhi; 2009 May;34(9):1137-40

62. Multiple studies on terminalia chebula from BioMedLib.com: http://bmlsearch.com/wlcm.asp?kwr=terminalia+chebula+&kwr=&ck=&cxts=10&fntszff=100&hghlght=maroon&srtrdr=relevance&annttn=none&pdthm=2010&hqryhstry=52dc9f572c14e50e01d5c5e6d9ed3f42&pgwdth=100&mld=&wft=wims&b4s=967461034&ifjs=ys&frmty=srchbx Retreived Feb. 10, 2013

63. *Quorum-Sensing Inhibitors and Biofilms* Kociolek, Martin G. Anti-Infective Agents in Medicinal Chemistry (Formerly Current Medicinal Chemistry - Anti-Infective Agents), Volume 8, Number 4, October 2009, pp. 315-326(12)

64. *Quorum Sensing in Gram-Negative Bacteria: Small-Molecule Modulation of AHL and AI-2 Quorum Sensing Pathways* Warren R. J. D. Galloway, James T. Hodgkinson, Steven D. Bowden, Martin Welch, and David R. Spring Chem. Rev. 2011, 111, 28-67

65. *Influence of polyphenols on bacterial biofilm formation and quorum-sensing.* Z Naturforsch C. 2003 Nov-Dec; 58(11-12):879-84.

66. Synthesis of Anti-Angiogenic Isocoumarins Current Organic Synthesis, Volume 1, Number 1, January 2004, pp. 1-9(9)

67. Research on *Haritaki* http://www.toddcaldecott.com/index.php/herbs/learning-herbs/361-haritaki Retreived Feb. 10, 2013

68. *The Natural Compound Ellagic Acid Reduces Biofilm Formation Specifically in S. Dysgalactieae strains NCTC 4671 and ATCC 27957.* Study posted to Springerimages

http://www.springerimages.com/Images/Chemistry/1-10.1007_ s00253-010-2471-0-0 Retrieved Feb. 10, 2013

69. *Research Update of Galla Chinensis.* MDidea Exporting Division Extracts Professional http://www.mdidea.com/products/herbextract/gallachinensis/ research.html Retrieved Feb. 1 2013

70. *Dietary plant components ellagic acid and tannic acid inhibit* Escherichia coli *biofilm formation* Hancock V, Dahl M, Vejborg RM, Klemm P. J Med Microbiol April 2010 59:496-498;

71. *Growth-inhibiting activity of active component isolated from Terminalia chebula fruits against intestinal bacteria.* Kim HG, Cho JH, Jeong EY, Lim JH, Lee SH, Lee HS. J Food Prot. 2006 Sep; 69(9):2205-9.

72. *Madhavi Gavini, ISEF 2006 Intel Foundation Young Scientist* by Amy Hodson Thompson *Cogito*, 12.12.2006 https://cogito.cty.jhu.edu/15951/ madhavi-gavini-isef-2006-intel-foundation-young-scientist/ Retrieved Feb. 2, 2013

73. *Pure Prescriptions Natural Health Solutions* http://www.pureprescriptions. com/ellagic-defense-extract-antioxidant-cancer Retrieved Feb. 2, 2013

74. *What is Carnivora?* Carnivora International website http://www.carnivora. com/about-carnivora.html Retrieved Feb. 2, 2013

75. *Venus Flytrap & Cats Claw Nature's Little-known Remedies for Chronic Disease* By Angela Garabo http://www.awarenessmag.com/sepoct0/SO0_ VENUS_FLYTRAP.HTM Retreived Feb. 2, 2013

76. *Why Do I Love Carnivora* °? by Dan Kenner Sunday, 11 January 2009 05:40 For the "Ormed Institute Newsletter" Alternative Medical Breakthroughs from Around the World, Special Carnivora Edition http:// www.dankennerresearch.com/kenner/index.php?option=com_ content&view=article&id=61:why-do-i-love-carnivora&catid=37:article& Itemid=28

77. *Increased production of antigen-specific immunoglobulins G and M following in vivo treatment with the medicinal plants Echinacea angustifolia and Hydrastis canadensis.* Rehman J, Dillow JM, Carter SM, Chou J, Le B, Maisel AS. Immunol Lett. 1999 Jun 1;68(2-3):391-5.

78. *A systematic review of the anticancer properties of berberine, a natural product from Chinese herbs* Sun Y, Xun K, Wang Y, Chen X Anticancer Drugs 2009 (9): 757-69.

79. *The alkaloid Berberine inhibits the growth of Anoikis-resistant MCF-7 and MDA-MB-231 breast cancer cell lines by inducing cell cycle arrest* Kim JB,

Yu JH, Ko E et al. Phytomedicine, Volume 17, issue 6 (May, 2010), p. 436-440.

80. *Berberine induced apoptosis via promoting the expression of caspase-8, -9 and -3, apoptosis-inducing factor and endonuclease G in SCC-4 human tongue squamous carcinoma cancer cells* Ho YT, Lu CC, Yang JS et al. (October 2009). Anticancer Research 29 (10): 4063-70. PMID 19846952.

81. *Chronic effects of berberine on blood, liver glucolipid metabolism and liver PPARs expression in diabetic hyperlipidemic rats* Zhou JY, Zhou SW, Zhang KB et al. (June 2008). Biological & Pharmaceutical Bulletin 31 (6): 1169-76.

82. *On the mechanism of antidepressant-like action of berberine chloride* Kulkarni SK, Dhir A (July 2008). Eur J Pharmacol. 2008 Jul 28;589(1-3):163-72.

83. *Golden seal* Herbal Materia Medica. David L. Hoffmann BSc (Hons), MNIMH Available at: http://www.healthy.net/scr/mmedica. aspx?MTId=1&Id=219 and http://www.healthy.net/asp/templates/article. asp?id=1906&HeaderTitle=Herbal+Materia+Medica&action=print. Retrieved Feb. 2 2013

84. *Advances in studies on antimicrobial activities of alkaloids* Li Y., Zuo G.-Y. Chinese Traditional and Herbal Drugs 2010 41:6 (1006-1014)

85. *Berberine Inhibits HIV Protease Inhibitor-Induced Inflammatory Response by Modulating ER Stress Signaling Pathways in Murine Macrophages* Weibin Zha, Guang Liang, Jian Xiao, Elaine J. Studer, Phillip B. Hylemon, William M. Pandak,, Jr., Guangji Wang, Xiaokun Li, and Huiping Zhou PLoS One. 2010; 5(2): e9069 http://www.ncbi.nlm.nih.gov/pmc/articles/PMC2817721/

86. *Berberine suppresses proinflammatory responses through AMPK activation in macrophages* Jeong HW, Hsu KC, Lee JW et al. (April 2009) American Journal of Physiology—Endocrinology and Metabolism 296 (4): E955-64.

87. Smart Supplementation: *Echinacea and Goldenseal* Huntington College of Health Sciences Literature Education Series On Dietary Supplements By Gene Bruno, MS, MHS—Dean of Academics, Huntington College of Health Sciences http://vivavitamins.com/literature/Echinacea%20Goldenseal.pdf Retreived Feb. 10, 2013

88. *New hope for liver disease: curcumin in tumeric spice fights liver damage and cirrhosis* Tuesday, September 28, 2010 by: S. L. Baker, featured writer http://www.naturalnews.com/029872_curcumin_cirrhosis.html Retrieved Feb. 10, 2013

89. *Curcumin* Article from All About Multiple Sclerosis website. http://www. mult-sclerosis.org/curcumin.html Retrieved Feb. 10, 2013

90. Articles covering the Antibiotic and Antibacterial
Properties of Turmeric / Curcumin http://spreadhealthfoods.com/ turmeric-research/antibiotic-antibacterial.php Retrieved Feb. 10, 2013

91. *In-vitro antimicrobial activity of the ground rhizome, curcuminoid pigments and essential oil of Curcuma longa L* Peret-Almeida, Lucia; Naghetini, Cristina da Cunha; Nunan, Elziria de Aguiar; Junqueira, Roberto Goncalves; Gloria, Maria Beatriz Abreu. Ciencia e Agrotecnologia (2008), 32(3), 875-881

92. *Sparganium and Zedoaria - Herbs Combined to Treat Solid Masses* by Subhuti Dharmananda, Ph.D., Director, Institute for Traditional Medicine, Portland, Oregon http://www.itmonline.org/arts/sparganium. htm
Retrieved Feb. 10, 2013

93. *How to Keep Lyme Fatigue Away with These Biofilm-Busting Herbs.* By Greg Lee LAc. Article on Two Frogs Healing Center website. http://www.twofrogscenter.com/busting_biofilm_fatigue.html   Retrieved Feb. 18, 2013

94. *Mirrh and Frankincense* by Subhuti Dharmananda Ph. D. Article on Institute for Traditional Medicine website. http://www.itmonline.org/arts/ myrrh.htm Retrieved Feb. 18, 2013

95. *Allying with Teasel Root* Lady Barbara's Garden. http://ladybarbara.net/ html/using_teasel.html Retreived Feb. 18, 2013

96. Ibid.

97. *Isolation of phytoalexin-deficient mutants of Arabidopsis thaliana and characterization of their interactions with bacterial pathogens* J. Glazebrook and F. M. Ausubel (1994). Proc Natl Acad Sci U S A. 1994 September 13; 91(19): 8955-8959.

98. Article on Allicin on www.allicin.com/ Retrieved Feb. 18, 2013

99. *Stabilized Allicin* Article from Allimed. http://www.allimed.us/pdf/S_ Allicin.pdf Retrieved Feb. 18, 2013

100. *Allimax Nutraceuticals US completes clinical trial for treating Lyme disease* James R. Walton, President Allimax Nutraceuticals US http://www. allimax.us/Lyme_NPI_Press.pdf Retrieved Feb. 2, 2013

101. *Antimicrobial properties of allicin from garlic* Microbes Ankri S, Mirelman D. Infect. 1999 Feb;1(2):125-9..

CHAPTER 12

Essential Oils

Lyme patients are always on the look-out for new ideas that will accelerate their healing, and are always remaining open for some new therapy that holds promise. Often we hear an anecdotal story that leads us to take a closer look to see what potential it may hold. This is how my interest in essential oils became piqued.

One day I was reading a post on a Lyme blog about someone that had tried something new. For some reason this person decided to do a fast eating nothing but oranges, lemons, and limes—except they ate the whole fruit, rind and all! I believe about two weeks later they said their Lyme symptoms were completely gone. I was scratching my head on that one trying to figure out how that happened. Although I suspected they were obviously not completely cured from this, it did leave me wondering. (I later learned that it may have been its combination with fasting that significantly accelerated the healing of Lyme. More on that later.)

Being the brave (or stupid) soul that I am, I decided, "why not give it a try". If you've never eaten a whole orange or lime with its rind, it's not as easy as it sounds. So also being the innovative genius that I am (scardy cat) I decided to buy a food processor to turn the fruit into mush, and eat it like a smoothie rather than eat the peels and rinds whole. Again, not as easy as it sounds! The taste is so terrible that you can't keep it down. So I quickly decided that medicines you can't keep down may not work quite as well as those you do.

But what that did was to get me to wondering what it could have been in the fruits that had such an effect. Who knows exactly what can happen in a person when one considers the many variables that are at work. That's when I realized that the eating of the rinds would have meant that the person would have been eating a part of the fruit not normally consumed. That would have been the essential oils. What I did not yet understand was that these particular fruits had a chemical (limonene) which is known to have powerful antimicrobial properties. Thus began my quest and development of a new therapy that would have dramatic effects on accelerating my healing.

Essential oils are generally either cold-pressed or distilled concentrations of a plant that contain the essence of the plant with all of its natural and chemical properties. They are volatile oils meaning they do not have the same oily or fatty properties as those found in animals, but can evaporate as a clear liquid without leaving a stain. Another reason they are called *essential* is because the oil contains the constituents of the plant that are essential for its survival. Whereas animals possess a distinct immune system which is made up of all the individual cells with their specifically designed functions, plants contain phytochemicals which act as its immune system by repelling insects and killing certain microbes that would infect it. Essential oils contain those chemicals which are known to possess very potent antibacterial properties in a highly concentrated form. This is what makes some essential oils ideal as natural antibiotics, far surpassing the benefits of some synthetic drug-based pharmaceuticals. For instance, many essential oils contain *farnesol* which was discovered to disperse certain bacterial and fungal biofilms, as well as possesses antimicrobial properties.

This area of research led to a real breakthrough and advancement in my own personal development of therapies for my Lyme. Having spent years searching for and experimenting with a multitude of products, I had reached a plateau and needed to find something that would allow me to go deeper. I needed to address an angle that none of the things I had already done were addressing, since some form or aspect of the infection was still persisting. This led to the exploration of essential oils. What I had learned about these oils was quite remarkable, in that the healing properties of these oils was so dynamic, in many ways they exceeded almost any other therapy I had tried.

Essential oils are well known for their applications in aromatherapy. However this seemed to puzzle me why they are mostly only known for this, since what I was about to learn was quite remarkable. EO's face the same problems as any other natural products in that much of what we know of them comes from traditional sources and historical usage. With government regulation limiting what a manufacturer can claim in the absence of scientific research, more and more companies that make and sell essential oils are doing their own research to discover what properties and chemical constituents are involved in their therapeutic effects. This has led to real advancements and the shedding of their reputation as being "fringe" medicines, as much of their historical uses are being discovered to be supported by scientific evidence. No longer will essential oils be regarded as "folk" medicine, as more and more research is proving their almost miraculous-like effectiveness in given applications.

It must be remembered over and over again, that all healthcare practitioners in this country are highly controlled in what they are allowed practice, claim, and even what they can tell their patients. Hence, any information that is derived from these sources must be interpreted through the filter of government approval. This means that what you are hearing of the benefits that natural products such as essential oils possess, is almost always coming from a manufacturer or seller of a product, or from a practitioner, both of which are being told what they can make known to the public by the government. Often times, we must go outside the US for sources of information where censorship and the deliberate withholding of information are not so regulated.

One such area of therapy suppression is essential oils. As one begins to research this subject, virtually all information that is available involves their use in the area of aromatherapy or external applications. When I began studying essential oils, almost no research could be found regarding their internal use. The few places that made mention of their internal application seemed to be in the form of a warning. Most essential oils are listed by the FDA as GRAS (generally accepted as safe). There are a few essential oils that are known to have some toxicity that should be avoided. However other than the fact that some oils can be irritating to the skin and mucous membranes, and should generally be applied combining them with a carrier oil to dilute them, very little information is supplied explaining why these warnings against their internal use are given.

For instance Australian tea tree oil, a very common essential oil used as an antiseptic, is often found on several websites with the warning, "not for internal use". Of course there are factors involving purity which could explain some warnings. But that doesn't sufficiently explain why so many give this caution. With all the research that I had done before beginning essential oil therapy, not one source had given a reason for the warnings. In fact, generally speaking, when one researches essential oils, they are almost never being touted or sold for internal use. Yet the literature is almost completely absent as to why this is. How can they be a non-toxic plant, generally accepted as safe by our own FDA, yet almost nothing is mentioned as to their internal use, especially in light of the incredible curative properties that essential oils hold? Tea tree oil possesses some of the most potent antimicrobial properties of all the essential oils, and in fact is one of the few substances known that can kill or inhibit the anti-biotic resistant staph bacteria MRSA.

I read an article that mentioned that one naturopathic physician, apparently trying to prove a point, took an entire ounce of tea tree oil internally every day for a month with no harmful effects whatsoever. That amount is tens of thousand of times the level any one would normally ever take. Most essential oils, when taken internally are normally in the range of a few drops a day. So why then would these products have a warning with no reason given? (We are not speaking of those oils which are known to have specific cautions.)

Certainly each oil will possess its own unique properties with its own particular potential dangers, as is true with anything else. And how any particular oil will affect an individual will be based upon their own health and condition. Some oils can be potentially dangerous and should be avoided, e.g. bitter almond, juniper, wintergreen, tansy, wormwood, rue, common sage, red thyme, savory, and sassafras are listed.[1] Some oils are labeled "emmenagogues" which theoretically can induce a woman's menstruation or cause bleeding problems. Although the list is long, these common oils are a few examples: rose, sage, cinnamon, fennel, ginger, jasmine, juniper, myrhh, peppermint, chamomile, rosemary, and eucalyptus.[2] All of these examples are dose dependent. However the general use of essential oils internally as a group have had a stigma associated with them that is completely unwarranted, and that is supported by very little, sometimes no evidence whatsoever.

A practicing aroma therapist in Australia, Ron Guba has had a special interest in research involving the topic of essential oil toxicity. He has worked with various government and industry bodies as well as with the general public. He wrote an article called *Toxicity Myths and the Actual Risks of Essential Oil Use* as it relates to the internal use of essential oils.[3] He lays out the historical philosophies as to the precautious outlooks of therapists over the past 80 years with regards to the internal use of essential oils. Even with his extensive experience he sees no apparent justification for the unqualified warnings given by practitioners of aromatherapy to discourage the general internal use of essential oils. He says:

> *What can be noted in many publications are statements that are based on the attitude: 'If I do not know about the possible negative effects of an essential oil, then, if any possible negative effect might be noted, I'm going to recommend that people not use such oils at all or else in very tiny amounts.*
>
> *To err on the side of caution may be considered laudable. However, we can notice that such exaggerated statements have led to a common perception that the therapeutic use of essential oils can be an extremely risky proposition, even amongst those who are purported to be highly qualified practitioners.* [4]

In fact MD's, pharmacologists, and even alternative health practitioners alike simply are not trained in the pharmacology of essential oils, or their medicinal uses. However in France the use of internal essential oils has had a long tradition, and is still used today. Penny Price, Director of Training at Shirley Price International College of Aromatherapy, Hinckley, UK, says

> *There was certainly no problem in using essential oils externally, internally, diluted or neat in those days. Even since that time, in France, the practice of all methods of using essential oils carries on, unchallenged and positively successful. In France,*

essential oils are administered internally by medical doctors and phytotherapists as an extremely effective method for treating disorders . . . [5]

The fact is, although technically speaking prescription drugs are poisons which need to be controlled due to their toxicity, they are obviously beneficial if used responsibly. So it is with most essential oils internally without the comparable toxic affects. The only logical explanation as to what may be driving the overly cautious warnings against internal essential oil use is liability issues. It is far safer to just say that the oils are for external use to protect yourself against any potential problems or misrepresentations associated with manufacturing and selling a product. And that is especially true here in the US where the FDA is duly feared.

Having said that, one word of general caution may be warranted. Regardless of the plant source, essential oils in general are considered volatile, and do possess a potential for certain cellular interferences at high doses. Again Ron Guba,

> *Most essential oil compounds have a 'non-specific' toxic effect, whereby the absorption of these lipophilic compounds into cellular membranes can eventually lead to disruption of membrane permeability. The primary toxic outcome is that of the disruption of ion channel function in nerve cells, first affecting the heart and central nervous system, leading to cardiac and respiratory depression . . . To create such effects, however, require huge dosages, in the order of 300mL and beyond.* [6]

That would be equivalent to drinking over 10 ounces all at once, many thousands of times beyond recommended doses. You can therefore see that such warnings against the prudent internal use of essential oils tend to largely be exaggerated.

I contacted a researcher at perhaps the most reputable essential oil manufacturer in the US with regards to the safety of their internal use. I asked her if she was aware of any negative reactions to their use. She told me only one story of a man that had gone to see his physician about a health issue. The doctor did some tests and returned to advise the patient that he was going to have to stop drinking since he had developed cirrhosis of the liver. The patient told the doctor he doesn't drink. After exploring the man's history it was found that he had been taking apparently large quantities of essential oils over time.

I share this with you to give a fair yet informative viewpoint. Comparatively speaking even the taking of aspirin or ibuprofen would be far more toxic, and can cause severe damaging gastrointestinal problems, making essential oils far safer than these drugs. However using small amounts of essential oils that are only going to be pulsed anyways do not represent anything close to dangerous or toxic levels. As a sidenote, some have considered taking essential oil hydrosols internally as they theorize they may be safer. However many hydrosols do not possess the same germicidal properties as the essential oils. Some may. I read one article that did a study and found that none of the hydrosols in that study had the same antimicrobial activity as their essential oil counterparts. Some are even contaminated with bacteria. A word of warning.

As for dosages, as a general safety rule, most essential oils should only be taken 2-3 drops at a time (although I have taken some oils many times that amount). Some may be more tolerable than others. But sticking with this rule should keep you within the margin of safety. Although I am not recommending nor advocating this or any amount, I have personally taken some 30 drops of mixed essential oils internally several times per day with coconut oil as the carrier for several weeks with no negative or adverse reactions of any kind. But remember, you are going to be rotating your therapies, including the essential oils. Therefore these will only be taken for several days, and certainly less than two weeks before taking a rest and switching to a different therapy. In this manner they are being optimized for their antimicrobial potential, while giving the body a rest to prevent any potential harmful effects. (Remember, even toxic drugs prescribed in conventional medicine violate this simple rule. That is the reason for so many deaths by conventional medicine. However essential oils in general are far safer than drugs.)

Essential oils are always taken with a carrier oil. A carrier oil is a non-volatile base or vegetable oil that is more compatible with the body when used either externally or internally. It is combined with the essential oils to dilute them to make them less volatile, less irritating, and more easily absorbed. This way one receives the beneficial properties of the essential oils, yet are buffered to make them more biocompatible, and allows them to be taken at higher doses. This is another reason why essential oils can be taken safely. Additionally, essential oils tend to very readily absorb into the skin or mucous membrane. Adding a carrier oil slows down this absorption allowing them to be taken deeper into the blood stream and dispursed throughout the body. Also, just as a precaution, taking curcumin or ursolic acid prior to the taking of essential oils internally would be beneficial as these herbs have liver-protecting properties. My advice: ***Always take curcumin or ursolic acid when taking essential oils. This gives you even more protection, and adds to the antimicrobial and anti-inflammatory benefits.***

LIST OF OILS

Australian Tea tree oil—This is one of the most well known of the essential oils. There are three oils called "tea tree oil". *Melaleuca alternafolia* is the common "Australian" tea tree oil sometimes called *Melaleuca Oil.* It is generally sold as an antiseptic. This particular specie is highly antimicrobial in a wide spectrum manner. It is considered to be one of the most antibacterial of all the essential oils. This tea tree oil has demonstrated some effectiveness at inhibiting or killing even the highly antibiotic-resistant staphylococcus areus.[7] Tea tree oil is also anti-inflammatory. As any essential oil can potentially cause allergic reactions in those that are susceptible, as can happen in a drug as well, tea tree oil seems to be well tolerated even when applied directly to the skin. However some may develop contact dermatitis.

Due to its popularity, and its common use externally, many have asked the question as to whether it is safe for internal use. It was mentioned earlier that many websites warn not to take the product internally. However I was not able to find even one single incidence of poisoning of humans. (By "poisoning" I mean an actual death.) Although the source is unconfirmed, earlier it was shared that a naturopathic physician is reported to have taken an entire ounce every day for a month with no negative side effects.[8] I have personally taken up to 1 ml (about 30 drops) taken as part of a carrier oil with no reactions of any kind. I did find a few sites that did in fact recommend taking tea tree oil internally if done so at low quantities along with a carrier oil.

I attempted to get to the bottom of this as there were too many inconsistencies and unfounded warnings as to oral toxicity issues. The reports that were warning against internal use simply were not giving what I felt were reasonable or balanced views. There are no reports of death or any permanent damage even when taken at high doses. The only references were related to young infants that accidentally ingested 10ml[9,10] and few adults.[11] The effect it caused was temporary ataxia (some loss of motor skills) and drowsiness, the same affect that was witnessed in rats when given in exceedingly high doses.[12] This is essentially equivalent to the condition one would see in someone that was drunk, and may in fact be related more to TTO's turpenes than from any toxic components. One report read "Incidences of oral poisoning in children and adults have been reported. In all cases, the patients responded to supportive care and recovered without apparent sequelae. No human deaths due to TTO have been reported in literature." [13] I suppose it depends on how one defines "poisoning".

In every instance I have found that tea tree oil was called "poisoning" in humans referred to an obvious allergic reaction, or when taken undiluted by a very young child. But in every case, recovery occurred uneventfully. And judging by the credentials of those reporting (those strongly associated with an allopathic background) it became clear to me that these reports were being made to deliberately insinuate that it is dangerous. (One can see the obvious prejudice when the sheer amount of deaths from actual alcohol poisoning are seldom reported.)

I have personally concluded that what is being called "poisoning" is far from being a poison or "toxic" in the sense that there is a component that causes death or permanent damage. Certainly at higher doses than is necessary some sort of negative effects may be seen. But the taking of essential oils or any substance for that matter is all about the taking of therapeutic doses that will not induce toxicity. To say that something should never be taken under any circumstances because it *may be* toxic is most certainly over-stating and exaggerating a problem. There are a few reported cases of people drinking too much water all at once that killed them. Or for that matter, wine or champagne could be called a "poison" since they contain a "toxic" substance called alcohol which can kill brain cells and cause liver damage at certain levels. And if using that same reasoning, many prescription drugs should never be taken since they are known to kill thousands of people each year even when taken according to "accepted" levels. Drugs can certainly be far more toxic taken on a dose per dose basis than tea tree oil, yet we are seldom warned to not take drugs because they can be poisonous. Even peanut butter can kill someone who is highly allergic. Again, as in anything, one must weigh the cautions of taking something with the potential benefits. This would apply to most essential oils, not just tea tree.

Substances are sometimes graded according to their toxicity levels by what is called LD50. This means that when testing against say rats for example, the LD (lethal dosage) that would kill 50% of the animals is given. 1.9 grams per kilogram is the approximate LD50 for tea tree oil. This would be equivalent to about 1 teaspoon for every 5 pounds. The grading is done on the basis of animals since few humans volunteer for this test. However making an approximate equivalence between animals and humans, that would mean that 50% of humans would die at 1 teaspoon per 5 pounds of bodyweight. So it would take about 30 teaspoons of tea tree oil to kill half of those in a group of individuals weighing 150 lbs. At this level one can see the enormous quantity of tea tree oil that would be necessary to kill someone, particularly when we are speaking of using less than 10 drops per dose in an average sized adult.

As a word of caution however, certain animals such as cats, dogs, and birds do appear to be more sensitive to tea tree oil. Certainly infants will also be more sensitive. But as for taking tea tree oil internally, one must weigh the facts and make personal decisions. No recommendations are given one way or the other. Personally, I have had no problems taking this oil internally when combined with a carrier oil, which is the *only* *way* these oils should be taken if ingested orally in my opinion.

New Zealand Tea Tree oil—This is a relative of the Australian version. *Leptospermum scoparium,* also known as *Manuka oil,* also possesses powerful antimicrobial activities, similar to Melaleuca oil. The Manuka plant has been used by the indigenous local Maori people medicinally long before European settlers. Its traditional use has been to speed the healing of wounds, ringworm, colds, sinus problems, hay fever, asthma, skin diseases, to reduce infection, eczema, painful joints, urinary tract infection and to reduce fever. What makes manuka oil different is that based upon much of the research that has been done seeking to identifiy its antimicrobial constituents, the plants possess widely varied properties from one location to another even though they are from the same plant specie. Dr. Alan Cooke of the Cawthron Institute researched and discovered that a specific location on the East Cape of New Zealand grew Manuka plants that possessed significantly greater antibacterial properties than other areas. Tairawhiti Pharmaceuticals was established as an outcome of this discovery. It exclusively produces Manuka Oil from this location. The results of the research are quite remarkable.

The oil was tested against 9 gram positive, and 6 gram negative bacterial varieties. It was discovered that in the gram positive group, Manuka oil possesses approximately 20-30 times the potency of Australian tea tree oil! The gram negative, although did not fair quite as well, showed remarkable bacteriocidal qualities.[14] This makes Manuka oil perhaps one of the most potent antimicrobial essential oils in the world. Although essential oils are generally safer used in conjunction with a carrier oil, applied externally it appears that Manuka oil may be somewhat more tolerable than Australian Tea Tree oil even without a carrier oil.

I have personally used Manuka oil applied externally both with and without a carrier with no problems. I have also used it internally combined with at a rate of approximately 6 drops per tablespoon of coconut oil with no problems. The most likely problems that are going to occur with most essential oils if there are any, is going to be the liver. So it is recommended that this organ be protected prior to taking these oils with curcumin, which is a good liver protector. Again, it is recommended that you always pulse and rotate Manuka, as well as any essential oil, particularly when using internally, so that they do not build up in the system just in case there are some sensitivity issues.

Although Australian Tea Tree oil is quite popular and well known for its antibacterial properties, it seems to fair better against gram-negative bacteria (of which Bb is a member), while the Manuka is far superior against gram-positive. Manuka oil has been successfully used against MRSA. A good research reference for a study of Manuka oil can be found. [15] Last checked Manuka oil is not yet listed in any category by the FDA. So there are no currently known toxicity issues with Manuka oil.

Melaleuca and Manuka oils are described first due to the fact that they may be among the most potent essential oils. Other oils also hold notable antimicrobial properties as well.

Thieves oil—This is a popular and unique blend of 5 oils: Lemon, cinnamon bark, eucalyptus, rosemary, and clove. It became popular for its antipathogen properties dating back to the period of the spread of the plagues that nearly desimated Europe during Medieval times. Four thieves had been caught stealing from the dead and dying. Their sentences were reduced in exchange for their sharing what their secret was for not contracting the disease in spite of continous contact with the sick. They shared that they were perfume makers who were familiar with the effects of certain oils to dispel disease.

Interestingly, as usually seems to be the case, traditional use has been scientifically proven to be true as studies have been done that demonstrated the germicidal effects of these 5 oils.[16]

However, this addresses another potential benefit of essential oils. They seem to block the transmission of disease. We explained in a previous chapter how that bacteria in particular communicate with each other called quorum sensing. This communication system would seem to be particularly important to Borrelia since its morphology would rely on autoinducers as a signaling mechanism. We know that its pleomorphic capacity is what gives it its advantage by constantly changing. By coordinating these changes within the colonies it can counter the effects of specific immune cell attacks as well as bacteriocidal substances. The use of certain essential oils seems to have an effect on the infectivity, defensive or offensive capacity of some pathogenic microbes. Since it has been discovered that certain essential oils have the capacity to disrupt biofilms and infectivity, it may be that the potency and specific chemical make-up of these oils disrupts bacterial autoinducers which are the small diffusible signals bacteria use which allows quorum sensing to take place. We will see a few examples of essential oils having antibiofilm potentials. By incorporating essential oils into therapies, we hold the capacity to weaken infectivity and reduce biofilm communication.

The following is a list of essential oils which are known to possess significant antimicrobial constituents; some have anti-biofilm potential. This is only a partial list. Most plant oils to some degree or another are going to possess the capacity to resist or kill microbes since their oils contain the properties to defend the plant. But those on the following list stand out as being some of the most potent. Many have been tested for research purposes to determine not only their ability to kill specific pathogens, but for their effect against biofilms. However keep in mind that these were not tested specifically against Bb. And so it cannot be assumed that the effectiveness against a tested pathogen will necessarily have the same or even a similar effect against Borrelia strains. Also, the effective dilutions may not be attainable to necessitate the desired effect. However it does give a starting point from which to experiment. It is extremely helpful to know that a particular oil was effective to some extent in the inhibition of biofilm activity. However my own use of essential oils led to herxes and a significant improvement in my symptoms which I can only interpret as being subjective proof that they are effective. Where a particular oil has specific cautions they are noted.

Cinnamon oil—Use caution to dilute, very strong. Has biofilm resisting properties against staphylococcus epidermis.[17] Cinnamon bark is also available as a powder in capsules, and may be taken conjunctively to potentiate its anti-biofilm benefits.

Clove—Very strong. Antibiofilm activity against candida.[18] One of the most powerful antioxidants known.

Melaleuca (Tea tree) oil—Reduced growth of biofilms of listeria monocytogenes.[19]

Lemon—Contains limonene, natural antibiotic properties.

Rosemary—Reduced growth of biofilms of listeria monocytogenes.[20]

Eucalyptus—Antibiofilm activity against candida albicans. [21]

Peppermint—Reduced biofilm growth against listeria monocytogenes.[22]

White Thyme—Highly antimicrobial, but is irritating to the skin and mucous membranes. Red Thyme should not be taken internally. White thyme only very cautiously used in a diffuser.

Lime—Limonene.

Orange—Limonene.

Sage—Dilute, very strong.

Niaouli—Combined with Manuka and Melaleuca oils for maximum antibiotic activity.

Palmarosa—Besides possessing extremely powerful anti-viral and bacteriocidal activity, this oil has a unique benefit of being cytophylactic, meaning it may actually stimulate and promote the growth of leucocytes and other defense system cells.

Lemongrass—Exhibited killing effect on s. aureus biofilm.[23]

Geranium—Often used together with Lemongrass synergistically

Oregano—Dilute, very strong. Not to be confused with oil of oregano which is a non-volitile oil.

Ravensara—Principally an antiviral oil for flu, herpes zoster, and other viral infections.

Japanese Red Pine Needle Oil—This is a relatively new available oil. Very little research is available to explain its constituents. However based upon the incredible anecdotal testimonials, time may turn out to reveal this to be one of the most powerful of all oils by far.

It is extremely well tolerated (somewhat higher dosages may be allowed than other oils), and has a very wide range of uses, including powerful antimicrobial properties.

Turmeric—Demonstrated to have similar antibacterial effectiveness as the antibiotic *chloramphenicol.*

Ideally you want to combine essential oils. Sometimes a particular oil alone may only inhibit bacteria and thus actually promote biofilm formation. However combining them allows multi-tier activity to interfere or kill some pathogens and their biofilms when used together.[24]

CARRIER OILS

There are a number of excellent oils that can be used to dilute when combining with essential oils for internal use. These are only a few good ones. Others include Hempseed oil, olive oil, and flax seed oil.

Moringa Oil—This oil has been discussed under the herbal section. It is included as a carrier oil. I have used this either alone or conjunctively with coconut oil when making essential oil tea.

Coconut oil—Coconut oil may be the ideal carrier oil for internal use. In it's own right coconut oil has been called by some "the healthiest oil on earth" because it has so many amazing properties, and should be taken on a regular basis whether with or without the essential oils.

Coconut oil is considered a saturated fat, which has led to some unfortunate misconceptions. Although saturated fats have long been considered unhealthy due to their ability to line the arteries and raise cholesterol, these bad saturated fats are called *long chain fatty acids* (LCFA). Due to their molecular structure, these kinds of oils are not well metabolized by the body, and are stored as fat. However coconut oil is *a medium chain fatty acid* (MCFA) which is processed by the body in a completely different manner. In fact MCFA is readily processed by the liver where it is converted as energy, so it actually increases the metabolism and aids in weight loss. I recall reading one story about how in the early days of learning about coconut oil being a saturated fat, some ranchers would add it to the feed in order to fatten up their cattle. To their dismay their cattle actually began losing weight. It is now known that coconut oil can actually contribute to losing bodyfat and reduce waisteline size.[25]

Coconut oil resists rancidity far longer than other food and vegetable oils, and is very heat stable, so it is ideal when used for cooking. It has a "freezing point" of about 76 degrees. Below this temperature it begins to form a semi-solid.

The list of health benefits is long. However it has been well researched and has been used in both industry and medicine. Due to its ability to increase absorption it reduces insulin resistance in diabetes; relieves stress on the liver, pancreas, and enzyme systems; protects against osteoporosis; increases calcium, magnesium, amino acid, vitamin and mineral uptake; increases digestion and reduces symptoms of gall-bladder disease; reduces symptoms of stomach ulcers, hemorrhoids, and Crohn's disease; supports tissue repair; supports healthy skin and hair; relieves chronic fatigue syndrome due to its ability to increase energy levels; has antioxidant properties, etc.[26]

**Coconut oil should here forward become incorporated into your overall diet if for no other reason than because it enhances absorption of supplements, and aids the body in processing biological functions to speed healing whether due to insufficiencies, damage, or infection.

A good general dosage may be 1-2 teaspoons 2-3 times per day. When used as a carrier oil with the essential oils, it can be placed in a cup of hot green tea which is then melted in the tea. The "oil tea" will be described later. Although water and oil don't mix, it can be stirred and drunk in this manner. Be certain you purchase the extra virgin coconut oil that has not been processed to preserve its potency. It is coconut oil's absorption properties that make it a good surfactant. A surfactant is a product that lowers surface tension of water making oils and fats more water soluble, like soap. So adding coconut oil increases the ability for other chemical processes to take place, making it a potential candidate as an antibiofilm therapy.

Although coconut oil has incredible seemingly endless benefits, its main benefit as an antimicrobial is found in its lauric content. Lauric acid is only one of some 9 fatty acids that make up coconut oil. It is a type of fatty acid which promotes good cholesterol or HDL, and makes up 47% of the total fatty acid content. Lauric acid is also found in mother's breast milk and is known as a natural germ fighter. Although lauric acid possesses powerful antiviral, antibacterial as well as antifungal affects, it does this by converting to *monolaurin* in the body thru enzyme action. It is the monolaurin that is the real power house of its antimicrobial activities. Due to the low conversion of lauric acid into monolaurin in the body, it would require large amounts of coconut oil to receive potent benefits from the monolaurin. So products have been developed that pre-converts the lauric acid into monolaurin thru a special process called *esterfication*, and is put into capsule or pellet form.

The manner in which lauric acid and monolaurin acts as both an antiviral and antibacterial is by disrupting the lipid layer of these germs which both prevents them from attaching to cells, and inhibits replication. Lipid coated viruses include: Herpes 1 and 2, Epstein-Barr, influenza, RSV, Rubeola, Newcastle's, Cytomegalovirus, measles, leukemia virus, syncytial, pneumonovirus, visna, human lymphotrophic virus (type 1), and HIV-1 or HIV+. Lipid coated bacteria include: listeria, H. pylori, hemophilus influenzae, staphylococcus aureus, streptococcus agalactiae, groups A, B, F & G streptococci, gram positive (bacillas anthracis—anthrax, listeria monocytogenes, mycobacteria) and gram negative organisms (if organisms are pretreated with a chelator) (Chlamydia pneumonia, Neisseria gonorrhoeae, helicobacter pylorus, mycoplasma pneumonia, vibrio paraemolyticus).[27] These represent pathogenic microbes monolaurin can affect.

Borrelia Burgdorferi is considered in the class of gram negative bacteria, however does not possess the same manner of lipid coating, although its lipoprotein may be partially vulnerable due to its high lipid content. However even more vulnerable would be its biofilm due to monolaurin's surfactant properties. As previously mentioned, surfactants reduce the surface tension of a liquid, lowering tension between two liquids, thus making them more readily dispersible and absorbable. Biofilms readily absorb and hold water due to its exopolysaccharide content. In fact exopolysaccharides can absorb many times its weight in water. Thus monolaurin, if used in conjunction with a chelator before administration, may readily bind to lipoproteins of Bb residing in biofilms, and may be an ideal treatment option. Oral EDTA with enzymes such as Interfase Plus or Essential Daily Defense may be ideal chelators to use in conjuction with monolaurin.

Essential Oil Tea

The following are examples of "essential oil tea" that I have used with great success. But you can develop your own recipes/formulas. Again, before proceeding with the entire recipe, remember to always begin taking only one product at a time to see how your body reacts, taking 1-2 drops per essential oil per dose. Then try another each day until you have determined you have no reactions. Although any reactions may be extremely rare, it is best to follow this guideline. Thieves oil would be an exception and a good place to begin since it comes as a combination of 5 oils.

Into the hot tea of your choice, add 2-3 heaping tablespoons of extra virgin coconut oil and 1 level teaspoon of Xylitol and/or Manuka Honey. Then add

1. 2-3 drops of Thieves oil, or
2. 2-3 drops Melaleuca (Australian) Tea Tree oil/ 2-3 drops Manuka oil/ 2-3 drops Niaouli oil, or
3. 4-5 drops Japanese Pine needle oil/ 2-3 drops Palmarosa oil/ 2 drops Rosemary oil, or
4. 4 drops Lemongrass oil/ 2-3 drops Geranium oil/ 2-3 drops peppermint oil.

Then stir completely while drinking. Depending on the combination, you may wish to take with a little food to enhance absorbtion. Remember to take curcumin or ursolic acid with your tea.

These are of course only simple examples you may try. In time you may wish to change the combinations you use, or increase the doses.

It is recommended to only do this therapy once per day depending on your tolerance levels. Remember, this is not, nor are any of the therapies described meant to be stand-alone therapies. Ideally they should be rotated as part of a larger program which will be described later. I personally used 3-4 times the volumes listed above with no problems. But these amounts are listed to be within a zone of safety, particularly in the beginning.

ENDNOTES

1. *Essential Oils to Avoid* By Corinna Underwood Article on Safe Alternative Medicine website. http://www.safealternativemedicine.co.uk/essentialoilstoavoid.html Retreived Feb. 18, 2013
2. *Fertility Awareness Planning Essential Oils Some listed To Avoid during Pregnancy* http://www.amandabears.com/essential-oils-avoid-during-pregnancy-toxic.html Retrieved Feb. 19, 2013
3. *Toxicity Myths: The Actual Risks of Essential Oil Use* By Ron Guba http://www.naha.org/articles/toxicity_myths.htm Retreived Feb. 18, 2013
4. Ibid
5. *Aromatology Its History and Uses* by Penny Price http://www.abundantlifeessentials.com/aromatology.htm Retrieved Feb. 19, 2013
6. *Toxicity Myths: The Actual Risks of Essential Oil Use* By Ron Guba http://www.naha.org/articles/toxicity_myths.htm
7. *Staphylococcus aureus and wounds: a review of tea tree oil as a promising antimicrobial.* Halcon L, Milkus K Am J Infect Control. 2004 Nov;32(7):402-8.
8. *Tea Tree Oils (Melaleuka/Leptospermum - Manuka) Article on* The Analyst website. http://www.digitalnaturopath.com/treat/t414585.html Retrieved Feb. 19, 2103
9. *Melaleuca oil poisoning in a 17-month-old.* Del Beccaro MA. Vet Hum Toxicol. 1995 Dec; 37(6):557-8.
10. *Melaleuca oil poisoning.* Jacobs MR, Hornfeldt CS. J Toxicol Clin Toxicol. 1994;32(4):461-4.
11. *Tea tree oil poisoning.* Elliott C. Med J Australia 1993;159:830-831.

12. *Melaleuca alternifolia (Tea Tree) Oil: a Review of Antimicrobial and Other Medicinal Properties* C. F. Carson K. A. Hammer, and T. V. Riley Clin Microbiol Rev. 2006 January; 19(1): 50-62.
13. Ibid
14. *Tairawhiti Manuka Oil.* Study from Tairawhiti Pharmaceuticals Ltd. Website. http://web.archive.org/web/20110902151851/http://www.manuka-oil.com/antimicro.html Retrieved Feb. 18, 2013
15. Studies on the efficacy of Manuka Oil. Original post (http://www.manukanatural.com/pages/Manuka-Oil-Antimicrobial-Activity.html) could not be relocated. Can be found as a DMCA complaint against google.com at http://chillingeffects.org/N/134671 Retrieved Feb. 19, 2013
16. Multiple Theives oil studies cited on secretofthieves website. http://www.secretofthieves.com/bacteria.cfm Retreived Feb. 19, 2012
17. *Effect of trans-Cinnamaldehyde on Inhibition and Inactivation of Cronobacter sakazakii Biofilm on Abiotic Surfaces* Amalaradjou, Mary Anne Roshni; Venkitanarayanan, Kumar Journal of Food Protection®, 2001 Volume 74, Number 2
   Effect of cinnamon oil on icaA expression and biofilm formation by Staphylococcus epidermidis Nuryastuti T, van der Mei HC, Busscher HJ, Iravati S, Aman AT, Krom BP. Appl Environ Microbiol. 2009 Nov; 75(21):6850-5.
18. *Prevention of Candida albicans biofilm by plant oils.* Vishnu Agarwal, et al. MYCOPATHOLOGIA. Vol.165; 1, 13-19,
19. *The in vitro antibiofilm activity of selected culinary herbs and medicinal plants against Listeria monocytogenes* Sandasi M, Leonard CM, Viljoen AM. Lett Appl Microbiol. 2010 Jan;50(1):30-5.
20. Ibid.
21. *Prevention of Candida albicans biofilm by plant oils.* Vishnu Agarwal, et al. MYCOPATHOLOGIA. Vol.165; 1, 13-19,
22. *The in vitro antibiofilm activity of selected culinary herbs and medicinal plants against Listeria monocytogenes* Sandasi M, Leonard CM, Viljoen AM. Lett Appl Microbiol. 2010 Jan;50(1):30-5.
23. *The effect of lemongrass oil and its major components on clinical isolate mastitis pathogens and their mechanisms of action on Staphylococcus aureus* Aiemsaard J, Aiumlamai S, Aromdee C, Taweechaisupapong S, Khunkitti W. Res Vet Sci. 2011 Feb 11
24. *Bioactivity of selected essential oils and some components on Listeria monocytogenes biofilms* South African Journal of Botany Volume 76, Issue 4,

October 2010, Pages 676-680 Chemical diversity and biological functions of plant volatiles

25. *The Amazing Oil That Trims Women's Waistlines* http://articles.mercola.com/sites/articles/archive/2011/06/22/magical-fat-that-increases-good-cholesterol-and-lowers-abdominal-obesity-in-women.aspx Retrieved July 22, 2011

26. *Coconut: Tree of Life* Article on Coconut Research Center website. http://www.coconutresearchcenter.org/ Retrieved Feb. 19, 2013

27. *Technical Information on Monolaurin* Antiviral and Antibacterial Actions of Monolaurin and Lauric Acid http://www.monoclean.com/MonoLaurin_Technical_Info.pdf Retreived Feb. 3, 2013

CHAPTER 13

Mixed Oxidants

It wasn't until I experienced first hand the failure of antibiotics, and began employing the conventional medicine model for my own Lyme disease, did I finally realize that this system of medicine was certainly no match for such a serious illness. In my humble opinion, despite many of their good intentions, allopathic medical doctors practicing the conventional model and their misguided "legal medicine" were doing more of a disservice to many of their patients than helping them. Conventional medicine has been hijacked by the FDA and holds them hostage by tying their hands and limiting what they can offer to patients. They have taken the evidence-based medicine model to an extreme by requiring that drug companies or even makers of natural substances "scientifically" prove their effectiveness before they can legally make a claim to cure your condition or treat a disease. The deception of this model is that even so called "proven" treatments are not proven at all to work for the vast majority of Lyme patients. Their philosophy of using one or even two drugs for one disease fails to address the complex multi-system breakdown that occurs in this illness. And the one or even two anti-biotic approach almost never solves the problem of chronic Lyme disease since pleomorphism and biofilm defenses can easily render them nearly useless in long-term applications. This system takes a unilateral approach in attempting to solve a multi-lateral problem. It is simply ill-equipped to deal with chronic Lyme disease. And that is why so many allopathic MD's deny the reality of chronic Lyme. It just doesn't fit into their paradigm.

Natural medicine holds a distinct advantage in that it at least addresses the whole person by taking a multi-faceted approach to address the many systems that breakdown, such as detox pathways, emotional and psychological stresses, anti-oxidant/ nutrient depletion, mineral deficiencies, allergies, pain, etc, and seeks to support these areas while at the same time uses it own unique anti-microbial herbal or non-drug applications to fight the infection. However natural medicine sometimes tries to mimic the conventional medicine model by simply replacing a drug or two with an herb or two when it comes to the primary battle of Lyme, which is to address the destruction of the infection itself. It uses different (non-drug) medicines, but takes the same approach. Try one or two products to kill the pathogen. If they don't work, try something else. Until you have a cupboard full of things you've tried that seemed to help a little, but never eradicated the condition. And so the journey continues.

In 2006 I had finished writing my first book which was titled, *Lyme Disease, Energy Medicine, and the Biochemistry of Borrelia.* It was a rather novel work at the time. But as is so often the case in today's modern internet age of information, what is news today is common knowledge tomorrow. However I made a rather interesting observation at that time which enabled me to see a way to kill Borrelia, in spite of its ability to both evade anti-biotics and herbal products, and to adapt to them. Bb's pleomorphic capabilities and propensity towards adaptation were self-revealing its own weaknesses. A general word of wisdom I learned long ago that seems to have more than one application is that a person's greatest strength is always a person's greatest weakness. We often become over-reliant upon our strengths, which can lead to unbalance and vulnerability. If you know what front a person is using to defend himself, then you know thru simple observation that that person may be attempting to hide a weakness. And watching how they maneuver will reveal their susceptibilities.

So it was with Borrelia. By constantly maneuvering and changing its forms, it had the conventional model by the gonads if you will. It knew that allopathic medicine prided itself in using one medicine for one illness. Sometimes it tried switching to another, then another. And each time it did so, Borrelia merely changed its form, all the while in the background it was colluding with other pathogens forming biofilms that were resisting those new antibiotics. This gave to Bb an even greater advantage, because once it changed its forms, it was able to deceive the doctors even more so because doing so reduced and/or altered the patients symptoms from very acute and virulent, to more sublte, yet deeper and more entrenched—i.e., chronic. This led both the doctor as well as the patient to believe he was getting better. But even more than this, Bb knew that it might fool a lot of those conventional medical doctors because of their propensity to use the "scientific method" of tests to determine the presence of disease rather than their God-given common sense and clinical observations. Bb loved this since it knew how to avoid detection thru those tests, as nearly half of even the best of them are incorrect. And those doctors that relied upon those tests as their primary diagnostic tool ended up sending their patients home without help. In many ways, conventional medicine became Borrelia's best friend.

BEATING BB AT ITS OWN GAME

The time has come to share with you a rather obvious observation that led me to develop a highly effective strategy against deep-seated Lyme infection after many other treatments had gone as far as they could. It is a powerful and innovative treatment for not only Lyme disease and its biofilms, but also viral, fungal, and some parasitic infections. I simply observed something already happening in an industry, and wondered what would happen if that same treatment were used in specific applications such as highly resistant pathogenic infections like Lyme disease, or mycoplasma, or even HIV? What would happen if a group of compounds already being used to disinfect tap water, or to treat swimming pools was used in a very specific and safe way to do the same thing in the human body?

There are five specific paths of resistance that need to be addressed that both alternative and conventional medicine alike find difficult to answer.

They are:

1. The stealth nature and ability for the microbe to adapt to most treatments.
2. Intracellular infections, which give the germ a safe haven within its host.
3. Molecular bonds that take place between a virus and a cell. (Lyme disease can often have a viral or mycoplasmal coinfection component).

4. Biofilms that allow entire infectious colonies to proliferate virtually unaffected by most antibiotics and non-drug treatments alike.

5. Remote penetration of connective tissues and bone for evasive harboring.

Unless a therapy at least in part addresses each of these, the infection may endure indefinitely, or remain what conventional medicine calls "chronic" at best, "incurable" at worst. All that is, is a term that was created from a paradigm that says, "Our toolbox doesn't have the tool needed to solve that problem." As has been stated before, if you choose to live in that paradigm, then don't complain if you have a leaky faucet with only a hammer and screw driver to work with. Leave the paradigm and you will find in it another toolbox that contains the tools you need to solve your problem.

For many years it was believed that the resistance seen in Lyme disease was exclusively from its pleomorphic capacity which allowed it to become stealth in the body. Each of the variable forms seems to possess its own defensive capabilities, which may be unique to that particular expression. For example a spirochete may find it extremely difficult to hide its presence due to its high profile and highly virulent outer surface proteins being so toxic. It is also highly susceptible to antimicrobials. But its advantage is its motility, or ability to easily move about in the body to evade immune cells. On the other hand, cysts are just the opposite in that they remain quiet and still, yet the shedding of outer surface proteins to expose a less alerting membrane makes it much less vulnerable to immune attack. The same could be said of L-forms, which also tend to hide inside immune cells, the very cells necessary for their destruction. Granular forms may be the most resistant of all. But no matter how Bb expresses itself, resistance is only a matter of constantly remaining a step ahead of an immune response initiated by adaptive immunity, or by whatever antimicrobial happened to be used. Bb simply alters its form or lipoprotein expression.

What we learned about plasmids and protein expressions was that although Bb may be in a constant state of flux and alteration as it makes defensive maneuvers in the body in order to protect itself, any individual bacterium can only express one bit of lipoprotein-altering information at a time. In order to change forms, it must alter its proteins. It doesn't take a rocket scientist therefore to understand that the taking of one or even two antimicrobials at a time will only affect whatever expression the bacteria happen to be vulnerable to at that moment. As it changes however, due to quorum sensing, an entire colony within an infected individual may morph into a completely resistant form or forms. Even the taking of some macrolide antibiotics which work by inhibiting protein synthesis to slow or prevent the morphing of Bb has not resulted in the eradication of chronic Lyme disease. So that is obviously not the answer either since antibiotics can only work when the bacteria are metabolizing the drug, which slows down when reverting to certain low metabolic forms such as granular, cyst, or biofilm forms.

I had shared earlier that Bb's greatest strength was its greatest weakness. And if you can identify and exploit that weakness, you can beat it at its own game. It was also explained how that in a fortress, its defenses are placed where they are needed most. But if there are not sufficient forces to reinforce all walls, those that aren't will be vulnerable to attack.

The greatest breakthrough in my Lyme treatments occurred when I realized that taking several antimicrobials which attacked the Bb from various angles all at the same time may actually short circuit its transcription process. (Although multiple therapies are not a new concept, one rarely sees this approach for Lyme disease being taken by conventional medicine for the reasons stated earlier.) In other words rather than slow down or inhibit the process which is what macrolide anti-biotics do, it was preferential to actually speed it up to force it to overload and self-destruct. Each form, lipoprotein or membrane expression is going to have its own level of discomfort to whatever antimicrobial it is exposed to. So even the "incubating" forms will be stimulated or forced to change based upon their vulnerability. This was the secret that Bb has been hiding. And that is exactly the opposite of how the conventional medicine model has been attempting to resolve chronic Lyme disease, and why it has been such a failure up until now.

When I learned that taking certain antimicrobial compounds concurrently as well as rotating them in such a fashion that their combined antimicrobial activities were attacking Bb simultaneously from various angles, it simply couldn't express all of its defensive forms or communicate properly with its own gene or plasmid-pool to retrieve the necessary defensive information. Thus it short circuited itself. This exponentially increased the speed of recovery from the illness.

Although taking a shotgun approach by indiscriminately using several different anti-pathogen non-drug products all at once would be a quantum leap compared to the traditional approach of simply using one or two products, later we will discuss a game-plan that uses specifically chosen products which are optimal. Natural substances do not have anywhere near the same interaction conflicts as drugs. Some herbal and other natural products may not however be ideal when combined. Although I have never personally experienced any negative combinations, in theory this is possible. So some caution would be advised when taken together.

Not an army of one

Now that we have identified Bb's weakness, and will later devise some protocols for monopolizing on its susceptibilities to certain combinations of therapies, there remains one final obstacle to finally being rid of the disease—biofilms. The good news is that the same strategy of using multiple or mixed therapies to deal with pleomorphic-based chronic Lyme disease, can also be used to slowly erode biofilms.

Currently, the primary therapy being used to aid in the destruction of biofilms is with the use of certain enzymes. Some of these have been discussed already under the heading of Healing Substances. As it was explained in the chapter on biofilms, each bacterium posseses its own characteristic exopolysaccharide matrix that would be vulnerable to highly specific enzymes. Since we don't yet know what specific enzyme would potentially dissolve Borrelia Burgdorferi biofilms, in general, the use of fibrinolytic and proteolytic enzymes seem to be having an effect on biofilms to varying degrees, regardless of the specie of bacteria. These enzymes may not have a direct killing effect on an individual bacterium by themselves. So they are taken on an empty stomach prior to taking antibacterial substances. This way the film is disrupted and immediately followed with germicides to kill the released bacteria. Some individuals and doctors have used certain enzymes such as serrapeptase, nattokinase, or lumbrokinase, as I myself have as well. However, theoretically using a more varied approach would seem wiser since it is not known which particular enzyme is going to be most effective depending on a number of factors.

Limited and mixed results have been reported by those taking these individual enzymes. Since, depending on how long a person has had Lyme disease, biofilms would have slowly formed over potentially many years, it is likely that the taking of enzymes to theoretically degrade biofilms would also take time to reverse. However enzymes alone do not address all components of biofilms, and are not ideal as stand-alone treatments.

LOOKING BACK

Until the development of broad-based Lyme disease treatments that incorporate varied substances that attack Lyme disease from different fronts, most of us Lyme sufferers didn't know any better but to play the game we were taught to play using the conventional medical model of using one or two antibiotics. Early on I learned not to play that game, and found success using a more natural approach. Of course the concept of chronic vs acute was not the focus of my thoughts. I didn't care what it was called. I only knew I was determined to rid myself of the horrid disease. As time passed I, like others, began to learn what worked and remained vigilant to pursue higher levels of success. However once the acute phase and its symptoms were more or less resolved and/or manageable, my subsequent attempts at addressing the chronic aspect of the disease seemed to be taking place at a snails pace crawl. Looking back over the years and many tens of thousands of dollars in treatment expenses, probably somewhere in the range of 25-30 doctors in total I have seen in one capacity or another, and the health food store owner's retirement plan I helped pay for, I still could not believe how resistant this infection was. Yet in other ways, hearing many of the testimonials of Lyme sufferers that after literally 15, 20 and 25 years on antibiotics and many still were deeply suffering, I felt that my progress was light years ahead of these folks. It had taken some 10+ years, and virtually all of my systemic symptoms were gone. No more chronic fatigue, head-aches, severe depression and Lyme-rage, profuse night sweats, neurological symptoms such as sensitivity to light, numbness and tingling in the hands and fingers, skin problems, joint pain, etc. And probably less than 5% of my therapies involved anti-biotics. Yet admittedly, most of those years were experimental and not nearly as productive as they could have been had I known then what I know now.

Yet something was still holding on that hadn't yet been completely resolved. In fact I had reached a point where no matter what therapies I employed, what combinations I used, and what dosages I took, I just couldn't progress any further. The infection had become entrenched so deeply in areas around old injuries, the lower back and sacrum, and up the spine forming a kind of Lyme meningitis, that nothing seemed to affect it. The original tendon tear injury in my lower back from 12 years earlier that set off my Lyme disease to begin with had become so debilitated and chronically painful, that I at times wondered if I had evolved into the Neanderthal man from the pain and limping.

I was convinced beyond any doubt that what had been taking place over the many years of Lyme treatments was that biofilms had formed around these old injuries, and moved up my spinal column into the lower neck. (And it was the manner in which I employed the conventional model that actually entrenched the chronic aspect of the disease.) The lack of systemic symptoms signaled to me that virtually all of the planktonic bacterial infection was gone. But that they had now accumulated into colonies along the old injuries of my knee, old tendon tear, spread into the adjacent sacrum area and up the spinal column, was rather apparent since I had never stopped taking some form of bacteriocide during the entire time. I, like many others had only recently taken a serious look at the potential of biofilms to be the contributing factor in this final stage of the disease.

However now it was all coming together to make perfect sense. Although I had known of biofilms for many years, I had never taken biofilms all that seriously since there were few treatment options available for them anyways. Up until these past several years, very little was known of the potential to degrade or erode biofilms. The only thing we knew was to continue to take our germ killing therapies, not knowing that we were only addressing a part of the problem, and actually making the infection more difficult to kill by doing so. However as biofilm research has been coming to the forefront as of late, attention is now being focused on treating these resistant fortresses. An understanding of biofilms and their development in chronic Lyme patients finally vindicates and explains the resistance experienced by those of us who have been in the battle for more than many years. Those pundits that have denied the existence of chronic Lyme disease since its discovery will finally have their mouths silenced once and for all, or be made known for the fools they have been making of themselves all along.

Now that my attention was focused on the real problem, I could divert my energies to finding the real solution. Although I had been aware of the potential for certain enzymes, as well as herbs such as Sanicle, Haritaki, Sparganium and Zedoaria, Carnivora, even Goldenseal to some extent to address biofilms, I wanted to open myself up to the possibility of a more potent therapy that would shorten the time necessary to resolve biofilms. What I learned may not be for everyone. But it was exactly what I was looking for. Here is how it evolved.

OXIDANTS

Approximately mid-2008 I first learned of a product called MMS being used by some in the Lyme community to try to eliminate Lyme disease. This was the name given for sodium chlorite which is a chemical commonly used to disinfect water. Except it had the added benefit of being activated with a mild acid which made it many times more powerful by causing it to release an even more potent gas called *chlorine dioxide*. Although many of us Lyme sufferers were showing some remarkable improvement using MMS, many beyond any former antibacterial medications previously used, it wasn't the ultimate cure for Lyme that everyone had been hoping for.

This was the second time in my life that I had been exposed to what some call *oxidation therapy*. This term encompasses many different applications of the administration of some form of oxidant. Many years earlier I had learned of hydrogen peroxide being used in IV's as well as taken orally, which I had also experienced first hand. So I was very aware of the effectiveness of using oxygen as a powerful anti-pathogenic.

I had also spent a great deal of time researching the use of ozone in medicine, as well as had many opportunities to apply its uses. In addition to owning my own ozone generator, I had experienced the benefits of ozone saunas, IV ozone therapy, insufflations, ozonating water, and inhalations thru oils. I was able to experience the effectiveness of ozone for my candida infection, as well as to clear the toxicity I had developed from my many years being over-exposed to toxic chemicals.

However with all I had learned about oxygen therapies, it was an observation I had made from the water treatment industry that lead me to explore a remarkable application for Lyme. One day I was on youtube doing a biofilm search. One video popped up that caught my attention. A company by the name of Miox had developed a device that was being used to treat the water in swimming pools and for use by municipalities in their water treatment plants. They were showing a before and after video. In the first, it showed a camera scanning the inside of a water recirculation pipe that was completely lined with biofilms. The water flowing thru the pipe was being treated with a common chemical normally used to clean swimming pools called *sodium hypochlorite*. Although this "chlorine" generally kills planktonic bacteria in the water, it seemed to be having no effect on biofilm formation. In fact, it may have been promoting its formation by driving the bacteria to protect themselves from the chlorinated water.

The next video showed that same water pipe 22 days later after having the water treated with what was being called *mixed oxidants*. The biofilms were completely eliminated. The exclusive use of sodium hypochlorite had been replaced by the mixed oxidants which had totally dissolved the biofilms. It was a rather dramatic demonstration that led me to question, what are mixed oxidants?

There are a number of different compounds and substances which are called "oxidants", or sometimes called "chor-oxidants". Some of

253

these are chlorine dioxide, chlorine, sodium hypochlorite, calcium hypochlorite, singlet oxygen, ozone, hydrogen peroxide, sodium chlorite, hydroxyl radicals, sodium hypobromate, and various combinations such as peroxone and peracetate, and others. Sodium hypochlorite possesses strong antiviral, antifungal, antibacterial, and antiprotozoa capabilities alone. However just as using a single antibiotic in medicine only attacks a bacterium from a particular angle, so any particular oxidant only "oxidizes" or transfer electrons to or from a microbe based upon its own limited capacity. And just as attacking a bacterium from multiple angles increases the odds of killing it, so using various or mixed oxidants also degrade the biofilm which is made up of various complexes.

Biofilms have been a very common nuisance in the water treatment industry. They resist chlorine, and so over time will build up along the water distribution lines. With the introduction of mixed oxidants, water lines become clear and free from recontamination once they have been treated. Additionally, mixed oxidants have been shown to have a much broader kill or deactivation capacity to a larger variety of microbes than chlorine alone. Also, since you are using a greater variety of oxidants, the dependence upon any one particular oxidant becomes reduced, and so reduces problems sometimes associated with the build-up of unwanted or dangerous by-products.

For instance, Trihalomethanes are a group of chemicals which are potentially produced as a by-product of chlorination. As chlorine reacts with various contaminants it can form any number or combination of chemicals in this group. According to some studies, these have potential carcinogenic properties, and have been criticized by some who say the use of chlorine in water is unsafe. However, there is a lot of controversy surrounding the topic of chlorination and the various citings of potentially dangerous by-products since virtually all of these have been animal studies using much higher concentrations than would be normally be considered relevant. One must always weigh the risks with the benefits. Most likely these potential risks might be considered pertinent only in the context of long-term and/or over-exposure.

These oxidants, when combined actually appear to be safer and more effective than when taken as individual treatments. Some of them dissipate very quickly, but are much more volatile and active against pathogens. For instance chlorine dioxide and ozone are both gases which only last a short time once activated. But they leave behind very little residual by-products. By using them in a mixed combination, individually much smaller amounts are necessary.

Beyond a single illustration of the effectiveness of using mixed oxidants against biofilms in water treatment applications, they have also been used in the paper making industry and water cooling towers for decades as well for this same purpose. However the reasoning behind using hypochlorous acid and other oxidants originates from our own immune system's use of what also happen to be common household disinfectants. Much the same way that mixed oxidants are extremely potent against pathogens and their biofilms, human white blood cells use a very similar process in the digestion of bacteria. So the idea behind this therapy parallels the processes of some of our own immune cells.

Upon learning of the potential for using chlor-oxidants, I began to consider the possibilities of using them internally not only for their strong capacity to kill all sorts of pathogens, but also for their powerful anti-biofilm activities. Since they had already proven to work against both of these problems, and since they were already being used internally in everyday applications in a safe manner, it seemed to be only a matter of increasing their amounts within safe levels to see if they held the same potential to destroy biofilms in disease conditions in the body.

There is a science behind the production of mixed oxidants. They involve dissolving salt in water to form a brine solution. Then an electrical charge is applied to the solution. At one electrode sodium hypochlorite and a number of mixed oxidants such as hydrogen peroxide, ozone, and chlorine dioxide are produced. At the other electrode hydrogen is released as a gas from the water, but is not part of the end solution. The end product is added to contaminated water for purification.

Upon first consideration of writing this book, it was my intention to describe individual chlor-oxygen based treatments that are currently being used for a number of applications, for instance, MMS (aka master mineral solution), ozone, hypochlorous acid, etc. This was done to make the reader aware how they work, and to share some of the benefits that have been experienced by others. However as my research advanced, I came to an understanding as to how to make these various oxidants work better together than as individual therapies. I am nonetheless providing them here for you to become aquainted with them to lay the groundwork for their use in a different manner than is described.

The following 4 products are not being recommended as stand alone therapies for Lyme disease even though they are being explained as if they were. This is only for descriptive purposes.

MMS, (formerly called Miracle Mineral Supplement, now changed to Master Mineral Solution) actually starts as a simple compound called Sodium Chlorite. It has been used extensively in industry for a long time as a powerful antimicrobial agent. It has also been used by consumers for water purification for years. So the efficacy of this product has already been established, and sodium chlorite by itself is already known for its potent antimicrobial effects. Jim Humble, a geologist discovered that Sodium Chlorite can be potentized exponentially by activating it using a small amount of citric acid. In the unactivated form it is alkaline in water, but when activated with certain acids such as acetic or citric acid it releases chlorine dioxide gas. Chlorine dioxide (ClO2) is a very powerful oxidant, used in disinfecting of water and many other uses in industry. It is this gas that gives off its characteristic chlorine smell, yet does not chlorinate the water itself. This is because ClO2 is very stable in solution and does not hydrolyze as chlorine gas does. So it remains in solution as a gas. This is what creates the highly potent affect. At the dosages suggested, the safety of this product does not appear to be in question as toxicity reports are non-existent at these levels. (However the FDA has recently told consumers to cease using MMS. This should be your first clue that it is in fact a very potent product. The warnings were the result of some that reported some nausea after taking the product. This has already been discussed. It is not a toxic factor or safety issue. It is listed for your information nonetheless.)

Quite a number of uses for a myriad of pathogen-based diseases have been reported with incredible results. For instance it had been used to treat some 75,000 people with malaria with reports that virtually every person recovered, many within literally hours of taking the product. It is being used in Africa to treat AIDS patients. When combined with Calcium Hypochlorite, most were reported to be symptom free with negative PCR tests for HIV within several weeks.

Reports have been given by thousands of people taking the product from all over the world testifying of incredible cures of all sorts of conditions. Many with Lyme disease have taken the product with good success. Although this therapy probably lists near the top of all Lyme therapies for its killing ability, there are too many variables to rely on MMS as a sole therapy, as there are no reports I am aware of that it has completely cured Lyme. Borrelia, being a *microaerophile* means that it is capable of existing only in small amounts of oxygen. Most bacteria do not possess antioxidant capabilities. However in rare cases some have developed this capacity. An example of a pathogen that has this ability is staphylochocus aureus, and is why it has become resistant to many antibiotics which attacks the cell wall. Given Borrelia Burgdorferi's complex plasmid system, it would not be unexpected that it may develop some capacity to inhibit oxidation at some level.

However I personally had far more benefit taking MMS than any antibiotic I have ever taken. Although for especially ill patients it is recommended to start out taking one drop or less, then work up slowly due to the strong herx it can give, I personally started taking 3 drops on the first day. The dosages and manner in which it is taken varies depending on the condition you are taking it for, and the recommendations have changed by Jim Humble since it was first introduced. But it seems that with the resistance displayed by Lyme disease it has been suggested it is better to take MMS in small consistent doses every hour or two, than single large doses taken a few times a day. This seems to have demonstrated the most benefit for nearly every application it has been taken for. This is because the chlorine dioxide gas which is released after being activated, once ingested, only remains active for no more than two hours in the body, after which it dissipates into harmless water and sodium chloride or salt.

There is a specific method whereby the MMS needs to be taken for optimum benefit.

I had taken MMS rather consistently for around 2 ½ months using this method, gradually increasing the dosage to higher and higher amounts. I suppose I had been averaging taking around 12 drops every 2-3 hours. The most difficult aspect of taking MMS is quite frankly the chlorine smell. You just don't ever seem to get use to it. It is not much of a problem at lower doses, but becomes more intolerable at higher dosages, even when putting them into capsules before drinking them down with water (optional). I will say that I did experience very pronounced herxes. And I think that due to the oxygen and chlorine released, not only does it have a direct killing affect, but probably also destroys much of the toxins as well. For several hours after taking MMS you will notice a pronounced feeling of being very alert, clear headed, and calm due to the high oxygen release. This probably explains why some people don't experience quite as a severe herx reaction as one would normally experience when killing off such a high bacterial load in such a short period of time. The antitoxin activity of chlorine dioxide appears to be considerable. But based upon the responses from others and the inability to completely eradicate the disease, it seems rather apparent that there are either some forms of Bb that are resistant to chlorine dioxide, or more likely that it resides in biofilms and cannot be reached.

I have a different take on Jim Humbles recommendation to take MMS consistently at lower levels rather than the higher levels, at least for Lyme disease, for this reason: chlorine dioxide, like many other kinds of anti-microbial substances is very much dosage dependent. Higher concentrations will do what lower dosages cannot. This seems rather obvious to understand. So no matter how often you take MMS, if the concentration is not high enough to penetrate the bacterial cell membrane, it simply needs to be raised until it does. I say this because I definitely experienced a comparable increase in herx reactions as I continually increased the dosages.

Sidenote: Dr. Joseph Burrascano MD, a prominent Lyme physician has spent many years treating Lyme patients and researching Lyme disease. One of the principles he observes with regard to antibiotic treatments is that "Kill kinetics indicate that a large spike in blood and tissue levels is more effective than sustained levels".[1] This principle is likely true with regards to most non-drug antimicrobials as well. The taking of single or pulsed high dosed substances seems to hold a greater advantage at the direct killing of Bb, particularly given what we know of its propensity to morph very quickly to evade or adapt to antibacterial substances.

One note of interest. It is reported that nausea being experienced while you are taking the MMS is a warning to back off because you are probably killing off too many pathogens all at once, as well as detoxifying too fast. I would agree that this is no doubt true, and was part of my experience as well. There is simply no reason to rush the therapy so fast that it makes you sick. However I will also say that not all the nausea was from die off. Although I experienced no negative or toxic side affects in any way in the 2 ½ months I took MMS, the very taking of the product with its release of chlorine dioxide gas is so distasteful that the body naturally cringes and wants to expel it. It can make you quiver even at the thought of it. At the higher dosages, it takes a lot of control to keep it down. And I personally experienced vomiting several times from taking too high of dosages too fast. You finally reach a level where the body simply won't allow you increase the dosage any further because it becomes intolerable. You just cannot process the high dosages without expelling them. It is just a natural reflex from being so distasteful.

I can recall returning home from Mexico having experienced no benefit from the therapy I had received there, the money I had wasted, and a deep feeling of hopelessness and depression that followed. I had hoped to be able to try MMS intravenously while there since I wasn't able to take it in high enough doses orally to receive much more benefit than I already had. Since they weren't willing to administer the MMS after I had already arrived, I felt like I wasted a trip. In fact I became so disgusted that when I returned home I threw caution to the wind and decided to take the largest dose of MMS I had ever taken hoping to receive some benefit—about 34 drops within a single hour taken in two doses 20 minutes apart (not recommended!) I am certain there have been others who have experimented with even higher doses than that in such a short period of time. But for me, it was all I could do to keep it down. And within a few hours I was experiencing a definite herx reaction. I did the same thing again a day or two later at about the same level. But this time the herx was barely noticeable. I was never able to exceed that amount again as my body simply became so repulsed by the smell and taste of such high doses of the chlorine dioxide, I had to stop the therapy, at least in the higher dosages. But the lower smaller dosages taken over longer periods of time seemed to have little ongoing affect. So I felt it necessary to search for newer therapies since the MMS appeared to have done all it was able to do. At least for me, it simply required doses so high in order to either oxidize the more resistant forms of the bacteria, or needed such higher concentration levels in order to go deeper into the tissues to reach them, that the body could not tolerate it. But by now my bacterial load had been significantly reduced, and I was feeling better than I had in 10 years.

MMS can be purchased online. Be sure to follow the instructions for mixing and avoid taking antioxidants such as vitamin C or juices containing them for around 4 hours before taking it. Then avoid them for around 2 hours after taking it. In my opinion, MMS is one of the most effective and safe products I have ever taken for my Lyme. But this has not been the experience of everyone taking the product.

Hypochlorous acid (HA)—Aka—Calcium Hypochlorite and MMS2. Hypochlorous acid is a compound naturally produced in the body. It is used by the innate immune system as a powerful bacteriocide. As white blood cells invade a microbe, they engulf it, and then release hypochlorous acid which acts as a powerful oxidizer to break down the germ. From a chemistry standpoint, HA is formed when calcium hypochlorite (CH) is added to water. In fact hypochlorous acid is actually a synonym for CH. HOCL is hydrogen, oxygen and chlorine. CH is not actually chlorine. But chlorine becomes available upon release in water. The product is actually a very low cost product that can be purchased at most neighborhood hardware or pool supply stores under the name "pool shock". This is actually what some people have mistakenly called "swimming pool chlorine". In the dry form it is called calcium hypochlorite. The solution form, what we call "chlorine", is sodium hypochlorite.

Upon first learning of this, I was a bit taken back and surprised to think that our immune systems actually make the same product we clean our pools and toilets with. We associate these with highly toxic and poisonous chemicals. And to think that someone actually came up with the idea of using it as a therapy seemed counterintuitive and down-right dangerous since calcium hypochlorite has warning labels on the product telling me to call the poison control center if swallowed!

Once I awoke from shock and picked myself up off the floor I learned all was not as it seemed. I learned that the manner in which it would be used is only in very small amounts put into a capsule. Calcium Hypochlorite and sodium hypochlorite are both already used in municipal water purification systems throughout the country as strong oxidizers of pathogens. This is what gives water its slight chlorine smell. The disclaimer placed on the product is for warning as an oxidizer and irritant, and for taking large amounts. However when taken in capsule form in tiny quantities with large amounts of water, in this safe manner, it can be extremely beneficial. In fact CH is readily used in survival situations to purify water, and is better to use than chlorine because it is more stable in the dry form. It should only be used in small amounts and when diluted. It can oxidize and irritate when taken in large amounts. But remember, the body has a certain capacity to shield itself against low level oxidation because cells utilize antioxidants as a form of defense mechanism, whereas most viruses and bacteria do not possess this capacity. Hence they are extremely vulnerable to oxidation from HA.

According to Jim Humble's website, he has been working with HIV victims in some clinics in Africa using activated Sodium Chlorite (MMS). He found that using MMS alone restored many to health and resulted in many negative PCR tests against HIV after about 3 weeks of continuous therapy. (They had no more symptoms of AIDS, and their tests were negative. You be the judge as to what that means.) However according to his testimony it didn't heal everyone. But when they added what he dubbed "MMS2" (calcium hypochlorite) to the therapy, in all the cases reported, everyone got well and all received negative PCR tests. He has also reported success in every case by those reporting back to him when using it for prostate cancer. I had personally used hypochlorous acid myself for about 3 weeks in conjunction with MMS therapy. According to reports it doesn't appear to interfere with medications.

Previously, it was mentioned that a company by the name of MIOX had developed water purification systems for swimming pools and municipal water treatment plants. This same company has designed a portable water purifier that has actually been tested and used by the US military. It is a small device that operates by using ordinary salt and batteries. A small amount of water is added to form a brine solution. This is then electrically charged and converted into—sodium hypochlorite—aka—hypochlorous acid and other mixed oxidants. (Both Calcium and Sodium Hypochlorite are reduced to hypochlorous acid.) This is then added to the unpurified water to kill germs.

Hypochlorous acid is taken by being put in a size 0 gelatin capsule. A very large glass of water is taken before administering. In this manner I have never experienced any kind of harmful effects whatsoever. However the chlorine smell is even far greater than MMS. The protocol, when taken in conjunction with MMS is: 3 drops of MMS every hour for eight hours. Concurrently 1 capsule of MMS2 is taken every 2 hours for eight hours per day. This was done for 3 weeks. Of course this was the therapy used in the HIV infected patients, and may not necessarily be optimum for Lyme victims should they so choose to experiment with the therapy. I personally did not do the therapy in this manner since it was too grueling, and work interfered with my ability to remain consistent. I took the capsules about 2 times per day for about 3 weeks on and off along with the MMS. However I wasn't consistent enough to give an honest and reasonable assessment of the therapy. Taking it in conjunction with MMS was simply too much for me personally. This therapy is not for the weak hearted, but may be one of the most powerful of all therapies. And I am not personally aware of any Lyme patients that have used this dual therapy. But it is listed here for informative purposes.

One additional note. Although taking anti-oxidants concurrently with activated sodium chlorite and calcium hypochlorite are contraindicated due to their ability to reduce the combo's effectiveness, they are recommended outside of the 2 hour window when not taking them. For instance if your last dose of the oxidants was at 8:00PM, you could take your antioxidants at 10:00PM before bedtime. In addition to aiding in sleep, melatonin is one of the most potent hydroxyl free radical scavengers known, even surpassing Vitamin C and E. So taking melatonin, astaxanthin, C and E would be good supplements at bedtime when doing this therapy.

H2O2—Hydrogen peroxide has traditionally been used externally to disinfect wounds and as a mouthwash. According to William Douglas MD, H2O2 in the body has many benefits given it is an essential metabolite. It stimulates the production of interferon for use by killer cells and monocytes,[2] lowers blood pressure,[3] is used by granulocytes to fight infections,[4] can act much like insulin by transporting sugar thru the body,[5] creates intracellular thermogenesis in the presence of CoQ10 for the generation of heat and activation of intracellular processes,[6] is a part of the process necessary for the production of prostagladins.[7]

However it has also been used in IV form by some physicians to oxygenate the blood and to kill pathogens in the bloodstream. IV Hydrogen Peroxide Therapy has been used by even conventional medical doctors for many years. I had this treatment many years ago to help with my allergy and candida infection. Physicians have used it for cancer and tumors, gangrene, sarcoidosis, Multiple Sclerosis, lupus, depression, candida, chronic fatigue, and a whole host of other diseases. Just as any other treatment, it is not a cure-all, but has shown remarkable improvement and in many cases complete cures of untreatable conditions.

Yet it has also been used orally by individuals for various infections. This is usually done by using food grade or 35% hydrogen peroxide diluted in water. (The 3% USP grade purchased at the grocery store may contain undesireable impurities.) Although the IV administration of H2O2 has it critics, the oral form has even more. This is due to potential dangers that are often cited. One Japanese study showed that the administration of oral hydrogen peroxide to mice caused some to develop erosion of the stomach lining, tumors, and even cancer.[8] What we do not know however is what the comparable human dosage that they were using would be. It must have been an extreme dosage for the mice. Animal studies are obviously often inconsistent with human studies. But even so, many thousands of people around the world are known to use hydrogen peroxide orally. Yet I have never heard of this happening in humans, nor have I seen any reports representing this. However this is of course theoretically possible at high enough doses or concentration levels. H2O2 is known to convert to damaging superoxide free radicals. Although they are very short lived, they can have a cumulative effect if not given sufficient recuperative time and protective antioxidants.

There are often two primary problems cited using hydrogen peroxide orally as a stand-alone therapy. First, the body produces *catalase* which is an enzyme which performs dismutation, or the separation of oxygen from the H2O2, leaving singlet oxygen and water. This deactivates the H2O2 very quickly in order to prevent oxidative damage. In intravenous administration, this occurs within 2 seconds of being injected into the vein.[9] So, orally administered, it will have similar decomposition rates. This doesn't leave much time to oxidize pathogens in the bloodstream, and it is not likely to have much affect on deeper pathogens.

This leads to the second problem with oral H2O2. In some pathogens, studies have been done which indicate that H2O2 inactivation for viruses and bacteria requires long contact times as well as high concentrations, putting oral H2O2 as a stand-alone therapy at a disadvantage. Also, H2O2 has been cited as being 50 times weaker than hypochlorous acid as an antipathogen.[10] This is the reason why our own immune cells convert H2O2 into mixed oxidants and hypochlorous acid rather than using H2O2 alone.

However, what is often ignored by those critics of H2O2 therapy is that the dismutation of oxygen from the H2O2 molecule does in fact raise oxygen levels in the bloodstream, which lasts far after the dismutation process has occurred. Thus the separated and gaseous singlet oxygen is utilized by cells for respiration, deactivation of toxins, acts as a free radical to oxidize pathogens, and is used in the conversion processes of many cellular activities.

Much remains a mystery with this therapy. Only very diluted amounts of H202 are ever introduced into the body. Yet oxygen has been both measured and observed following the administration of H2O2 for far longer than would be expected. Dr. David G. Williams in an article, "The Many Benefits of Hydrogen Peroxide" wrote:

> *The small amount of oxygen present couldn't be solely responsible for the dramatic changes that take place. Dr. Charles Farr, a strong proponent of intravenous use, has discovered another possible answer. Dr. Farr has shown that hydrogen peroxide stimulates enzyme systems throughout the body. This triggers an increase in the metabolic rate, causes small arteries to dilate and increase blood flow, enhances the body's distribution and consumption of oxygen and raises body temperature.*[11]

So it appears that the benefits one receives from HP therapy goes far beyond simply raising oxygen levels. It stimulates cellular systems and enzymes to raise metabolic functions far beyond the oxygen benefits alone.

When taking H2O2 orally, one experiences an activation of senses, is more alert and awake, feels more energetic, yet calm. However, as is the intended use as an antimicrobial, it can be followed by herx reactions. A long list of uses and benefits have been experienced by those using the therapy including diabetes, viral infections, periodontal disease, allergies, sore throat, liver problems, asthma, insect bites, detoxification, all sorts of microbial infections, etc. It can be applied full strength (35%) directly to skin as a wart remover. (Guard healthy skin.)

As a protocol, it is suggested to use only diluted 35% grade. This grade is very potent, and should be kept in a glass bottle in a freezer to keep it stable longer. It will oxidize the skin white and slightly sting. Rinse for several minutes if this occurs. Usually it is started slowly at several drops in 12+ ozs of water. Then slowly build up to three times per day. The same guidelines as taking MMS apply to H2O2. It should be taken on an empty stomach, and away from antioxidants. I personally used this therapy when I had candidiasis and experienced no gastrointestincal side effects of any kind. However I personally would not exceed 20 drops per dose. Even that is high for most people. As in every other kind of therapy, each individual is different, and is responsible for his/her own actions. So do your research, and put safety first.

There is a tremendous amount of research on the use of hydrogen peroxide therapy. There are books written about it as well as countless articles on the web. This is one of those therapies which you will often see being derided even by physicians who warn of "dangers" of "unproven" cures along with the hundreds of other effective and safe therapies they scoff at. A good book on the subject was written by William Campbell Douglas MD called *Hydrogen Peroxide Medical Miracle*. However the topic of oral H202 as a stand-alone therapy is not being recommened here for Lyme disease since in my opinion it would require unnecessarily high doses, and still would not match the effectiveness of mixed therapies, which require much smaller amounts of each oxidant.

Ozone—Ozone may be the granddaddy of antimicrobial treatments. Its third oxygen molecule is readily released and oxidizes dangerous and radical toxins, microbial and chemical molecules which themselves could damage healthy tissues and cells if not neutralized. It has been used as one of the most successful treatments for fungal, viral, and bacterial infections of all sorts. These germs simply do not possess natural defenses against such radical oxidation.

Many have used ozone to varying degrees to reduce their bacterial load, and symptoms for their own Lyme disease as it can be used in many forms. It is readily absorbed thru the skin in ozone saunas, rectal insufflations, autohemotherapy, direct injections into the blood, oil-bubbled inhalations (not recommended), ozonated water, and other means. Small portable ozone machines can be purchased inexpensively.

Ozonated water can be an effective means of getting it into the bloodstream, albeit in small quantities. The internet is flooded by testimonials of users having testified of using nothing but ozonated water as an effective means of improving their Lyme symptoms. However ozone is not readily retained in water long. Therefore the use of an ozone diffuser is highly recommended. This will atomize the bubbles to make them much more dispersed in the water and allow a significantly higher concentration than just using the larger bubbles from the end of the hose. Colder water also holds the ozone longer. So adding ice to the water while bubbling increases its potency. Drinking ozonated water continuously throughout the day will advance any therapy you are currently using.

Ear insufflations are another effective way to get ozone into the bloodstream. I had been aware of this method of administration and actually used it during my several year bout with candida infection many years ago, but didn't realize at the time that the ozone was actually being absorbed into the bloodstream. I learned of this when I heard the story of a man that had been given several months to live by his oncologist for cancer. He used this method to cure himself of the cancer.[12] The end of the ozone air hose is placed about an inch from the ear canal. The gas is introduced thru the ear drum. Due to the drum being semi-permeable, it is absorbed into the bloodstream. The major concentration areas affect the eyes, sinuses, and the brain, although small amounts will be circulated throughout the body. Only do this several minutes per ear. Then build up slowly to 10 minutes per day if tolerable.

Books, research articles, and the internet are rich with information about ozone. The real difficulty is that once again the FDA has attempted to restrict its use by denying it has any medical value. It seems pointless to address the reasons for this since we already are aware of the crimes against US citizens and God this organzition is guilty of. An excellent paper, *Scientific And Medical References Proving Ozone's Validity As A Medical Treatment,* written by Ed McCabe verifying and documenting the history of the medicinal use of ozone in the US is worth reading.[13]

The use of ozone is another weapon that can be added in your battle against Lyme. A number of people have used ozone in various forms to significantly improve their symptoms and return to normal lives. It is now being used more and more as a standard therapy. However this is one that won't be available from your conventional practitioner any time soon.[14]

IMMUNITY'S USE OF MIXED OXIDANTS

We have also known that our own immune cells use various oxidants to destroy pathogens. Hydrogen peroxide, or H2O2, is naturally generated by antibodies and T-cells as a means to deactivate or destroy pathogens.[15] One example is the white blood cell, also called a leukocyte. These cells actively migrate to areas of trauma and infection. There, a certain type of leukocyte called a neutrophil, attempts to engulf bacteria using a process called *phagocytosis*, by forming an evelope or what is known as a *phagosome* to enclose the germ within itself. Then several different processes or means by which to kill the bacteria can occur. However one primary action is oxidation.

Areas of infection and injury are often low in oxygen due to impaired cellular respiration. This places stress upon leukocytes which require higher amounts of oxygen during the phagocytosis process. Leukocytes begin taking in oxygen for the production of hydrogen peroxide. This has been termed the "respiratory burst". Then as the bacterium becomes engulfed within the phagosome, other members of the cell migrate into the phagosome called *lysosomes*. These contain an important catalyst called *myeloperoxidase*. This myeloperoxidase combines with yet another chemical induced into the cell called a *halogen*, which is an element that possesses a certain ionic charge which allows a catalytic process to occur. When these three: H2O2, myeloperoxidase, and the halogen combine, a chemical reaction occurs wherein they form various oxidants and hypochlorite, aka—hypochlorous acid.[16] These various or mixed oxidants then drench the bacteria and kill it. This is the primary function of these white blood cells.

Part of the problem we mentioned in a previous chapter was that often areas in the body where injuries occur are very low in oxygen, and become a sort of safe haven for bacteria. This is because circulation becomes impaired, and cells become starved for oxygen. As neutrophils comb the area, they too require larger amounts of oxygen, sometimes as much as 50 times more than normal in order to generate H2O2. However since oxygen levels here are low, significantly less H2O2 is able to be produced. Subsequently myeloperoxidase is used up without a comparable conversion of hydrogen peroxide to hypochlorous acid and oxidants, thus creating a downward cascade effect called *myeloperoxidase deficiency* which can be acquired during times of acute or chronic infection. Dr. A. True Ott, PhD, ND also describes this as hypochlorous acid deficiency.[17] (Dr. Ott may also have been involved in the rediscovery of the lost Koch glyoxilide, and may explain the effectiveness of his 02 therapy.)

This means that the effectiveness of neutrophils becomes significantly impaired particulary during chronic infection, as both the necessary production of hydrogen peroxide and its required myeloperoxidase becomes depleted. Subsequently the oxidation-based phagocytosis process can become dramatically impaired, and bacteria are now no longer constrained and are less threatened. This enables them to chronically reside within the infected, injured, or biofilm invaded tissue. (This in my opinion is a prime contributor of chronic Lyme disease.) Therefore the importance of oxidants in the process of bacterial destruction used by leukocytes is vital. One can see from this that it is not just oxygen itself that is having a direct oxidizing affect against pathogens. But by oxygen being released when taking hydrogen peroxide, ozone, and other oxidants, our own immune cell's capacity to destroy microbes becomes significantly enhanced by increasing availability of oxygen to be converted for use in the production of mixed oxidants.

As a special note, oxygen therapies of various sorts have had their critics. Perhaps the greatest criticism is the fear-mongering by accusations of unsafe and "dangerous therapies." And yet interestingly one virtually never hears of these dangers actually occurring. Of course caution should always be taken when using any kind of therapy. But given the hundreds of thousands of deaths each year by conventional medicine, it is the pot calling the kettle black, when the kettle is not actually black.

And of course seldom are these warnings ever backed up by any scientific proof or even examples of actual dangers. The few examples that are given, are almost always by some who have used dosages and/ or frequencies that exceeded rational or safe guidelines, or were done with animal studies that don't always react the same as humans. They are simply called unproven and unsafe. Perhaps someone needs to tell our bodies that its use of oxygen in this manner should not be used, because it is unsafe and unproven. In fact, the concentration levels of these oxidants used by our own cells must be high enough to destroy bacterial cell membranes and components, while at the same time within the margin of safety against self-destruction.

To my knowledge, no one has observed an actual Borrelia biofilm in vivo. However Lyme biofilms are known to exist due to the fact that they have been observed in vitro, what is known of their behavior, and the conditions in the body that develop that are consistent with this model. Additionally, due to the complexity of Borrelia and its adaptive capabilities, and due to its high antibiotic resistance once the major symptoms have been reduced, there appears to be few other explanations. Those critics of chronic Lyme who suggest "post-Lyme disease" being an autoimmune condition have an even more difficult time explaining this condition since this argument doesn't align with reality. How does a disease that no longer exists relapse? In fact one of the names given to one form of Lyme disease is "relapsing fever", wherein the condition periodically returns again and again. This only occurs if it was never resolved in the first place. Post-Lyme theory is based upon an unverifiable assumption that anti-biotics have completely killed the bacterial infection. This does not take into account the agility that is known of pleomorphism. Given that we also know that biofilms aid in bacterial resistance against antibiotics, and that by and large it is the planktonic bacteria that are going to promote systemic symptoms, which become significantly reduced after antibiotic therapy; these facts are completely consistent with the chronic Lyme disease model. In fact, it is rather astonishing knowing what we now understand of Bb that post-lyme syndrome is actually accepted by anyone at all.

Having given a description of biofilms in an earier chapter, and having now demonstrated an example of one type of immune cell that would be involved in the attempts to eradicate these bacterial colonies, it is easy to see why it would be difficult for immune cells to remove biofilms. Phagocytes represent a group of different immune cells that have the capacity to engulf and devour bacteria. However this would be no easy task with biofilms due to the shear size. Although they attempt to do this, some non-lyme bacterial biofilms have been observed to fight back by paralyzing attacking enemies.[18] Biofilms may represent the most difficult form of Borrelia for our immune systems to challenge. In fact it may be that immunity is mostly ill-equipped to resolve this aspect of Lyme disease at all on its own. And so intervening using some of our own body's methods, only on larger scale, may be a valid option.

As one can see, the development of mixed oxidant therapy closely resembles the process used by our own immune cells. It has also become a highly valuable process used to disinfect one of the most important resources we have, water. And so is not just some made up out of thin air idea. It is based upon human immunity as well as proven disinfection processes that go on every day.

> You recall in an earlier chapter we described how the FDA has historically persecuted and jailed doctors that have attempted to use various oxygen therapies. We now know why this is. The accomplishments of oxygen therapies surpass drugs so effectively that some of their accomplishments included the actual elimination of HIV, and the heretofore unheard of cures of cancer beyond anything that pharmaceutical drugs have been able to touch. This is because the FDA is also aware of the enormous potential that oxygen therapies hold. They fear that the use of inexpensive cures such as oxygen therapies will topple the pharmaceutical empires that the FDA has sought to protect, and thus would lose their significance, importance and revelance. Please excuse the editorial opinion here, but the gravity and danger that the FDA poses to US citizens is beyond any enemy this country has ever faced. This is a rather obvious observation, not an accusation. We do not seek to demonize this organization. They have already done this on their own. Sometimes the truth needs to be spoken, even when it hurts.

Various or mixed oxidants have been used not only in industry for the elimination of biofilms, but our own immune cells destroy bacteria using a very similar process. Industry uses a special chemical process to produce mixed oxidants on demand for large scale purposes. However, to simplify and produce a solution that could be standardized and more easily prepared, I came up with my own version of mixed oxidants from products already available. I then combined them in water to be consumed. Below is an explanation of the process.

Needed:

- 28% sodium chlorite and a 50% solution of citric acid. (Aka MMS, available on the web.)
- Preferably 78%+ calcium hypochlorite powder. (Aka MMS2, also on the web.)
- 35% food grade hydrogen peroxide, although a weaker 17% solution could also be used by increasing the amount.
- Magnesium Oxide (Homozon with citric acid). (Activated to release oxidation with magnesium as a buffer).
- Himalayan Sea Salt
- A small portable ozone generator (can be purchased for as little as $75).
- Singlet oxygen (such as Vitamin O) could be added (optional)

**The following is only a sample formula and would need to be adjusted to each person's level of tolerance.

In a large tumbler or glass, fill 1 1/4 cups of spring water, add ¼ teaspoon sea salt and some ice cubes, and begin bubbling with the ozone generator. Depending on the ozone output, bubble for at least 3-5 minutes. 15-20 minutes or longer is even better. Remember to use a diffuser to significantly increase the ozone levels. (Ozone dissipates from the water very quickly. So keep this bubbling until immediately ready to mix and drink. Use cold water and some ice to increase ozone concentration.)

In another smaller glass prepare the MMS/sodium chlorite by putting 3 drops of 28% sodium chlorite solution in a dry cup or small container, then add 1 drop of 50% citric acid for every drop of sodium chlorite and lighly mix. Let stand for 3 minutes while it catalyzes into chlorine dioxide. (Note that some MMS formulations include 10% citric acid. In this case use 5 drops citric acid for every drop of sodium chlorite.)

Take your calcium hypochlorite powder and fill a size "0" gelatin capsule about half full. Also, you may want to keep the 35% Hydrogen Peroxide in a dropper bottle until ready to use in the freezer to preserve it (it will not freeze). Keep the bottle upright so as to keep the rubber from the dropper bottle dry. (Keeping the rubber wet with H2O2 may cause the rubber to expand.)

After the 3 minute activation period for the MMS, add about 1/2 cup of spring water to the MMS. Put 4 drops of 35% Hydrogen Peroxide into the same cup.

Now take this solution of activated MMS and Hydrogen Peroxide, and add 1 teaspoon Homozon. Pour them all into the 1 1/4 cup bubbling ozone water. Take your Calcium Hypochlorite capsule and drink it down with this 2 cup solution.

In a separate glass, add about 15 drops of 50% citric acid to ½ cup of water and immediately drink. This is to activate the Homozon. (The directions on the can say to drink the Homozon in a glass full of water followed by part of a squeezed lemon. This is so the citric acid in the lemon will activate the magnesium oxide much like it does to the MMS. However lemon also has vitamin C which will act as an antioxidant and actually reduce the effectiveness. This is why we say to use citric acid in place of the lemon.) Then sit down and relax.

A few words about the protocol. This is a powerful solution and you should only begin with a very small amount of each. In fact, I would only recommend using this therapy after you have used some of the other therapies first for some time in order to reduce your bacterial load to a minimum. Then graduate to this mixed oxidant therapy later. Start out with a very small dose. For instance one drop of the activated sodium chlorite and hydrogen peroxide to start with. Then build up slowly over time. Keep in mind that you may experience some nausea. If you do, you took too high of a dose. At lower doses, it is tolerable and usually causes little problem. However the chlorine smell is naturally strong. It is not a toxic affect that is going to harm you at these low levels. It is such a completely distasteful experience that the body simply wants to vomit it up if taken in too high of a dosage. This does not mean it is dangerous, and it is not a problem if you keep the dosages low and within a tolerable range. It is far better to take several small doses throughout the day, than only one or two large ones. After all, what good is a medicine if you can't keep it down?

Do not take this with food. I personally found that food can react with the oxidation process and actually make you more nauseated. It is best that you wait ideally for at least 3 hours or more after eating before taking this. Also, do not take with juices or any kind of anti-oxidants since they will neutralize the oxidants. Do not take antioxidants for at least 4 hours before taking the therapy. Once you have taken the mixed oxidants, wait at least 2 hours afterwards before taking food or antioxidants again. By then most of the oxidants will have dissipated in the body.

Ideally you would want to work up to three times per day. It can either be spread out or taken in 3 consecutive doses waiting a minimum of 2 hours between doses. Safety precaution: I have not received any negative side effects from using this, other than taking in too high concentration can make you feel nauseated. Sit or lie down after consuming for around 20-30 minutes to give time for any queezy feeling to subside.

Warning: Oxidants are strong free radicals. So long-term exposure can theoretically damage cells, although I personally never had any problems. Although our cells possess antioxidants to protect us from oxidation, this is a therapy you absolutely need to maintain high amounts of antioxidants between doses, preferably liposomal vitamin C to other forms, astaxanthin, vitamin E, glutathione, and melatonin at night. Over time, you may need to rest from this therapy to give your cells time to recuperate. (Although I did the therapy for nearly 4 weeks, 2 weeks would be optimal for most people. Then rotate by switching to another therapy while the body recuperates.) You will likely herx from this in the beginning stages. The advantage of this therapy is that it not only holds the potential to reverse biofilms, but acts as a biocide as well. As a long-term therapy, it should be rotated on a regular basis as any therapy addressing biofilms will necessarily take time.

Every therapy has its limitations. Any kind of oral therapy whether as a pharmaceutical drug or herbal product will obviously become less potent the deeper into the connective tissues it goes. That's were Borrelia likes to reside. Therefore, even though this therapy holds potential, it too is limited to its ability to penetrate deeply enough to remain active as it oxidizes. Once you take it and it enters the bloodstream, you want it to circulate as much and as deeply as possible, since oxidants by nature do not last long in the body before they dissipate. One thing I have found useful to do is to do some light activity such as walking or riding a bike, just enough to increase the circulation so that the oxidants are drawn into the tissues and cells more aggressively than if you were inactive and immobile. This should increase the effectivenss of the therapy. But remember to wait as least 20 or so minutes to let the stomach absorb the water into the bloodstream. This will additionally reduce nausea. Don't overdo it. It is more important to keep comfortable while doing this therapy and to keep it down, than to be overly active and nauseated. Listen to your body, and stay relaxed. That way you can receive maximum benefits.

Some of the advantages of this therapy are:

1. Not only is it effective against bacteria, but also is highly effective against viruses. This one therapy alone may eradicate most of the viral factors that contribute to chronic illness.
2. Oxidants are highly anti-inflammatory.
3. Since they are also effective against fungi and yeast, they hold a distinct advantage over antibiotics since they will not contribute to yeast over-growth and candidiasis. In fact, they will do just the opposite by reducing fungi colonies and protozoal infections which are often seen in patients on long-term antibiotics.
4. Although oxidants can temporarily create oxidative stress in the body, ceasing them periodically and allowing time for regeneration can actually reenergize immune cells by reducing anemic cells and stimulating the body to develop newer and stronger more potent immune cells.
5. Neutralize toxins making it easier for the immune system to do its job.

6. Increases energy availability and relieves fatigue. It will heighten senses and increase alertness, thereby acts to address chronic fatigue.
7. Has distinct antibiotic as well as anti-biofilm properties.
8. Alkalizes the blood.

While mixed oxidants hold a strong potential as an adjunct therapy against biofilms, alone they may not completely resolve Lyme infection (as no therapy is yet known to do this). Mixed oxidants anti-biofilm therapy is but one of the many therapies addressing biofilm reduction. It should not be used as a stand-alone therapy, but should be rotated along with the other biofilm reducing treatments mentioned in the next chapter.

ENDNOTES

1. *Advanced Topics in Lyme Disease Diagnostic Hints and Treatment Guidelines for Lyme and Other Tick Borne Illnesses* Sixteenth Edition Copyright October, 2008 Joseph J. Burrascano Jr. M.D. http://researchednutritionals. com/FactSheets/Burrascano's%20Advanced%20Topics%20in%20 Lyme%20Disease%20_12_17_08.pdf Retrieved Feb. 19, 2013
2. Douglas, W. C. *Hydrogen Peroxide Medical Miracle* Atlanta, Georgia Second Opinión Publishing, 1996 p. 16.
3. Ibid. p. 11.
4. Ibid. p. 19.
5. Ibid. p. 19.
6. Ibid. p. 20.
7. Ibid. p. 20.
8. Meyer, et al, J. Clin. Gastro., 3:31-31,1981.
9. Douglas, W. C. (1996). *Hydrogen Peroxide Medical Miracle* Atlanta, Georgia Second Opinión Publishing, 1996 p. 15.
10. *The phagocytes: neutrophils and monocytes.* Dale DC, Boxer L, Liles WC. Blood. Aug 2008;112:935-945.
11. *The Many Benefits of Hydrogen Peroxide* Dr. David G. Williams (Proceedings of the International Conference on Bio-Oxidative Medicine 1989, 1990, 1991). Posted July 17, 2003 http://educate-yourself.org/cancer/ benefitsofhydrogenperozide17jul03.shtml Retrieved Feb. 19, 2013

12. *Ozone: A Quick Overview* Ken Adachi http://educate-yourself.org/ozone/ Retrieved Feb. 3 2013

13. *Scientific And Medical References Proving Ozone's Validity As A Medical Treatment* Ed McCabe http://www.understandingozone.com/docs/Scientific_References_Ozone_ Therapy.pdf Retrieved Feb. 19, 2013

14. *The power of Ozone* Video series on youtube.com http://www.youtube.com/ user/thepowerofozone#p/a/u/2/4OwnT9XrCMY Retreived Feb. 19, 2013

15. *Mechanism for antibody catalysis of the oxidation of water by singlet dioxygen.* Wentworth, P., Jones, L. H., Wentworth, A. D., Zhu, X. Y., Larsen, N. A., Wilson, I. A., Xu, X., Goddard, W. A., Janda, K. D., Eschenmoser, A. & Lerner, R. A. (2001) Science 293, 1806-1811]

16. Guido Majno, Isabelle Joris. *Cells, Tissues, and Disease: Principles of General Pathology* Oxford University Press 2004 pp 419-422

17. Dr. Ott's Oxygen (02) Treatment and Therapy Scientific Data Sheet and Summary A. True Ott PhD, ND http://www.restandrepair.com/template/ research/oxygen-therapy/data_sheet.pdf Retrieved Feb. 3, 2013 also, http://www.meminerals.com/catalog/NewsLetter.asp?RecordID=7%2F9% 2F2009+12%3A57%3A48+PM

18. Sapi, E: *Biofilms: A New Hideout for* Borrelia burgdorferi? Lyme Times 2009 February p45.

CHAPTER 14

Anti-Biofilm Substances

Throughout these writings are mentioned substances that hold potential to address biofilms on some level. After all, chronic Lyme disease will never be resolved unless there is a resolution to the biofilm problem. One of the things I have personally observed both in others and in myself is that the taking of antibacterial agents, whether drug-based or alternative, may hold the potential to worsen biofilms. This is not to imply that anti-Lyme medicines are to blame for their development. After all, through culturing, biofilm formation has been observed in vitro in the complete absence of antimicrobial agents. But the very presence of Borrelia residing in vivo may be all that is necessary for this morphology to express itself. However, exposing bacteria to threatening substances is all that is necessary for biofilm advancement to progress. It is a two-edged sword.

With our understanding of biofilms, the entire face of Lyme disease has changed. As this phenomenon becomes even clearer over time, more and more Lyme-educated doctors will hopefully begin employing antibiofilm strategies as part of standard Lyme disease protocols. This will bring us one step closer to shortening the long-term nature of this illness in those new victims, and hope for recovery for those already chronically afflicted.

With the recent understanding of the magnitude of the biofilm problem, not just in Lyme disease, but other chronic bacterial-induced conditions, research is now turning en masse to explore this new frontier. Thus far, as for therapeutic regimens, we will examine what is currently being employed to see what benefit we might gain.

Some of the enzymes being used include, serrapeptase, nattokinase, lumbrokinase, glucoamylase, cellulase, pectinase, beta-glucanase, chitosanase, protease, peptidase, lysozyme, and others. Rechtsregulat, Wobenzyme, No Fenol are a few enzyme products showing some potential. Additionally, some specific herbal and non-drug products have been identified which also have antibiofilm activity such as haritaki, sparganium and zedoaria, sanicle, goldenseal (berberine), gallium nitrate, mixed oxidants, sodium chloride (salt), mannose, xylitol, and certain essential oils. Of these we will be briefly examine a few. However it should be pointed out that unless a thorough study is done on each of these, the importance may not be truly appreciated as to their potentials.

As was mentioned previously, biofilms by their very nature are highly resistant and protective which will not quickly resolve even with the best of therapies. Therefore as difficult as finding success gaining a foothold over systemic, planktonic-based Lyme may be, resolving biofilms could take years to resolve if ever. This is because biofilms can be almost tumor-like in that they can grow in a mass in and around tissues and bones; they can metastasize (by released bacteria forming new films); they can continue to grow over time, and are resistant to most therapies. What makes biofilms even more difficult to treat than tumors however is their low metabolic processing which makes it difficult for germicides to penetrate.

Of the products that are mentioned, some have been observed to prevent or slow the formation of biofilms. They work by reducing or preventing the initial adhesions to internal tissues and bones. These same products however may have little or no affect on already formed biofilms. Some may have the capacity to penetrate the outer-most layers of the biofilms to kill the surface bacteria, but may be ineffective against the fibrous or exopolysaccharide structure itself. While others may have no killing affect at all, but may have a direct dissolving action against the structure. So although some products may have "anti-biofilm" activity, exactly what that means depends on its mode of action. Once its action is understood, a more complete protocol can be created.

A general look at the overall development of biofilms was described earlier. However in order to see how we may design a battle plan of attack, let's break down the components. Generally speaking, first, there is the adhesive element described as the sticky substance that is used to initially attach the bacteria to the substrate. This mucous-like exopolysaccharide goo is used to also bind the film together. Then there is a structural aspect to the biofilm. This is a protein weive-like matrix called *fibrin*. The goo holds this fibrin together. And much like the construction of a building, there are building blocks that are supporting the fibrin. These are the (positively charged) calcium and magnesium minerals and metals mentioned that are released from the bacteria, or gathered from the environment that cannot be incorporated into living tissues. They are repelled and act as free radicals. The mucous-like exopolysaccharide then acts as a glue or cement, the fibrin like the rebar, and the minerals like the building blocks. Thus the biofilm has the same basic components as a building. So therapies that are developed to break down biofilms will ideally contain substances that affect each of these individual components.

Some interesting work by Peta Cohen, M.S., R.D., founder of Total Life Center in Northern New Jersey gives us a good model to work from due to her work with autistic children. She found that pretreating many children suspected of having chronic infections had some interesting affects.

> It's standard knowledge that biofilm bacteria sequester calcium, magnesium and iron to help build that matrix. Minerals give the biofilm integrity—as if you're building a wall . . . To address this, first you use fibrinolytics to help dissolve the fibrin, then you use EDTA to chelate out the minerals. And guess what? We started getting huge dumps of toxic metal. Now why is that? I think the answer points to something so huge, whether we're dealing with autism or lyme disease or multiple sclerosis or lupus or even cancer.[1]

So addressing biofilm components is a good strategy and finding excellent clinical success. Here we examine various substances which have the potential to inhibit, damage or destroy biofilms. Zedoaria and sparganium combination, Sanicle, Haritaki, Gallium nitrate, mixed oxidants, various essential oils, to a minor extent curcumin and other herbs have already been mentioned in Chapter 11. The following are additional substances which are known to have anti-biofilm characteristics.

Serrapeptase—This is an enzyme derived from the silkworm. It uses it to dissolve the cocoon in order to emerge as a moth. The worm also uses it to digest the leaves upon which it feeds.

This is a protein digesting enzyme used in many applications that involve inflammation, as it possesses strong antiinflammatory actions. It can replace some NSAID's and asprin. However its selective ability as an enzyme in the body is to digest non-living tissue. Thus plaques, blood clots, cysts, fibrin and mineral deposits are potential targets for destruction. It has been demonstrated that serrapeptase when taken together for bacterial infections makes the antibiotics more effective. This is probably due to its ability to digest protective biofilms and enhance susceptibility.

> The mechanisms of Serrapeptase consist fundamentally of a reduction of the production of the inflammatory reaction within tissue and an inhibition of the release of inflammatory mediators (histamine, etc). It induces the breakdown of fibrinose tissue and reduces the viscosity of exudates. Serrapeptase breaks these substances down into harmless amino acids which are then dealt with by the body as normal waste products. The enzyme quite literally digests the inflammatory tissue.[2]

It also may reduce excessive old scar tissue over time.

One of the advantages of this enzyme is the lack of serious side effects, even at high doses, enabling it to be taken in combination with other enzymes which may have other pathways of function.

Nattokinase—This is another fibrinolytic enzyme which is extracted by fermenting soy with the bacterium called *Bacillus natto*. It possesses similar activities as serrapeptase by reducing excess fibrin that is known to promote atherosclerosis in blood vessels. Studies have been done comparing nattokinase with lumbrokinase. It has been found to be far less effective. But every person is different and may find some benefit. A product called Neprinol has combined serrapeptase and nattokinase into one supplement in addition to a number of other fibrinolytic enzymes.

Lumbrokinase—This is a fibrinolytic or fibrin dissolving enzyme. It is derived from earthworms, and is actually made up of 6 different enzymes which are collectively called *lumbrokinase*. This has been used for hundreds of years in China as a traditional medicine. It is well researched with many studies having been done including clinical trials. A large study was done in China involving 16 hospitals where it was shown to be very effective and safe.[3] It has been used for hypercoagulation of the blood, which means excessive clotting. This is a problem often associated with chronic diseases such as pulmonary disease, diabetes, malignant tumers, unresolved injuries and infections.

However fibrin is used in the clotting process and lumbrokinase helps dissolve the fibrin as an anticoagulant. Its application for biofilms is for the dissolving of fibrin material associated with these formations. It has been compared to nattokinase in studies and found to be far superior. Boluoke brand Lumbrokinase is being used by many Lyme patients testifying to its effectiveness.

No Fenol—This product was developed based upon the idea that some people have a difficult time digesting phenols, which are constituents found in all foods which give them their color, flavor, smell, etc. Certain carbohydrates associated with these phenols are believed to be involved in the problem of digestion. These carbohydrates are plant polysaccharide-based. As a result an enzyme called *xylanase* is believed to aid in the digestion of these polysaccharide components. Since biofilms use polysaccharides as the goo that holds them together, it is believed that this sugar-dissolving enzyme may benefit. Most microbes derive their own unique polysaccharide. So it is not known what specific enzyme(s) affect Lyme biofilms. As has been said, at this point we are so early in our understanding of Lyme biofilms that no particular enzyme has been definitively matched to Borrelia's exopolysaccharide. However it is hoped that using enzymes that have known associated properties will show benefit.

Rechtsregulat—Biofilms can form around chronic injuries. These injured sites become areas of poor circulation due to inflamed tissues, and due to blood clotting which can act to close off small capillaries. Just as fibrin forms inside blood vessels as clots, biofilms act to block necessary enzymes from reaching the source of the infection. Thus higher concentrations of enzymes than are normally produced by the body are sometimes required in order to help dissolve biofilms.

Rechtsregulat is a very powerful form of enzymes that have been created from vegetables, nuts and fruits from a special process. The developer's website provides very little information beyond this, and no clinical benefits are provided. The product is made in Germany whose law prohibits the mentioning of any benefits provided by food products.

However some clinical applications and benefits have been provided by Dietrich Klinghardt M.D., Ph.D. Dr. Klinghardt is Founder of the American Academy of Neural Therapy, Medical Director of the Institute of Neurobiology, and lead clinician at the Comprehensive Medical Centre, all located in Bellevue, Washington. He has worked extensively with Lyme patients, and has successfully treated over nine hundred Lyme patients. Dr. Klinghardt has developed his own Lyme protocols. As part of these therapies he uses Rechtsregulat as a prime agent to address biofilms. It appears to be superior than the other enzymes. In his article, *A Look Beyond Antibiotics*:

> *Rechtsregulat ("right rotatory fluid") is an enzyme rich extract of fermented fruits and vegetables. It has outperformed the s.c. injection of heparin in our own trials and frequently leads to rapid subjective improvement. Lumbrokinase is far more effective than Nattokinase. Both appear weak when compared to Rechtsregulat . . .*

> *Mycoplasma responds well to enzymes when it is treated in sequence with the other microbes as outlined here. The most effective strategy is the German product Rechtsregulat. This simple drink has been extremely effective in eradicating mycoplasma and other cell wall deficient microbes. It also has a heparin like anti-fibrin effect that surpasses injected heparin by far. It has just like heparin, a strong biological effect against Babesia as well.*[4]

Cis 2-decenoic acid—A March 2009 study in the Journal of Bacteriology posted a remarkable discovery.[5] A fatty acid messenger from the bacterium pseudomonas aeruginosa, called *Cis 2-decenoic acid* was discovered that actually disperses existing biofilms in vitro. And not only that, but it performed this action in gram-positive and gram-negative bacteria, as well as Candida biofilms—meaning it acts as a cross-specie cell to cell communication molecule that signals dispersion to a broad range of pathogen biofilms. What's more, this fatty acid messenger is also contained in Royal Jelly, which is the substance fed to queen bees and larvae, and is commercially available on the internet as well as health food stores. Some research indicates that this same cis 2-decenoic acid in the Royal jelly also acts to inhibit and reduce biofilms.[6]

It was mentioned earlier that Manuka honey also possesses antibiofilm activity. Whether this is the same ingredient as found in Royal Jelly remains to be seen. Royal Jelly is an energy booster as well as a natural antidepressant, which makes it an excellent all-around supplement for Lyme.

Xylitol—This sugar substitute is a member of a class of sugar alcohols known as *polyols*. They are naturally contained in some fruits and also in fermented foods. Xylitol is a five carbon sugar with similar taste as sucrose. However it possesses fewer calories than the 6 carbon sugars of fructose and is a non-fermentable sugar. For this reason it has been used in gum and candies to reduce and even prevent caries (cavities). It is also used as a low calorie sweetener which is more suited to diabetics as it has approximately 40% fewer calories than sugar. Generally sugar alcohols have been used as food additives due to their sweet taste similar to sugar, however they are more slowly absorbed. There is no known toxity level, although at higher levels than can be absorbed, a laxative effect can occur.

It is this molecular similarity to sucrose that induces some pathogenic bacteria to attempt to utilize xylitol as a food source. Xylitol is readily taken up thru cell walls of these bacteria where it is transformed into *xylitol phosphate*, a substance that is not able to be metabolized. Over time as xylitol phosphate accumulates in the bacteria, it interferes with digestion and acts much like a toxin, and so starves them. Interestingly, sugar alcohol does not have this affect on human cells. (Xylitol on the other hand does appear to be toxic to dogs.)

Having similar properties as sugar, xylitol is preferentially taken up by bacteria without a benefitial use as fuel leading to eventual starvation. For this reason xylitol has been the focus of research for its potential against microbial proliferation, particularly against oral bacteria that can cause cavities, and other pathogenic bacteria. Researchers in one study found that children given xylitol gum by their mothers had a 70% reduction in cavities when they reached 5 years of age, compared to those that did not.[7]

Sugar fermentation leads to an acidic environment not only in the mouth, but the body as a whole, which not only is preferential to pathogenic bacteria, but also reduces mineral absorption for teeth and bones. This ability for xylitol to affect mineral aborption is not just isolated to the oral cavity however. Researchers in Finland discovered that rats fed a diet which included xylitol increased bone density and mineral absorption.[8] Although exactly how Xylitol increases bone density is not known, it is believed that perhaps it acts to increase ph levels in the body thereby increasing mineral absorption. Xylitol has also been demonstrated to increase newly formed collegen in the skin.[9] So its benefits are not isolated and may act on a broader level as other saccharides by affecting cellular communication, transport, and absorption.

Oral studies have demonstrated that xylitol not only reduces pathogenic bacteria, but also has the ability to reduce plaque and biofilm formation.[10, 11] It does this in many different species of bacteria known to cause biofilms. It is for this reason it has been used in products to reduce oral biofilms.

However it is theoretically possible that long-term exposure of bacteria to xylitol can develop a certain resistance. In order to do this, mutant bacteria must alter gene expression to accommodate tolerance to xylitol phosphate. These would then become xylitol-resistant strains. As time goes by, the bacterial colony would by natural selection produce greater numbers of these mutants. However in doing so, it has a double-edged sword effect in that mutant bacteria also tend to lose their virulence factors, which may also affect their adhesive properties. Xylitol has been shown to demonstrate in many studies biofilm inhibiting or destruction properties. So the taking of this sugar on a regular basis may have a long-term affect of not only reducing the numbers of pathogenic bacteria, but also reduce their biofilm development and advancement.

Although taking Xylitol at excessively high doses can cause intestinal discomfort, this will often subside in time as tolerance develops. Erythritol possesses similar properties as Xylitol; however appears to be more tolerable. So it may be used as a substitute if intestinal absorbtion to the latter causes problems, although erythritol may not be as effective. This sugar can be added to virtually any therapy, and when taken on a consistent basis may contribute to the overall decline of biofilm formations and inhibition of infection. It is an ideal conjunct when added to salt/C therapy.

ORAL CHELATION

The subject of oral chelation has been controversial since MD's were taught that EDTA is not easily absorbed by this method. Absorption of oral EDTA is on average approximately only 10% compared to IV EDTA, and therefore would require extremely high dosages to be effective. However according to Dr. Robert J. Rowen who wrote an article, Oral Chelation—Hoax or Heart Protector?,[12] an average IV dose of 3 gm twice per week would be approximately equivalent to 7.5 grams daily orally. Taking this level throughout the week would allow one to absorb roughly the same amount as IV EDTA. However when compared on a cost basis, 8 IV administrations per month may average around $800 per month, whereas the oral cost would be closer to $60, making oral EDTA much more affordable.

Additionally, with the introduction of liposome technology which we have learned can significantly increase the rate of absorption of most supplements, and given that we have learned to cost effectively employ this technology in our own homes, the possibilities using oral EDTA are now quite remarkable, and may even in time, depending on the dosage, be found comparable to or even exceed IV EDTA.

Some physicians have been using EDTA to theoretically address the biofilm problem. EDTA binds to heavy metals such as cadmium, lead, mercury, as well as positively charged minerals which are implicated in and contribute to biofilm infection. These minerals have been likened to the building blocks of the biofilms, and heavy metal ions would add an additional level of toxicity. Incorporating chelation as part of overall antibiofilm protocols, may add an additional step in the process of their slow degradation over time, which may not be affected to such a degree by any other treatment method. EDTA is well tolerated even at these high doses.

Not all EDTA formulas are the same however. For instance EDTA does not chelate aluminum which would be a significant culprit since it would potentially be found in the body at high levels due to our modern use of this metal. But some formulations may add additional properties which may be beneficial such as malic acid, which according to Dr. Rowan may dissolve aluminum. Dr. Gary Gordon of Gordon Research Institute has developed a high quality oral EDTA product. And other brands offer ready-made liposomal EDTA formulas which are now available for purchase should one choose that method.

Since only a physician can administer IV EDTA, which is generally followed by antibiofilm substances along with targeted antimicrobials when treating Lyme or other biofilm-based diseases, this would be a very expensive therapy to employ especially since even IV EDTA needs to be a long-term therapy to experience noticeable or significant results. However with our current ability to consume liposomal oral EDTA, it can be taken on a continual basis as part of an overall therapy regimen to address biofilm reduction over time, which would be an invaluable addition to our antibiofilm arsenal.

Carnivora has already been discussed extensively, but is mentioned here again since its enzymatic potential to catalize undifferentiated cells may also possess strong antibiofilm potential.

A word about co-infections—

The topic of this book is about chronic Lyme disease. It would be difficult to discuss Lyme disease without also recognizing co-infections since they are often an integral part of the over-all infection. One word of importance will be mentioned. It was once held that bartonella, Ehrlichia, and babesia were the most common co-infections, and have traditionally been included in Lyme serological testing. As has been previously stated, it is actually mycoplasma. Garth Nicholson PhD,

> We have found that the most common co-infection with Borrelia are various species of Mycoplasmas. Approximately 60-70% of Lyme disease patients also have mycoplasmal infections (Mycoplasma fermentans > Mycoplasma hominis > Mycoplasma pneumoniae, M. genitalium, M. penetrans, other species). In some cases multiple mycoplasmal infections can be present in Lyme Disease patients. The presence of mycoplasmal infections complicates the diagnosis and treatment of Lyme Disease, and some of the generalized signs and symptoms found in Borrelia-positive patients are also found in mycoplasma-positive patients.[13]

Dr. Eva Sapi of the University of New Haven performed research that discovered that 84% of ticks they examined carried mycoplasma.[14] The symptoms of mycoplasma overlap and are similar to Lyme, and is also extremely difficult to eradicate, requiring very long treatment time.

With the emergence of biofilm research, it has been learned that many mycoplasma species also develop biofilms.[15-18] With mycoplasma bacteria also being pleomorphic, this makes both Borrelia and mycoplasma share the similar categories of resistance.

Three particular substances that address Borrelia may also be ideal for mycoplasma.

Rechtsregulat enymes (biofilm), monolaurin (cell-wall), and PC-Noni extract (intracellular infection).

Since the topic of co-infections is vast and would involve an entire book in and of itself, we will leave that topic to the reader to explore on his own since there are now many excellent sources on the topic. However we would be remiss if we failed to point out that a great deal of evidence has been pouring in which implicates parasitic and protozoal infections being very often associated with Lyme infection. In fact some medical doctors are first addressing the parasite problem before dealing with Lyme since often times these infections, which can also be systemic, are known to significantly impede progress in Lyme treatments. Therefore, although traditional Lyme co-infections certainly may play a role in the furthering of the disease process, to a much larger extent than has previously been known, parasites should be strongly considered and treated along with Lyme infection. I personally found remarkable progress when I learned this one fact. Ironically, many of the same therapies that address parasites also seem to have an effect on the cyst form of Bb infections. I personally discovered remarkable benefits by adding Wormwood Combination (which contains a blend of herbs that primarily targets parasites) to my Lyme therapies. Artemisinin extract is also a prime supplement to deal with parasites as a whole, as well as the cyst form of Bb, but has traditionally been used to treat Babesia, also a known Lyme co-infection.

ENDNOTES

1. *New Enzyme Complex Isolated From Earthworms is Potent Fibrinolytic* Edwin Cooper, Ph.D., Sc.D. In Focus Nutricology Newsletter March 2009 http://www.nutricology.com/infocus/pdfletters/InFocus_2009Mar_Earthworms.pdf Retrieved Feb. 3, 2013

2. *Serrapeptase - the 2nd gift from the Silk Worm* Article from The Haven Complimentary website
    http://www.haventherapies.co.uk/10226/info.php?p=4&pno=0 Retrieved Feb. 3, 2013

3. *Healthy Coagulation & Biofilm Defense* Boluoke™ Lumbrokinase product description from Researched Nutritional Solutions
    http://researchednutritionals.com/FactSheets/Boluoke.pdf Retrieved Feb. 3, 2013

4. *Lyme disease: A Look Beyond Antibiotics* Dietrich K.Klinghardt, MD, PhD Article from website
    http://www.klinghardtacademy.com/images/stories/Lyme_Disease/Lyme_protocol_Jan06.pdf Retrieved Feb. 3, 2013

5. *A Fatty Acid Messenger Is Responsible for Inducing Dispersion in Microbial Biofilms* David G. Davies and Cláudia N. H. Marques Joural of

Bacteriology J. Bacteriol. March 2009 vol. 191 no. 5 1393-1403 http://jb.asm.org/content/191/5/1393.full - aff-1#aff-1

6. *Royal jelly's effect on glucosyltransferase expression in Streptococcusmutans* 19th European Congress of Clinical Microbiology and Infectious Diseases Helsinki, Finland, 16 - 19 May 2009 Abstract number: P1628; also, ISME J. 2007 Jun;1(2):149-55.

7. *Policy on the Use of Xylitol in Caries Prevention* American Academy of Pediatric Dentistry. (2006) http://www.aapd.org/media/Policies_Guidelines/P_Xylitol.pdf Retrieved Feb. 3, 2013

8. *Improved bone biomechanical properties in xylitol-fed aged rats. Metabolism.* Mattila PT, Svanberg MJ, Jämsä T, Knuuttila ML. Metabolism. 2002 Jan;51(1):92-6.

9. *Effects of a long-term dietary xylitol supplementation on collagen content and fluorescence of the skin in aged rats.* Mattila PT, Pelkonen P, Knuuttila ML. Gerontology. 2005 May-Jun;51(3):166-9.

10. *Effect of xylitol and other carbon sources on Streptococcus pneumoniae biofilm formation and gene expression in vitro.* Kurola P, Tapiainen T, Sevander J, Kaijalainen T, Leinonen M, Uhari M, Saukkoriipi A. APMIS. 2011 Feb;119(2):135-42.

11. Effect of xylitol on an in vitro model of oral biofilm. Badet C, Furiga A, Thébaud N. Oral Health Prev Dent. 2008;6(4):337-41.

12. *Oral Chelation - Hoax or Heart Protector?* Article from Dr. Robert J. Rowen's SECOND OPINION newsletter. Article found on http://www.arthritistrust.org/Articles/Chelation%20-%20Oral/index.htm?vm=r&s=1 Retrieved Feb. 3, 2013

13. *Diagnosis and Therapy of Chronic Systemic Co-infections in Lyme Disease and other Tick-borne Infectious Diseases* Prof. Garth L. Lyme Disease Diagnosis & Therapy Suggestions 2006 ACAM Meeting The Institute for Molecular Medicine http://www.immed.org/treatment%20considerations/NicolsonLYMEdiseaseACAM_06.rtf Retrieved Feb. 3, 2013

14. *Bacterial Biofilms and Lyme Disease* Richard Longland interview with Dr. Eva Sapi August 28, 2009 http://www.youtube.com/watch?v=AmvgOfIN_8c&feature=related Retrieved Feb. 3, 2003

15. *Differences in biofilm development and antibiotic susceptibility among clinical* Ureaplasma urealyticum *and* Ureaplasma parvum *isolates* María García-Castillo, María-Isabel Morosini, María Gálvez, Fernando Baquero,Rosa del Campo, María-Antonia Meseguer. Journal of Antimicrobial Chemotherapy Volume 62, Issue 5 Pp. 1027-1030.

16. *Mycoplasma Biofilms Ex Vivo and In Vivo* Warren L. Simmons and Kevin Dybvig. FEMS Microbiol Lett. 2009 June; 295(1): 77-81.

17. *Biofilm film formation by mycoplasma species and its role in environmental persistence and survival* Laura McCauliffe, Richard J. Ellis, Katie Miles, Roger D. Ayling and Robin A. J. Nicholas Microbiology April 2006 vol. 152 no. 4 913-922

18. *Biofilms Protect Mycoplasma pulmonis Cells from Lytic Effects of Complement and Gramicidin* Warren L. Simmons and Kevin Dybvig Infect Immun. 2007 August; 75(8): 3696-3699.

CHAPTER 15

Antibiotics

Because the focus of this research is to learn what we can of non-drug treatments available to Lyme patients, little time is being spent discussing antibiotics. Due to what has become an unbalanced and unhealthy reliance upon drugs by conventional medicine, not only for infectious diseases, but in general, natural substances are regaining much of their historical importance. However this is not to imply antibiotics do not hold an important place in healing. It is my own personal conviction that drugs should be the medicine of last resort, or where there are no natural substances known (yet) that can address certain kinds of conditions. They simply have a tendency to work against the natural chemistry of the body and produce toxicity placing an even greater burden on an already taxed liver, lymph, and cellular systems. Having said this, there are times when drugs certainly have their place.

Antibiotics are usually the first medicine of choice against not only early stage Lyme disease, but then as a longer term ongoing therapy. This is problematic for this reason: The most acute and symptom producing aspect of early Lyme is generally accepted to be sourced from the Bb spirochete. It has been repeatedly observed that spirochetes are the most highly virulent form of the bacteria. Comparatively speaking, spirochetes are highly susceptible to many antibiotics. Since the spirochete infection is the most intolerable aspect of Lyme disease, addressing that form of the infection is top priority for both the Lyme patient and his/her doctor. So antibiotics are aggressively administered in order to resolve this aspect of the infection. However as a trade-off, spirochetes can be driven into cyst forms which are highly resistant to abx. Although the symptoms of cyst-based forms are not nearly as acute, they are far more resistant to antibiotics, are more representative of longer-term infection, and can of course later release spirochetes from their encapsulated "cacoons".

A FEW INSIGHTS

It has been mentioned that Multiple Sclerosis very closely resembles Lyme disease, and that early Lyme vaccinations were based upon one particular outer surface protein OspA. The vaccination project was discontinued due to the fact that it was feared that myelin sheath proteins (the proteins supposedly the target of autoimmunity) may become a victim of molecular mimicry. That is, myelin sheath was so similar to Bb spirochete proteins that creating a vaccination that stimulated immune cells to attack Borrelia proteins may also unintentionally stimulate those same cells to attack the body's own protective nerve coverings. It was also discovered in the early part of the nineteenth century that spirochetes were identifited as being a causative agent of MS.

Now new facts seem to support that idea. Research presented in *Medical Hypothesis* demonstrated that the geographical distribution of MS nearly exactly parallels the distribution of Lyme disease. We have been told that MS is an autoimmune disease. But what are the mathematical probabilities that an autoimmune disease is going to exactly match the same geographical area as a bacterial infection that also happens to possess a protein that mimics the same nerve complexes in the human body as MS symptoms? Some now believe that unresolved Lyme-related disease can result in the formation of multiple sclerosis. The point of the research was to hypothesize that two specific antibiotic combinations might be a potential cure. They were tinidazole and minocycline.[1] This information is presented for your consideration.

A recent study done by Dr. Eva Sapi at the University of New Haven demonstrated that any particular antibiotic will have a different affect depending upon the form of bacteria it is being used against. This was an in vitro study. However it gives us a comparative to which to understand how antibiotics can affect different bacterial forms in various degrees. Here were the results of that study:

> While Doxycycline was able to kill some 90% of spirochetes, it forced many into cyst forms and actually doubled the amount of cyst forms. Amoxicillin killed off around 85-90% of spirochetes while reducing cyst forms by

68 %. Metronidazole led to a spirochete decrease of 90% with cyst form reduction around 80%. Tigecycline and tinidazole affected both spirochetes and cysts by 80-90%. As to biofilm colonies, doxy, amoxicillin, metronidazole, tigecycline and tinidazole all decreased actual bacterial colony formation by 30-55%. However with regards to the actual killing of bacterial forms within biofilms, tinidazole was 90% effective, while the other antibiotics 70-85% were still detected in the biofilm colonies.[2]

No observation is made of the CWD forms. Antibiotics seldom affect CWD form bacteria in the same manner as spirochete infections.

It can be observed that clearly some antibiotics used to treat spirochete infections do have the capacity to actually increase the more resistant forms and hence entrench the disease even deeper by using them. This is what has been historically observed in conventional medicine. This is likely the case with certain antimicrobials as well, as has been observed by some users of Samento e.g. However, as has been stated, many non-drug therapies tend to attack bacteria from more than one angle, and so may not have the same effect as do drug-based antibiotics with regards to forcing one form into another. However by and large, natural or non-drug therapies hold a huge advantage vs drug-based antibiotics.

One cannot assume that the above research is universally applicable to all strains of Bb, nor that antibiotic effectiveness will remain constant. As we discussed in chapter 4, plasmids allow Bb to develop resistance. Over time as the vast majority of spirochetes are killed off, those that remain develop resistance by altering gene expression and variable proteins to avoid the effects of any particular antibiotic's activities. This is what has been historically observed in many Lyme patients. This is why it becomes important to use a varied approach when using both antibiotics and antimicrobials. Using any single therapy for any amount of time will increase the likelihood of resistance, which may eventually eliminate that substance from your arsenal. Rotating medicines and using combinations can inhibit the plasmids from developing a single defensive posture in the first place, since Bb's attempts to defend itself against multiple antibacterial activities will be like trying to hit a moving target. In other words, the more varied your treatments are, the less capable the bacteria will be to develop resistance. You recall that Bb's greatest strength is also its greatest weakness. By countering using variable therapies, we can use its strength against it.

One of the most effective antibiotics mentioned was tinidazole, which not only reduced bacterial numbers, but also seemed to affect biofilm penetration (but not necessarily the biofilm itself). Tinidazole is primarily an anti-parasite/anti-protozoa medication, similar to metronidazole, yet is taken for a shorter period of time, hence is less toxic. Both Tinidazole and Metronidazole have also been used against some bacterial infections as well, and appear effective against cyst forms to various degrees. Tinidazole however seems to be somewhat more effective. Tinidazole primarily markets itself against protozoa infections such as amoebas, giardias, and trichomonas (parasites), but also against certain anaerobic bacteria.

Protozoa possess a different cell wall than bacteria. The unique nature of protozoa is that during stressful environments they can protect themselves against toxic chemicals, lack of oxygen, and nourishment deprivation by encapsulating themselves with a protective coating called a cyst. Although not a protozoa, Bb has developed this same capacity to protect itself, which is also what makes the Bb cyst form so resistant to most antibiotics. So it only makes sense that medications that would be effective against protozoa may also affect Bb cyst forms. These would include certain herbal preparations as Wormwood Combination, Artemisinin (artemisia extract), and garlic. These herbs may hold a similar capacity (particulary when taken together with cayenne pepper to increase absorption and circulation) as tinidazole with regards to cyst eradication. Many Lyme sufferers including myself have used anti-protozoa herbs with good success against cyst forms. These would also affect Babesia, another intracellular parasite co-infection.

After spending much time examining the various antibiotics used against Lyme disease, a common thread began to appear. Although certain antibiotics certainly seemed to be more effective than others depending on the patient, most of them to one degree or another still had resistance developed against them. This was the problem we discussed in chapter one. Too much reliance upon a given drug can lead to resistance, and ultimately strengthen the microbe. This is much more common in Lyme disease than most other pathogenic bacteria due to its variable proteins, plasmid system, and pleomorphism. I personally experienced that the antibiotic ciprofloxacin completely knocked out Lyme arthritis in my knee when I first used it. However several months later, it had no affect on my Lyme symptoms, and never did again.

So to those choosing to use antibiotics as their primary therapy be certain to discuss with your doctor alternating or rotating them periodically. But they are best used in combinations to reduce both the resistance factor, as well as to affect multiple forms of the bacteria to inhibit or prevent the morphing factor.

Obviously antibiotics have been the primary medicine of choice for most with Lyme and other infectious diseases. Although the choice is up to the individual, it seems to me that due to the damage that long-term abx can cause, it would seem to make far better sense to address spirochete infections using natural antimicrobials while preserving for last resort cyst killing abx such as tinidazole, and that only after biofilms have been dispursed to a degree. The reason is quite simple and makes a tremendous amount of sense. Spirochetes are easily killed using specific natural substances and some antibiotics alike.

But since resistance to antibiotics is a very common phenomenon, in part because they generally have one mode of action, Bb is much more easily able to adapt; whereas non-drug antimicrobials often directly affect bacteria from several different angles, many which are not even completely understood. (It may sound redundant to constantly reiterate this point, but it has become so instilled in the minds of people that antibiotics are a superior form of medicine, that even with some after decades of antibiotics having failed them, they still accept this as fact.) By using non-drug therapies, drug resistance will be held to a minimum and will be able to be used in extremely resistant last resort applications. If you use a nuclear weapon to fight every little battle, what happens when your enemy figures out that by hiding underground it can endure even the worst of onslaughts? You deliberately push your enemy underground where they cannot be eradicated no matter what weapon you use. (In this case the metaphor of a nuclear weapon is not being used to describe the effectiveness of antibiotics, but rather their ability to universally destroy everthing in its path, including the good bacteria.)

Before moving on I would like to point out something regarding these experiments by Dr. Sapi. First, because they were performed in vitro, the biofilm formation is not necessarily going to be representative of the same structural make-up as it would if it was done in vivo (in the body). This is because what we know of the biochemistry make-up of Bb is that it expresses different genes and plasmids when being challenged by immune cells, which would not necessarily be present in vitro. That means that they are going to potentially be far more resistant to antibiotics in the body.

Next, biofilms in the body will likely have incorporated human fibrin, and other dead human cells or debri, as well as any minerals that have become incorporated as scavenged from the body which will either aid in the structure, or be used as a defensive camouflage. All these will play a role as an additional resistance factor that would not be represented in this experiment. So to expect these same results in the body would be taking the experiment farther than it was intended. It does however demonstrate distinctions between the effectiveness of the various antibiotics, which is what the experiment was intended to demonstrate. The real test, in my opinion is how these substances affect biofilms in the body. If patients and their doctors were able to experience these same results using antibiotics alone, there would be no reason for them to be pursuing more effective substances and protocols in order to affect biofilms. But at least now they are beginning to realize that the paradigm that they have been using is not sufficient to address chronic biofilm-based infections.

I will conclude this chapter with an interesting observation. Note that the highly effective use of tinidizole in the above study which demonstrated a 90% kill rate, seems to nicely coincide with the highest degree of healing most Lyme sufferers can expect to experience. This is exactly the point of this book. Seldom do even the best of conventional medicine's antibiotics bring the Lyme victim to a higher level of healing and eradication of infection than 90%. Not only does this model not address the comprehensive killing of the bacteria, but antibiotics alone will not restore the damaged immune system, but actually weakens it. So although some may see experiments such as these as an overwhelming success, I see it as confirming the failure and inability for the conventional medical model to bring the Lyme patient to the deeper healing that is possible when using a different paradigm.

ENDNOTES

1. *Chronic Lyme borreliosis at the root of multiple sclerosis--is a cure with antibiotics attainable?* Fritzsche M. Med Hypotheses. 2005;64(3):438-48.
2. *Evaluation of in-vitro antibiotic susceptibility of different morphological forms of Borrelia burgdorferi* Dovepress Journal: Infection and Drug Resistance Sapi E, Kaur N, Anyanwu S, Luecke DF, Datar A, Patel S, Rossi M, Stricker RB Published Date May 2011 , Volume 2011:4 Pages 97-113.

CHAPTER 16

Putting it All Together

We now come to the important task of taking what has been learned, and creating practical strategies and therapies that can be used to develop treatment protocols. Having come to understand Bb is a unique microorganism which possesses agility beyond almost any known living pathogen, it then comes to no surprise that its resistance to virtually anything man or nature can throw at it is almost mind-boggling. It is not only cunning, but also possesses the necessary ability to survive and even thrive inside the most complex and advanced creature given dominion over all others—man. Yes, we must admit, it has outsmarted even the most genius among us. But one thing is for certain: Although many battles may have been lost, Providence has always placed within man's reach weapons that will allow him to rise up again when so many have fallen. It is only necessary to look both within ourselves for the strength and determination to fight when we feel like giving up, and take hold of a plan of action which when implemented and followed will assure the greatest chances for success.

Lyme disease represents 6 different levels of infection. They are:

1. Cell wall deficient forms (CWD)—This level can be the birthplace of Lyme disease in some people. It can be a benign form of the bacteria which has not begun expressing the virulent lipoproteins seen in the spirochete. However when stressed or challenged by immune cells, it can begin to morph into a more defensive and offensive posture and give rise to spirochetes.

2. Spirochetes—This cork screw shaped form represents the most pathogenic form of the bacterium whose proteins are highly toxic and virulent. They can be vectored by ticks and other insects, or arthropods including spiders, or they can arise from existing CWD forms already inhabiting the body.

3. Pleomorphic forms—As the spirochete becomes challenged either from antimicrobial substances or immune cells, it begins to

express gene-like plasmids which further enable the spirochete to morph into more stealth or evasive forms. These are represented by cyst, granular, and bleb forms. However L-forms (also called variant forms) can also become intracellular by infecting immune cells.

4. Fibrin/fibronectin bonding—spirochetes and other forms begin penetrating and bonding to tissue and cells to which it possesses a certain affinity for such as the fibronectin or fibrin within the extracellular matrix of epithelial cells, but also can infect nerve, muscle and connective tissue.

5. Biofilm formation. As the infection builds upon and within these cells and tissues, the bacteria in a sense trap themselves within this web of fibril, (and mineral deposits which can additionally form), and begin to become incorporated into the growth of the tissues themselves. As they accumulate and multiply, and as an additional layer of defense, Bb forms protective colonies. These emit their own exopolysaccharide coating or slime which then binds to tissues within the body further anchoring the infection on a more localized level.

6. Cellular bonding and DNA damage—As the infection persists, cells which are directly exposed to and interact with the bacteria become damaged and altered. But in order for human cells to survive as Bb proliferates unchecked by immune cells which have become down-regulated, they must accommodate the germs in order to survive. Some molecular microbiologists have witnessed a fusion of Borrelia DNA with human DNA. Thus DNA within human cells would become permanently damaged. This represents the deepest form of infection most resistant to healing.

Note that these various levels of infection do not even include the layer of infection that almost always occurs, which is the development of secondary and/or co-infections that form since the immune system becomes severely compromised. These can include viral, fungal, protozoal, and bacterial infections. We know AIDS (acquired immune deficiency syndrome) to develop from the HIV virus. But Lyme disease in essence forces the body into its own version of immune deficiency syndrome, thereby making the body susceptible to secondary infections much the same way as AIDS. And this is why seldom does addressing Bb infection alone lead to complete healing.

These 6 different levels could be broken down into further sublevels depending on how many steps in the process you wish to represent. But these include the major manifestations of infection. Of these various levels, conventional medicine has historically only addressed the level of the spirochete.

Depending upon the severity of the infection, the length of time a person has had the infection, and the degree to which the bacteria have imbedded themselves in the body, each person's capacity for healing will be different. That's why some people heal with no further symptoms, while others may face a lifetime of uphill battles.

However this is the hope we are giving to those that have up to this point been suffering chronically and deeply within a seemingly never-ending spiraling cycle of illness. Many Lyme sufferers never even get passed the level of planktonic spirochetal infection, let alone the deeper levels. This is because the conventional medical model, by only temporarily suppressing the spirochete infection and not going any deeper, sets up the condition, like a rubber band, to constantly snap back. This cycle must stop.

In order to confront chronic Lyme disease, all six levels must be dealt with to some degree, making this significantly more complex than a "simple spirochete infection". Therefore when developing healing protocols each of these levels must be considered. However, since the infection itself causes secondary damage to the body and immunity, additional support must be included in the equation, and each of the damaged systems of the body ultimately brought back to normal. Connie Strasheim, a long time sufferer of Lyme disease has written a book, Beyond Lyme Disease, which delves into the many systems of the body that secondarily can become affected. She educates the reader with strategies for dealing with and managing them.

THE NEW PARADIGM

We have lain out in this book the argument against the manner in which conventional medicine has historically viewed and treated Lyme disease. At almost every level it seems they have gotten it wrong, and has often left the patient worse off as a result. There is of course a learning curve to everything in life. And those doctors that choose to act like true scientists they are suppose to be periodically re-ask questions with the introduction of new information, or look at topics in a different way in order to constantly monitor and improve their ability to heal their patients. However, the subject of Lyme disease and its treatments has for far too long been entrapped in a system that denies the truth, and at times deliberately interferes with the normal scientific process at the deference to and beckoning of government control and manipulation. By taking the power out of the hands of physicians, and placing it in the hands of multibillion dollar drug companies, corruption has taken place at the deepest levels in order to maintain the fascist-like relationship where government can control corporations through law, and in doing so, can manipulate society as a whole making we the people pawns and slaves to their tyranny.

However we the people have been guilty of allowing this to go on unchecked by our own silence and fear of reprisal. The government and particularly the FDA functions with impunity and controls through instilling fear in the hearts of doctors, patients, and the entire health industry as a whole. With this new information we can take back our own power by seeing the truth for what it is.

Lyme disease does not have to be a life sentence. We can choose to divorce ourselves from the paradigm that has infected and corrupted conventional medicine. That is not to say we throw out the baby with the bathwater and stop seeing our doctors. Rather, it arms us with information so that we can make the right choices for ourselves, and not surrender our decision making power blindly into the hands of physicians that have succumbed to the manipulation of a system which by its very nature has enslaved Lyme disease patients to a lifetime of suffering.

Therefore, the new paradigm which is unfolding seeks to bring to light aspects of the disease, and the manner in which it will ultimately be viewed and treated. We have therefore introduced these new ideas and sought to explain them using traditional, anecdotal and scientific information to demonstrate the divide that has been taking place between the old and new paradigms. Many of these are of course experimental. The practical application of using multiple substances and antibiofilm protocols has tremendous advantages over conventional medicine which has prided itself in discovering and using individual substances and/or therapies in an effort to treat Lyme disease.

The degree to which you choose to employ the following may be as narrow or wide as your ability allows depending upon your motivation, finances, personal circumstances, your own personal abilities, etc. But this is not difficult to understand. Once you understand how this works, and depending on your own experience using natural and non-drug methods, you may creatively design your own therapies, work with your health care practitioner utilizing some of these ideas, or choose to use some of the protocols pre-designed in this chapter.

A point should be made once again regarding the manner in which natural or non-drug supplements should be viewed when designing treatment protocols. The entire basis of this new paradigm that has been developing in recent years regarding Lyme therapies, is that reliance upon any one particular substance for any length of time runs contrary to the premise that has been laid out which is to constantly attack Bb from various angles simultaneously. This will address at various degrees and levels: 1) pleomorphism, its ability to shift from one form to another; 2) plasmid expression which is what allows its proteins to become altered to evade antibody coupling; 3) lateral gene transfer, which is what allows antimicrobial resistance to occur primarily due to plasmid exchange between microbial species, and which can significantly increase virulence factors; 4) horizontal gene transfer which takes place by altering and transferring virulence factors from one generation of bacteria to another. This can change the genetic information and its affect on each subsequent bacterial colony that may accumulate in different levels of biofilms which change over time. Thus different levels of biofilms may carry bacteria and other coinfectious microbes which possess different gene and/or plasmid encoded information. All of these factors address the level of the microbe with regard to using different/ multiple substances or therapies simultaneously or periodically changing or rotating them.

However the other advantage of shifting, rotating, and regularly employing different therapies is to avoid or reduce the tendency for the human body's natural process of homeostasis from reducing the effectiveness of any one particular substance in your arsenal. In time the body has a tendency to biochemically and/or immunologically self adjust as the constant exposure to one substance can eventually cause a shift in order re-balance itself chemically and slowly reduce that substance's effectiveness over time. (This for example is one reason why you will often see a warning label on the herb echinacea, which states that it should only be taken for a period of about two weeks when being used for colds. It loses its effectiveness as an immune support herb over time.) This is theoretically possible with virtually any herbal product. This would be especially possible when taking products such as niacinamide, which has been shown in experiments to increase neutrophil activity by as much as 1000 times. It doesn't seem logical to assume that even immune cells would be able to indefinitely maintain that level of activity without periodic rests. So for example one may shift to using beta glucan after a period of relying heavily on niacinamide and/or carnivora (which has been shown to dramatically increase white blood cell activity within one hour of consuming the product) since each substance will have its own unique mechanism by which it functions.

Additionally, each substance will add its own particular manner in which it stresses the body, for example the liver, GI tract, or kidneys. By periodically discontinuing and changing to a different substance and/ or therapy you prevent them from becoming too taxed and burdened. For example conventional medicine seems wholly and overly dependent upon using individual drugs for certain health conditions, which often raises liver enzymes to dangerously high levels, requiring them to be monitored by yet additional tests requiring more visits, and more expense on the part of the patient; or the over reliance upon certain antibiotics which can wreak havoc inside the intestinal tract, or in the case of fluoroquinolone, serious tendon tears or CNS toxicity. By rotating or allowing time to rest when taking certain substances, this will significantly reduce the stress any particular system in the body may be experiencing.

This is why we defer to a completely different paradigm of thought when addressing Lyme disease. It seems that the entire approach of conventional medicine has distinct disadvantages from the approach presented in this book. And I personally experienced healing at an exponential rate once I began employing this new paradigm.

Certainly a case can be made that this book simply provides too much information, or over complicates things by putting the reader into information over-load. We now live in the internet age which can actually make our lives more difficult by giving us too many choices, hence we aren't able to take a simple approach. In fact it is often the simple approaches that work best. So we will attempt to take the information that has been presented in this book and funnel it all down to some simple ideas. However, keep in mind that dealing with a complicated illness such as Lyme disease requires a more insightful approach. By understanding how the complex Borrelia Burgdorferi bacteria survive in the body, that in and of itself will simplify our approach to developing protocols and dramatically speed the healing process that up to this time may have been taking place at a snail's crawl.

There are several ways to design therapies. One would be for example to take multiple herbs (say 4or 5) at the same time for a long period of time. By using different herbs which may each individually address a different pleomorphic form, and continuing on that for a long period, at least we are making a dramatic shift from a previous approach of say one or two herbs. There are now ready-made herbal concoctions designed synergistically to address Lyme disease.

The other would be to use varied herbal concoctions for a shorter period of time, but then to constantly be changing and alternating them. This would add an additional layer of challenge to weaken the infection. However, introducing antibiofilm substances as well as immune support are additional and necessary factors which are adding a completely new dimension to treating Lyme disease.

One of the most important observations I have made over the years experimenting with anti-Lyme therapies is that there must be a balance between the need to take substances, whether natural or drug-based, to directly kill pathogens, and the need to maintain our own internal integrity. Many of the substances used that have anti-germ capacity may also seem to have the affect of not only stressing the liver and the stomach or gut lining, as well as the beneficial flora obviously, but also immune cells. In our haste to use either natural and/or drug-based antibacterial therapies alike, sometimes they can be over relied upon and actually in the process weaken the immune system they are intended to aid. For instance many of the oxygen therapies, in addition to having powerful antibacterial and antibiofilm effects, if used long-term may also damage immune cells by oxidizing them. Also, long-term treatments utilizing drug-based antibacterial medicines can lead us to think this is the best approach.

If there is not a commensurate stabilizing of the body's pathways that allows it to both maintain itself in order to continue to endure such therapies, but also to eventually take over, all the germ-killing medicines in the world will not make you whole by themselves. This is why it had been mentioned earlier that the taking of probiotics should be at the top of your list as one of the most important supplements that should be maintained throughout your anti-Lyme journey. Probiotics, transfer factor, colostrum, Defense (by Native American Nutritionals), antioxidants, beta glucan 1 3/1 6 glucan, anti-inflammatories, and mineral intake all need to remain part of the over-all program that will stabilize all the systems of the body in order to be able to continue to endure your ongoing treatments.

Do not become so preoccupied with your desire to kill the germs that you neglect your own internal needs to maintain the health of your gut, organs such the liver and kidneys, and your immune system. They are integrally inseparable. We mentioned before that nearly 80% of your immune system resides in your gut, and is stabilized by the help of beneficial bacteria. Once these become significantly weakened, so goes your immune system's ability to fight not only bacteria in the body, but other opportunistic parasites, protozoa, fungus, etc. You start out thinking your battle is with Borrelia Burgdorferi, but end up developing other secondary infections as a result of your primary battle. (Although the weakening of beneficial bacteria is significantly less likely to occur with natural substances than with antibiotics, maintaining their health will also keep immune cells optimal.) Therefore, we will include in the following treatments a balance of pro-immune factors along with focus on the central cause of killing off the bacterial infection. I believe this is one of the primary reasons so many fail to get well despite aggressive anti-Lyme treatments.

> An interesting insight was made by Paul Jaminet PhD in an interview with Dr. Joseph Mercola regarding the taking of antibiotics. We already know that beneficial bacteria aid in digestion and in the production of certain nutrients, for example B vitamins. But they also actually impair opportunistic and potentially disruptive microbes which would wreak havoc on the health of the body. Since the vast majority of immune cells align the intestinal walls, one of the functions of these immune cells is to release antimicrobial peptides for purposes of not only killing pathogenic bacteria, but to control the population of beneficial bacteria as well so as not to overwhelm the body. However, when abx indiscriminately kill beneficial flora as well as the pathogens, immune cells naturally relax or ease their aggression. But what's more, because of the reduction of the population of beneficial bacteria from abx, in an effort to allow them to repopulate, immune cells cease or significantly reduce their release of the antibacterial peptides. Thus whereas the intention for the taking of abx in Lyme disease was to aid the body in the killing of Borrelia burgdorferi in any of its forms, the unintended consequence was to further weaken the very immune cells they were intended to aid. This is yet another reason why the long-term taking of abx will virtually never cure chronic Lyme disease. The immune system simply cannot regain a foothold as it remains in a perpetually weakened condition as long the abx are continued. It also illustrates why relapse is often the rule rather than the exception. http://articles.mercola.com/sites/articles/archive/2012/01/07/dr-paul-jaminet-interview.aspx?e_cid=20120107_DNL_art_1

As one scans many of the pages of the internet reading many of the practitioners using some of the newer treatments which involve using anti-biofilm substances along with the traditional drugs and/or herbal medicines, you read of some of the successes they are having which is helping to verify that we are on the right track taking this approach. Some of the biofilm-dissolving and inhibiting therapies being used often take a single or even dual product approach. For instance serrapeptase may be taken along with or followed by some antibiotic or GSE with limited success. Or lumbrokinase may be followed with Kalmegh. But many of these approaches are still in the experimental stages since the idea of taking biofilm-busting products along with the traditional antibacterials is so new, standardized protocols that consistently work for most patients is still a hit or miss proposition. Some may even conclude after a trial or two using a particular approach this simply isn't the answer since they find little noticeable benefit. Many may therefore conclude that this whole biofilm theory is just another scam or dead end road, like so many others they've walked. Or sometimes the benefits are so subtle, the treatments are stopped before the real benefits kick in.

MY OWN EXPERIENCE

Using these therapies was slow and methodical; listening to the body as I continued to try one treatment after another. Each one seemed to have its own capacity to address some layer of infection, and some aspect of biofilm decomposition. Rarely are biofilms inhabited by one specie. Oftentimes colonies will have many different bacteria and even fungi living in the same biofilm. Even the same specie of bacteria however may have different gene expressions and resistance factors depending on the layer. So each level of a biofilm colony that is razed may release different varieties of microbes, hence toxic reactions may vary as ongoing treatments continue to dissolve subsequent biofilm "strata".

Keep in mind that on a continual basis for years I had been self-treating with multiple anti-Lyme therapies which had nearly completely eliminated planktonic bacteria, and a host of systemic Lyme symptoms. (Remember I became a prestigious member of the 95% Club.) But once this level had been reached, ongoing antibacterial treatments I was using were exhibiting very little noticeable results. Regardless of the dosages and varieties of antimicrobial substances I was using, they simply were offering no further demonstrable benefit.

Yet it was obvious that there were still deep-seated and unresolved inflammatory symptoms not being affected by the ongoing bactericidal therapies I was employing. Perhaps what many doctors had been saying about chronic Lyme not existing was true. Perhaps the taking of antibiotics or antimicrobials beyond a certain point was a waste of time. Maybe ongoing symptoms being attributed to some other factor other than Bb infection was also true. Maybe auto-immune factors becoming "turned on" as a result of the now-eradicated Lyme infection were in fact the underlying cause to persistent and antibiotic-resistant symptoms. Maybe the lack of any further improvement from the taking of antibiotics was evidence that in fact what the IDSA medical society found (as a result of their $75,000,000 grant from the US government) was true after all—antibiotic therapy beyond an initial course or two was non-beneficial, or was proof that the infection had been eradicated! If there was any doubt as to this being true, my own results would soon put to rest such non-sense.

I now began deliberate and aggressive trials with the anti-biofilm substances I was researching. My first therapies involved using the mixed oxidants. Since this was the first group of therapies I experimented with, it was unknown the kind of reaction I would have. This particular therapy was both anti-biofilm as well as antimicrobial at the same time. So it offered a dual-potential in one therapy.

My response to the mixed oxidants was that depression began to set in due to the releasing of toxins. These were symptoms I had not experienced in over a year. In other words the killing off of the top layer of biofilms and the released bacteria were now causing a distinct reaction and set of symptoms that I had not experienced for a long time. I wasn't sure what to make of this since this experimental treatment was now affecting me in ways that handfuls of antibacterial pills had stopped affecting me long ago. It became necessary to take a break since the herx was too much to continue for the time being. I soon understood that this was working. And so I continued to adjust the treatment and experimented to see what was optimal.

However oxygen therapies possess weak chelating or fibrin dissolving abilities. So it was not going to do as a stand-alone therapy, due to the fact that although very powerful, it may overwhelm the body's immune cells through oxidation damage over time unless sufficient breaks were allowed for recuperation. Especially given the intensity with which I was using them.

When employing anti-biofilm substances, it is important to use them as a form of pretreatment prior to taking antibacterial agents. The idea is to take them first to do whatever affective, dissolving, or chelating ability they possess. Then as the layer of film is damaged and frees the inhabitants into the environment, they now become vulnerable to antimicrobials. So the biofilm dissolving substance would be followed by antimicrobials shortly after being consumed to kill them off as they are released. This would then be followed perhaps within several hours with zeolite, chlorella, beta sitosterol, or burber, to clean up the toxic waste which results. In this manner a specific order of damage/kill/clean-up would be your optimal and most effective method when developing your treatment therapies.

However some anti-biofilm products may not have actual dissolving abilities. Some may merely inhibit the further development of films, perhaps by impeding their adhesive properties, or disrupting their signaling pathways to interfere with their ongoing development. Haritaki may represent such a substance. These then would be taken along with the dissolving substances to inhibit the further advancement of damaged biofilms and to reduce the possibility of released bacteria from mobilizing and attaching to remote substrates in the body.

Next the essential oil tea was incorporated. The tea containing coconut and/or moringa oil and the anti-biofilm essential oils were taken twice daily. (Although I later reduced this to once daily.) Since the essential oils are very strong antimicrobials in addition to possessing biofilm-damaging affects, there was no need to add a separate antibacterial substance to this therapy. By adding this oil-tea therapy to the mixed oxidant therapy already being used, this contributed additional pressure on the biofilms. The mixed oxidant therapy is taken several hours apart from other anti-biofilm therapies, not concurrently.

Slowly other protocols were added and rotated in and out in addition to the current strategies. Zedoaria and Sparganium were then incorporated and taken three times per day. These herbs (in theory and according to their traditional eastern medicinal usage) seek out anything creating a blockage or out of place in the body. An interesting affect began to take place. A deep aching began to developing along the nerves in the leg where considerable past injury had caused the body to seek to develop fibrous formations and mineral deposits. These to me represented the formation of vast deposits of biofilms all along the tendons and ilium along the lower back and pelvis. The lower back seems to be a favorite place for Borrelia infections, as significant lower back inflammation is a very common symptom of Lyme disease. From there it loves to travel up the meninges often causing a form of Lyme meningitis, and stiff neck at the base of the skull.

By now several layers of antibiofilm therapies were beginning to have a snowball effect by building on each other. Pain was increasing as they were directly targeting those specific areas where chronic unresolved inflammation had been slowly spreading over the years. It was almost like a volcano that was rumbling given warning signs that is was close to erupting. It was also like the clock was being turned backwards as I was now experiencing pain and symptoms I had not had for years. We are often told that when you go through a healing crisis and begin to resolve long-term infections, the onion effect begins to move backwards. That is, you find that your disease is almost like rewinding. Your symptoms can sometimes go backwards or in reverse order from how they developed. This seemed to be what was happening.

The final explosion was set off when I added sodium bisulfate and xylitol. (The sodium bisulfate I used as a powerful chelator, followed by monolaurin to attack cationic minerals in the biofilms. The pre-chelated biofilm is then attacked by the monolaurin. However I do not discuss nor recommend sodium bisulfate in these therapies due to it being very strong. Humic or fulvic acid, or sodium borate would be a better choice). But the xylitol seemed to be the straw that broke the camel's back. With the building of the various anti-biofilm therapies, an enormous release of symptoms suddenly emerged.

All along the way the anti-biofilm substances were followed by antimicrobials. So the internal release of bacteria was building while toxins were building up faster than the body could eliminate them. Remember too, Dr. William Koch MD the original developer of glyoxilide, observed that all pathogenic microbes were poisonous to one another. So as toxins are released they have a secondary effect of enhancing the virulence factors of other pathogens in the body or in biofilms, which makes the destruction of films and their subsequent release of infectious microbes more dangerous than a single source of infection alone. I know of no one that has used such an intense and aggressive approach to biofilm targeting as I did. This was done as an experiment to observe if in fact these would be effective, but also to what extent. Since this was never done to my knowledge by anyone before, there was no way of knowing the degree to which these therapies would be successful.

The pain became excruciating. I nearly lost the ability to walk for several days since the biofilms having formed along the nerves were being attacked and extremely painful. The entire lower back was so painful, I was not able to lie down or stand in any position without being in agony. The toxic release spread throughout the pelvis and groin area so that severe rashes and cyst-like infections formed in and under the skin from the toxins and dying biofilm-released bacteria. This was so painful for several days there was no way to sleep, and to even touch the area was so painful I almost began to hyperventilate. I was actually in fear since I didn't know what was happening to me, and since I had never experienced such a severe herxheimer reaction in my 11+ years with Lyme disease. It was something like a localized toxic shock. Every effort imaginable was made to alleviate the pain. I was quite literally at the point of tears. At this junction I decided to significantly reduce the anti-biofilm substances, and focus on simply relieving the symptoms.

Due to the infectious and painful "cysts" under the skin that were being released apparently from the biofilms, and due to the fact this was one of those extreme situations, I had a few days supply of tinidazole that I took to see what benefit an "anti-cyst" medicine would have to relieve the condition. Tinidazole is actually an anti-protozoal medication that is also often effective against Lyme cyst forms that was mentioned earlier. Upon taking the medication dead skin began to massively fall for days as the tinidazole apparently was taking affect. The symptoms very slowly began to subside. After about 3 days my supply ran out, and I substituted Wormwood Combination, Garlic, Artemisinin and cayenne pepper for the Tinidazole. This seemed to have virtually the same affect as the Tinidizole, as these herbs are known to also have anti-protozoal activity. (Since then I added MSM—methyl sulfonylmethane—to this cocktail which is also considered to have anti-protozoal activity as well as potentially aids in enhancing absorbtion.)

It took several weeks for the condition to subside as I began to aggressively employ different strategies once I was able to discern what was actually happening. Purely as an observation, it appeared that over the years the taking of traditional anti-Lyme herbs, although clearly was highly successful in killing off certain forms of Bb in addition to other co-infections, seemed to correlate with Dr. Eva Sapi's research in that Lyme cysts must have developed inside of and were released from the biofilms, as the film-busting treatments were revealing. This massive release was subsequently followed by an incredible herxheimer reaction so powerful, it was excruciatingly painful and caused the eruption of infection that was quite intolerable. Never in all my years of having Lyme disease did I ever experience such a dramatic outcome as when employing the antibiofilm therapies along with the antimicrobials. And I must once again repeat, this was long after 95% of my Lyme symptoms had disappeared, the point at which most Lyme patients consider themselves "healed".

I want to reemphasize this point because it is very important to reiterate in case there are skeptics. Antibiotics had stopped working for me long ago. And I had been on quite a few during the course of my illness. This even led my doctor to suspect that maybe I didn't have Lyme disease. It is the classic story we hear time and time again that antibiotics very often fail due to the many forms of Borrelia constantly altering themselves to adapt, and eventually develop the biofilm forms to fortify themselves against any further antibiotic or antimicrobial threats. But when anti-biofilm substances are introduced into the equation, the entire story changes. Not only was the bacterial infection revealed to still be there all along, but a massive killing began taking place the likes of which I had never experienced. This is why our understanding of biofilms has completely rewritten the Lyme narrative, and will forever change the way this disease is treated in the future.

One never knows how an experiment will turn out. In hindsight it was too aggressive. However my concern was that if not aggressive enough and no noticeable herx resulted, it may not be noteworthy. Keep in mind too that the anti-biofilm substances that were used were only a small handful of those discussed in this book. And so the potential options that are available for even the most resistant conditions seem only limited by one's ability to employ them. Let this be a warning that these are serious therapies that can actually be so effective, the herxing can be dangerous. And so caution should be taken to remain responsible. Although non-drug therapies tend to be significantly safer than prescription medications, their effectiveness can have the same and even superior results. In Lyme disease, it is more the effects of die-off than the therapies themselves that are a major concern. However no conventional medical treatments are available (that I have ever heard of or seen) that could even remotely compare to the effectiveness of these treatments.

What was learned through this was that even when a Lyme patient reaches a level when he/she feels they have nearly completely beaten the disease, as no further progress can be made through the taking of antibiotics or natural antibacterial agents, biofilms can persist usually completely unbeknownst to them. They act as bunkers hiding the enemy from view. Anti-biofilm substances can act like bunker-buster bombs. And you never know the extent of the hidden infection until they are exposed.

Biofilms take time to develop and will take time to resolve. Although these particular intense therapies took place over a two month period for me, and a huge step forward was taken toward deeper healing, this was only the beginning. It is interesting to hear the testimonies of so many Lyme patients. I am now very skeptical of many who claim to have "cured" themselves. Not because I don't believe this is possible, but because the elimination of *most* symptoms does not equate to the complete eradication of infection. Unless biofilms are addressed, those unresolved symptoms are probably not the result of left over damage caused by the Lyme disease, but simply a reduced level of infection being hidden. Unfortunately for us victims, the war may go on longer than we had anticipated. But at least we are offered hope by seeing the truth for what it is, and can move forward with a real possibility for healing if we choose to remain committed.

Obviously there are many factors that determine the extent to which biofilms will have developed in any particular Lyme patient. The length of time would no doubt be a major contributor, but not the only factor. And of course the less biofilms are a contributing factor in any particular person's infection, it seems logical to assume that the odds for a potential cure is significantly greater. The question then is not, "Is there a cure for Lyme disease?" as if to imply that there is a single therapy which when followed will ultimately lead to the eradication of the disease. But rather, "What is the true nature of this illness, and what methods are available to give me the best chances of complete healing?"

For me, relative to the length of time I have had Lyme disease, this two month long experiment was but a short beginning to the treatments that would continue until completely resolved. It is like a new chapter is being written that has up to this time been a mystery. I could have waited to write this book and made available its information after many months or even years after employing its strategies. This way the audience would know the extent to which these therapies hold the potential for a complete cure, or if this is just another Lyme book. But since each person's illness is going to resolve differently, not just in reference to the time it will take, but because of the treatment options chosen, as well as the extent and depth of their infection, it would be a disservice to those truly interested in gaining this knowledge to wait and withhold it when it has already been proven to be beneficial to myself and others.

The following are broad based protocols that truly need to be individualized for each person. The extent of healing and the level of treatments having already been experienced are but a few factors that will determine what therapies any person will ultimately adopt. But this will present a starting point to act as a guide. When it comes to direct anti-biofilm/antimicrobial therapies, **damage/kill/clean-up** is the formula to keep in mind. The medicines that are chosen should be taken in a specific order that will first damage biofilms; second, kill the released bacteria; third, clean-up the toxins that result. This will be the most important part of any Lyme treatments that are developed. One can see how this method differs greatly from the approach that has traditionally been taken by conventional medicine. Up to this point *kill* has been the only focus. But *kill* cannot occur when biofilms form. And without *clean-up*, the body reprocesses the toxins creating a greater burden on the lymphatics and liver, as well as the immune system by forcing immune cells to do all the cleaning up, thus significantly slowing the healing process.

SAMPLE THERAPIES

When beginning any therapy program, remember the important point to begin slowly. Since many Lymies have already developed gut damage due to sometimes many years on antibiotics, sensitivities and even allergies can be a common problem. Your body simply may not be able to handle the therapy you choose, or the particular combination you develop. Not only do you not know your body's reaction to the substance itself, but any healing crisis it may invoke, as had occurred in me.

Another point I would like to make. Although I am highly critical of the conventional medical community for reasons already discussed, I do highly encourage the participation of good Lyme-aware medical professionals and doctors that will help you, especially during the most acute phases of therapies, as well as to help discern both the best approach to take when deciding to employ some of these strategies; but also dosages and to monitor your condition.

With the addition of anti-biofilm substances, you may begin to experience a dimension of healing not previously known. Remember too, it appears to be an all too common practice to fall into what I call "passive therapies". This involves the taking of just enough medicines to feel like you are taking action against the infection, but have ceased being aggressive enough to be gaining on the disease. This often happens once we reach a level of healing where we feel comfortable. We feel like we have come a long way from where we were, have become "weary in well-doing", start to sluff off and become lazy. We psychologically feel like if we continue our therapies or remain at this less aggressive level, the disease will in time eventually go away. This is because that is in fact often the coarse that other kinds of infections take. We go thru an acute phase, followed by intense therapy—experience some relief; continue the therapy—feel better; lower the therapeutic levels—disease symptoms decline; nearly stop the therapies—illness goes away completely. However when biofilms become a part of the equation, this normal process becomes interfered with. The films themselves are much more difficult to eradicate, and the inhabiting microbes can continue to proliferate at a rate equal to or even surpassing the level of wearing down of the biofilm. So maintaining diligent and consistent treatment levels becomes important if your goal is a deeper level of healing.

The following is intended merely as a starting point. If you have already been involved in various treatments, you may wish to be more aggressive by adding additional or larger doses. But this should be done only after you have begun using the therapies long enough to see how you will react. At the first sign of a reaction, let off and wait. Then begin again slowly building up to a tolerable level. Lyme disease requires a long term treatment anyways. No sense pushing yourself to highly uncomfortable levels.

Here are some general categories. Many of these are not "proven" in the sense that conventional medicine recognizes them. Frankly, and in that regard, we don't care what conventional medicine approves or disapproves of. Sorry to be blunt. But unless you find a doctor that is incorporating these new ideas, in matters of chronic Lyme disease, most of the practices of conventional medicine have already generally proven themselves to be an utter failure. Rather, most of these are "potential" and are based upon research that gives to us an idea as to what their intended use may be, and how they have been successfully used by others. You may add your own to these lists.

Biofilm Inhibitors:

Humic/fulvic acid, zeolite, xylitol, Haritaki, curcumin, essential oils.

Biofilm dissolvers/dispersers:

Oral EDTA, Lumbrokinase, serrapeptase, Rechts Regulat, mixed oxidants, Sanicle, Carnivora, Sparganium/Zedoaria, No Fenol, Royal Jelly, Gallium Nitrate, essential oils (cinnamon, clove, tea tree, rosemary, eucalyptus, and peppermint.) Banderol, berberine.

Anti-spirochete:

Kalmegh, Cumanda, Samento, Allicin, Olive leaf extract, mixed oxidants, Carnivora, essential oils, grapefruit seed extract (GSE).

Anti-cyst:

Wormwood combination, Allicin, Artemisinin, garlic, MSM (is active against a number of cyst-forming protozoa and may affect Lyme cysts), cayenne pepper (to stimulate deeper circulation).

Anti-CWD form:

Rechts Regulat, noni-extract, Marshall Protocol.

General Antibacterial support:

Berberine, moringa, garlic, monolaurin/coconut oil, manuka honey, essential oils.

Immune support:

Liposomal C, humic acid, coconut oil, colostrum, transfer factor, beta glucan (Defense by Native American Nutritionals), gallactomannans, Sutherlandia frutescans, niacinamide.

Anti-oxidants:

Olive leaf extract, astaxanthin, liposomal glutathione, melatonin, curcumin, krill oil, vitamins C &E.

Toxin scavengers:

Humic acid/fulvic acid, zeolites, chlorella, spirulina, alfalfa and other green super-foods, burbur, cilantro extract, beta sitosterol.

Anti-inflammatories:

Ursolic acid, gallactomannans, curcumin, mangosteen, Nopal juice, Rechts Regulat and other enzymes, Gallium nitrate, MSM (methyl sulphonyl methane, not to be confused with MMS), niacinamide, sodium borate.

Anti-depressants/anti-anxiety:

High dose niacinamide, Royal Jelly, berberine, Destroxin, colostrum, camu camu, SAM-e, squalene, B-12/folic acid, mixed oxidants, sutherlandia, Passion Flower extract, Goji juice, Zormus homeopathic remedy.

Absorption enhancers:

Cayenne pepper, bioperine, DMSO, coconut oil, MSM, essential fatty acids (Krill and flax seed oil), soy lecithin.

Stand alone therapies:

Certain combinations of essential oils in tea/curcumin, mixed oxidants, salt/C/xylitol, Teasel root/GSE.

Liver support:

Curcumin, ursolic acid, Haritaki, milk thistle.

The following are sample therapies. They are based on the formula damage/kill/clean-up. You will likely develop your own treatment protocols based upon your current level of healing and unique biological needs. Each therapy may be taken 1-3 times per day based upon your tolerance level. "Slowly" should be the rule rather than the exception. The idea is to rotate and vary the treatments to reduce resistance and adaptation. You will likely require time off between some therapies to recuperate from herxes or allow time for the body to rest, as some of these therapies can be intense. The dosages are left up to the individual and/or his health practitioner to develop as each individual's needs and requirements will be unique. In addition to the following, except when taking antioxidants, ozonated water should be drunk throughout the day to further detox the body as well as contributing to the bacteriodical benefits. *These are very intense therapies by design, and may need to be reduced to accommodate each person's circumstances. This represents a 30 week program, but may need to be extended considerably. Remember, the first substance(s) represent damage to biofilms followed by a forward slash "/", the second substance(s) represents the killing herbs followed by a forward slash "/", the third represents the clean-up substances.

For example, in the following Week 1, Carnivora/ represents the biofilm damaging substance, samento/ represents the killing substance, and Destroxin and spirulina represent the clean-up substance. This is followed by over-all supportive therapies.

Warning: It is strongly recommended that anyone considering the following therapies see a healthcare practitioner that is knowledgeable about using them. Although their use in the manner being described is new, being monitored and receiving feedback is invaluable to your progress. Even more valuable is a plan that can be developed using kinesiology testing by a highly trained practitioner using this method to create customized treatment options. I have personally used all of these products and in various combinations with no adverse reactions except when taking in too large doses. Usually only temporary discomfort resulted.

Into the following oral EDTA may be added or used on a continual basis preferably away from food. If not taken in liposomal form, taking along with lecithin or other fatty acids will increase its absorbtion. Continuously drinking ozonated water on a regular basis is an additional step to speed your recovery and reduce herxes.

Week 1—Carnivora/Samento, garlic capsules/Destroxin, spirulina. Support—Gallactomannan, ursolic acid, antioxidants, minerals, and probiotics.

Week 2—Same, but add coconut oil to support.

Week 3 and 4—Haritaki and Regulat/Allicin, GSE, moringa, cayenne pepper/Alfalfa. Support—Squalene or krill oil, gallactomannan, antioxidants, minerals, probiotics, coconut oil.

Week 5—Curcumin/essential oil tea (Thieves oil)/humic/fulvic acid. Support—Gallactomannan, ursolic acid, sutherlandia, antioxidants, mins, probiotic, coconut oil.

Week 6—Same but add bioperine and/or MSM to curcumin. Add oil of oregano to essential oil tea.

*Note—If at any time neurological/emotional symptoms increase, you may add/increase your intake of Destroxin, burbur, and/or niacinamide, and if necessary add galactomannans with ursolic acid. But these may need periodic rests to remain potent.

Week 7 and 8—Sanicle/Carnivora, MSM, Wormwood Combination/chlorella. Support—Colostrum, liposomal C, antioxidants, mins, probiotics, MSM.

Week 9 and 10—Regulat and serrapeptase/GSE, olive leaf extract, berberine, cayenne pepper/humic acid or beta sitosterol. Support—Krill, Passion Flower extract, antioxidants, mins, probiotics, coconut oil.

Week 11—Lumbrokinase/samento, GSE, SSKI/Chlorella. Support—B12, noni or mangosteen, antioxidants, mins, MSM.

Week 12—Lumbrokinase with serrapeptase/Wormwood combination, Allicin, cayenne pepper/Destroxin. Support—Noni extract, antioxidants, mins, probiotics, coconut oil.

Week 13 and 14—Mixed oxidants/Essential oil tea (with tea tree, lemon, lime)/Alfalfa. Mixed oxidants can be taken back to back. That is, wait 1-2 hours after taking 1st dose before taking 2nd dose. Two hours after last mixed oxidants take essential oil tea. Support—Antioxidants taken 4 hours before and no sooner than 2 hours after taking mixed oxidants. Up to 3 mixed oxidant treatments can be done within a day. Glutathione, krill, mins, probiotics, MSM.

Week 15—Sanicle/Teasel Root with GSE/Destroxin. GSE should be taken about ½ hour after teasel root. Support—Antioxidants, mins, probiotics, coconut oil.

Week 16—Same but add olive leaf extract to GSE.

*Note: For those that work during the day, it can be difficult to remain consistent with these therapies. For this reason it is advantageous to use/add salt/C/niacinamide/Haritakie/xylitol therapy during the day. This would involve bringing a bottle of C tablets or liposomal C, along with a pre-mixed bottle of water/salt/Haritaki/xylitol which can be taken throughout the day until the recommended dosage is complete. Then resume that week's regular therapies in the evening.

To any of these therapies (except mixed oxidants) can be added berberine or Haritaki as support along with coconut oil. These have well tolerated antimicrobial/biofilm inhibiting properties. Moringa may also be added as supportive nutrition.

Week 17—Interfase Plus/monolaurin with cayenne pepper/humic and/or fulvic acid. Support—Antioxidants, liposomal C, mins, coconut oil, MSM, probiotics.

Week 18—Same but add serrapeptase approximately ½ hour following Interfase Plus. Add allicin to monolaurin with cayenne pepper.

Week 19 and 20—Interfase Plus followed by serrapeptase, lumbrokinase and no fenol/Allicin, garlic, olive leaf extract, Kalmegh, bioperine/Chlorella. Support—Antioxidants, mins, probiotics, coconut oil.

Week 21—Rechts Regulat with serrapeptase/Artemisinin, Garlic, MSM, bioperine, GSE/zeolite. Support—Antioxidants, mins, xylitol, probiotics, coconut oil.

Week 22—Same but add curcumin to support.

Week 23 and 24—Zedoaria and Sparganium with Sanicle/Cumanda and Samento/Burbur. Support—Coconut oil, antioxidants, probiotics. Zedoaria and sparganium taken 3 times per day.

Note: Zedoaria and Sparganium can be taken on a continuous basis for several weeks as this is a longer term supplement that will work more effectively and deeper over time.

Week 25—Interfase Plus, serrapeptase with lumbrokinase/ monolaurin with essential oil tea (manuka or tea tree, rosemary, lemon, peppermint)/Destroxin, humic acid, or chlorella. Monolaurin should not be mixed in the same glass as the tea. It should be taken separately mixed with cold water or juice. Support—Galactomannan, MSM, antioxidants, mins, probiotics. Continue taking zedoaria/sparganium 3 times per day.

Week 26 Same but add Sanicle taken with zedoaria/sparganium.

If biofilms seem to be resistant, do the following for an additional 3+ weeks.

Week 27 Rechts Regulat, serrapeptase, lumbrokinase. Wait 1 hour, then add no phenol and Royal jelly/Ursolic acid, curcumin, Wormwood combination, GSE, cayenne pepper/chlorella. Support—coconut oil, noni extract, galactomannans, probiotics.

For additional support may be rotated colostrum, mangosteen or gogi, liposomal C, Defense, MSM, liposomal glutathione, niacinamide. In addition to essential oil teas, xylitol and/or Manuka honey may be added to most therapies for their bacterial/biofilm inhibiting ability.

Additional antimicrobial herbs may be added or replaced with kalmegh, artemisinin, allicin/garlic, and any others mentioned as part of Dr. Cowden's protocols.

Anti-lyme cocktail: (Warning: This is a very intense therapy intended for those who have already experienced an advanced level of healing, and have had a good degree of experience with herbals already. It will have a "shock affect", will go very deep, and will produce massive herxes. **Work up slowly in small amounts until it is determined that it can be tolerated.** Some herbal combinations in some people are not biocompatible. You have been warned!)

First take Royal Jelly. This is to aid in the initial theoretical dispursement of the biofilm. Wait 1 hour.

Take ¼ cup of 1% gallium nitrate solution added to glass of water on empty stomach. Wait another ½ hour. Then take 10ml Regulat and/ or your choice of serrapeptase or lumbrokinase. After 45 mins:

In a glass, mix two ounces mangosteen juice, 1 teaspoon xylitol, 1 scoop monolaurin, 1 level teaspoon Haritaki, ½ teaspoon Kalmegh, 8 drops super saturated potassium iodide (SSKI), 1 teaspoon MSM (methylsulphonylmethane, to enhance absorption). Mix well and drink down with 3 capsules allicin supplement or garlic, 3 capsules Wormwood Combination, 1 capsule cayenne pepper. (Kalmegh may be taken by capsule or extract, as this is a very bitter tasting herb). As you progress and are able to tolerate them, you may add GSE, Olive leaf extract. (**You need to take this therapy with an apple or a little food to** *avoid nausea which can occur, and to increase absorption. Again, this is extremely potent!)* Also, you may wish to substitute capsules where possible rather than mix the powered herbs in water, as many of these are extremely bitter. Drink lots of water.

After 2 hours take chlorella. Later galactomannans taken with probiotics.

During the day between treatments do the salt/C/niacinamide/xylitol therapy.

For advance therapies, as a second therapy for the day, take Interfase Plus on empty stomach. Wait 1 hour. Then take no fenol and xylitol. After 45 mins:

Monolaurin and 3 capsules cinnamon bark. After 1 hour take essential oil tea.

After 1 hour take chlorella.

As you can see, any number of combinations can be developed, as well as the dosages. These were only examples. And since chronic biofilm-based Lyme disease by its very nature can be very resistant, expect this to be a longer term healing process; although this may not always be the case. Areas of old injuries will be the most resistant to therapies.

WHAT TO EXPECT

Sometimes the only way to know if a therapy is working is to observe any immediate reactions to treatment. But these are not always apparent when addressing biofilms.

I have been using all of the biofilm-affecting substances listed in this book to various degress and combinations. Each has provided benefit. And sometimes the response can be dramatic as observed in my own experience. However, generally the removal of biofilm-based infections is a very slow and involved process. In fact it may require the most diligent and persistent commitment on the part of the patient that may necessitate a very long term approach. And so whereas therapies which target planktonic and surface bacterial colonies with little to no biofilm development often are rewarded by rapid and sometimes dramatic results, biofilms will of necessity require much longer term treatment. Over time this should translate into an over-all improvement of symptoms and especially inflammatory responses. Often it is not known what specific therapy or combinations of substances will be most beneficial in any particular individual, and will require trials and sufficient time to tell if it seems to be working. Biofilm therapies are still in the infancy stages, whether speaking of Bb infections, nanobacteria particles, mycoplasma, or some other bacteria or fungus based structure. How their construction has formed and the microbes that contribute to their formation will affect the outcome of any particular treatment options that are chosen. However at least now we are beginning to understand the resistance factors these systems confer to the overall disease process.

Also, be alert to the often confusing response that can be experienced when incorporating substances which possess anti-inflammatory properties. Sometimes these substances can lead to reduced symptoms, leading one to interpret this as a commensurate reduction of biofilm. However some substances which have strong anti-inflammatory affects such as enzymes, ursolic acid and galactomannans, niacinamide, nopal juice, and curcumin, especially when used synergistically in various combinations, can so reduce inflammation, they almost seem to have healed the condition by themselves. But symptoms often return upon ceasing their use. While it is extremely important to reduce inflammation if for no other reason than the body will seldom be able to heal properly if at all while inflammation is occurng, taking a balanced approach allows for the body to heal and help to resume a normal life while at the same time slowly over time reduce the biofilm-based infection.

I shared with you the response that I personally had to the therapies that I applied in this book. My initial reaction was unexpected. In fact, I really didn't know what to expect, although I suspected it would be unusual and would take time. In the beginning my reactions were very intense and dramatic. This was probably due to the fact that the most susceptible and easily accessible biofilms were being destroyed first.

These first waves of acute herxes were quite intolerable, and beyond my ability to cope with them while still maintaining a normal life. As a result I had to stop them completely for several weeks just to recuperate. But I am probably a little more willing than your average patient to push the envelope with these therapies. I am also probably a bit more aggressive than I should be. In part this is due to my own type A personality and temperament. But also because I am testing these therapies; I needed to know if and how well they worked. Without a very distinct and noticeable response, I simply couldn't be certain that they were working. Also, when you are "feeling" what is happening inside you, it is easier to measure your response than if you are taking a slow and easy approach. I don't share this as a recommendation since it goes directly against what I advise in this book. But someone had to be the guinea pig. And now I know how the process works.

Biofilm destruction and the herxing that follows do not follow the same pattern as when you are killing off planktonic infection. During a systemic infection, your body's response to antibacterial therapies will also be systemic. That is, you will generally "feel bad all over". Although the releasing of bacteria from biofilm destruction can also have a systemic reaction, it will usually be more intense locally in the areas where the biofilms have formed. And while the systemic response will be mild comparatively speaking, and subsides quickly, the local response can be difficult to ascertain since it seems to never want to go away. That is, you wonder if the antibiofilm substances are actually eliminating them since the local pain keeps returning to an intense level with each successive wave of treatments. This can lead you to believe that this is a waste of time and that they are not working.

Biofilms by their very nature are very resistant. The frustrating thing about developing therapy strategies for biofilm-related infections is that it is difficult to gauge the progress. As an illustration, biofilms can be like mountain ranges in the body in that they come in all shapes and sizes. Some may be small like a rolling hill, hence, depending on the intensity of the therapy, the amount of time necessary to reverse and dissolve them may be relatively short compared to those that are extensive, complex and massive that took a long time to form. These may take exponentially more time to resolve than less developed biofilms. Also, just as geological strata that makes up a mountain may be multi-layered with different hardnesses, so response to treatment by any one layer of biofilm which is made up of not only different species of pathogens and gene expressions, but different exopolysaccharide, mineral, and fibrin components may represent varying levels of resistance. The body is going to maintain an immune response no matter what degree of progression the film has developed. So unless and until the biofilm is completely eradicated or dissolved, one may continue to experience symptoms leading to the belief that the therapies being employed are not being effective. This may therefore also lead the patient to decide it is not working and simply stop the treatments altogether, which if left unhindered can only lead to the further advancement and deepening of the infection.

However, one needs to be encouraged to maintain these therapies especially when they notice changes taking place either good or bad. The herxing, improving or lessening of symptoms over time is your reminder that you are moving in the right direction and slowly finding success. You may be moving along in your therapies and suddenly experience what you believe to be a significant setback due to an increase in symptoms. You may have reached and razed a level of biofilm that is particularly symptom-inducing that has released long buried toxic bacteria. In fact this repeated process may take place for a long time, again leading you to wonder if you are taking the right approach. But remember, those that have had Lyme disease that have eventually found success have experienced this process also. So it should not be discouraging, but should be understood that it is part of the process, and that in time you may be rewarded for your persistence.

However by doing nothing but accepting them they will inevitably do nothing but become worse. Until a time comes when someone has discovered a pill that will eliminate biofilms very quickly, which is not very likely any time soon, we must remain comforted knowing that over time, and with persistence the disease process is reversing. Think of the length of time you have had the disease, and how much time the biofilms have had to develop. In theory, the less time they've had to develop, the sooner it will take to recover. But for those of us with many years in the making, it will remain a long uphill battle. But what are the alternatives?

I have reached a point in my many years of Lyme treatments that from all outward appearances Lyme disease appears to be virtually gone. I have no more systemic symptoms. To the average person who doesn't know any better, he might say he has beaten the disease and cured himself. After all, do we not gauge the disease process by the symptoms of the disease? When they are gone, we feel well. But to many, they never seem to feel completely the way they did before the disease. I have read time and time again many Lyme sufferers who believed themselves to be cured say this is due to some left-over damage done to the body that will take time to heal. But I understand the nature of the beast. For me this is not so.

In the past, upon stopping all strictly antimicrobial medicines, in time I could sense a slow and sublte reemergence of fatigue and slight symptom increase. But if I had been cured of Lyme completely as some say they are, this should not be happening. To this day the only remaining sign of Lyme is a slight chronic arthritic pain in the right lower back from an old injury that remains somewhat painful, although at a much reduced level. Sometimes the pain is almost imperceptible. This is compared to only 2 years earlier when for many years I was walking and limping hunched over like a cripple. Some may say this is just ordinary arthritis that happens to everyone who has had a chronic injury. This is exactly my point. In contrast to osteoarthritis where the cartilage and bone wear down over time, pathogen-based arthritic conditions, much of the new research suggests, is often biofilm formation that has not resolved, even when all other systemic Lyme symptoms are virtually gone.

However as further evidence that Lyme has not been totally eradicated even in many of us that no longer even display Lyme disease symptoms, and as subjective proof as to the efficacy of these therapies, the reaction to these therapies coincides completely with the way one would expect to see in those infected with biofilms. Because the systemic bacterial infection is virtually eliminated, one would obviously not expect to see much further improvement of the condition. However my experience has been that upon receiving antibiofilm therapies, it's like the disease is reawakening (because it was never completely eradicated to begin with.) The constant exposure to antibiofilm substances causes a continual "leakage" of the bacteria into the body that can cause mild headaches, stiff neck, and some emotional agitation, etc. These will subside as the therapies are stopped to give the body time to rest and clear out the released toxins. In my own experience however, as the biofilms were reversing it seemed as though I would periodically hit some "pocket" of a biofilm that seemed to be especially reactive as the pain became particularly intense once again. To those not understanding the entire biofilm-reversing process, this can be confusing and leave you wondering why this is taking place. Remember, although your constant onslaught of antibacterial substances may have eradicated almost all systemic spirochetes, the razing of biofilms will release long-hidden and deeply buried spirochetes and other pathogens which will inevitably not only seek to burrow deep down into the same joints and other hidden areas where they saught refuge long ago, but will almost on a continual basis stimulate the release of pro-inflammatory cytokines. So until these are completely eliminated, your therapies must never let up.

So to answer the question, how are these therapies working for me, the answer is "very distinctly and slowly". To many who use semantics in describing the healing process that takes place in Lyme disease, one might say I have "beaten disease" long ago. However, when biofilms form in chronic Lyme disease, a more accurate use of words would be I am "reversing the disease". I would now describe my condition as being 99% healed. As I continued to mature in these therapies, and learned even more, it seems to have melted away.

Note: As this book goes to publication, it is now over a year since I began my initial highly intense therapies. One level after level has been exposed, and the healing has grown deeper. There are no signs of my systemic Lyme illness whatsoever. One of the lingering, annoying and persisting symptoms very common in Lyme disease, stiff and chronic neck pain is gone. The pain in the knee that seemed to never go away is now almost non-perceptible.

As I continue to administer these antibiofilm therapies, I have sensed an over-all deepening of the healing process. I would love to be able to tell any one person, "do this, and you will be cured of chronic Lyme disease". But that would be dishonest, no matter how well intentioned, or even how effective these will be for any one person. The truth is, it is all subjective to each individual. I remain convinced that in time eventually these therapies will eliminate the last remaining vestiges of Lyme that so many have experienced seems to "anchor" them to chronic disease. "Knowing your enemy" when it comes to Lyme disease can mean the difference between victory and defeat.

The development of chronic Lyme disease requires long-term therapy to reverse the process. Once deep entrenchment from biofilms and subsequent development of sequestered fibrin, accumulations of heavy metals and positively charged minerals has occurred, no one "anti-anything" medicine will solely eliminate the damage. Many medicines whether herbal or otherwise, appear to be significantly more effective against soft tissues and organs where they are fed by the vascular system; but are much less efficient in avascular or less vascular areas such as bone, joints, or the extra-cellular matrix within tissues. Pathogens and subsequent biofilm development naturally gravitate to these areas for refuge for this reason. This is also one of the reasons why intense antimicrobial therapies demonstrate significant herxes early on in the disease, but then become increasingly less effective as the more accessible microbes die off.

Therefore, in order to address these deeper and less accessible areas, methods which increase absorption of these medicines in order to continually and slowly over time dissolve, disperse, bind, and decompose these accumulations must be administered on a continual basis. That is the reason why and how *chronic* Lyme disease differs from its cousin Lyme disease, and why a distinction must be made between the two. The methods employed to reverse them both although overlap, are distinct in their ultimate goals.

FINAL THOUGHTS

Lyme disease remains one of the fastest spreading infectious diseases in this country. It seems as though nearly every single aspect of Lyme has some mystery attached to it, whether we are speaking of its origins, how it is diagnosed, what strains cause Lyme, how it is spread, what role testing plays in the process, what coinfections are involved, how it evades the immune system and antibiotics, whether or not it is curable, and the list goes on. This is one disease you simply cannot definitively define and clearly understand. So it stretches the imaginations of men, and like a chess game challenges men to reach deep within themselves to find a way to outmaneuver their opponent. But the stakes are much higher. Men and women suffer deeply and usually without rest. But a victor does not see himself as a victim. It is a challenge to become better and stronger. It is an exercise in excellence. It means falling down a thousands times, but getting up a thousand and one.

As Lyme disease sufferers, we are required to use all available tools given to us by the Creator. But unless we choose to utilize them creatively and aggressively, this is one battle whose end is decided largely by our own degree of commitment. We often think that illnesses bring out our worst. But in fact, these afflictions can often make us realize what we are capable of when we are challenged to be our best in spite of what we are facing.

You have in your hands knowledge of tools never before compiled in one source to aid you in your quest for healing. And every day we are learning more and more. There is hope for deeper healing for every person. The limits of that healing are determined by your own capacity to apply what you now know.

BONUS CHAPTER

CHAPTER 17

The Fasting Factor: Achieving Level 6 Healing

The ultimate goal of chronic Lyme sufferers is to reverse their Lyme disease to the point where they are finally free once and for all from the suffering that has plagued them for so many years. Unfortunately there is no cure for chronic Lyme disease, at least not as it would be viewed by conventional medicine. Remember, conventional medicine creates incurable illnesses by the very paradigm from which they operate, which says that only drugs can cure. Since they have not discovered a drug that can cure chronic Lyme disease, in their world, there is no cure for this illness. Let them live in their world while we move forward in our new paradigm to find healing.

In the world of natural healing, the possibilities are nearly endless. Where some practitioners of natural medicine have failed however, is that they, in their effort to compete with conventional medicine, have attempted to take that model, and replace it with natural substances, yet have retained the same paradigm. This too has resulted in a wrong approach to healing. It is only when we look deeply into the biochemistry of the body and the microbe, and examine the many complexities that are intertwined that essentially forms what at first appears to be a permanent condition, do we realize there are solutions—we just weren't looking in the right place for the answers. Albert Einstein once said, "You cannot solve a problem from the same consciousness that created it. You must learn to see the world anew." Hence, conventional medicine only sees solutions through drugs. That is the only consciousness they possess. What a sad world they live in if that is their only viewpoint.

However Einstein also said, "If you can't explain it simply, you don't understand it well enough." Up to this point we have attempted to explain and to see deeply into what is actually happening in the body at the level of the microbe. We have deepened our understanding not only as to the different levels of healing that are necessary to be addressed, but have suggested strategies or protocols that have been effectively used by others. None of these is a perfect solution. But by combining them into powerful combinations, they can become more effective than the sum of their parts since Bb hates this approach. It cannot defend itself against it, and will ultimately die off, or find an even deeper place to hide. But we must always remain a step ahead of this enemy. Where it hides, we must find it.

Well, perhaps we have arrived at a place where we feel we have done all we know that we can do. After all, one can only take so many different medicines, in so many combinations before we understand that even the best of them have their limitations. There have been so many Lyme sufferers that have reached a level where they just couldn't seem to find any further healing, yet they knew they still were not at the level where they were before their disease. As one can see from the last chapter, I too had arrived there, only to dramatically experience that deeper level I didn't even know was possible.

It is my intention to be as honest about my efforts as possible. I have been so tired of so many writers of Lyme books who themselves share a great deal of information, but at the end of their story you are left wondering if they still have Lyme disease, or what were the end results of all their efforts. This will not happen with this author. Because Lyme disease inflicts different levels of resistance in different people, 100 people can arrive at as many levels of healing. I think it is fair to say that I have been a member of a group of Lyme victims whose Lyme has been so severely entrenched due to not only ineffective antibiotic therapy, but also, and particularly not understanding in the early years that the conventional model approach actually forces Lyme to become far more resistant and chronic over time. But not only that, because I have suffered for years from chronic injuries, these became the perfect breeding ground for even further biofilm formation than would be expected in the typical Lyme patient, and thus set up the conditions for a perfect storm to "permanently" entrench chronic infection. This is the reason my own personal journey of healing was so slow. But when

I finally saw what was happeining, and realized there existed the means to reverse the infection over time, no longer was I wasting my efforts by throwing medicines at a condition and finding no improvement—the pattern experienced by the vast majority of Lyme sufferers. In fact, just the opposite. As you read, my success was beyond my wildest dreams, so much so I finally had to stop just to recover. My reason for saying this is that to whatever degree your body will allow it, there is hope for reversing even the most unyielding and defiant condition.

But now it is time to go deeper. Now we will address the final and deepest level of healing.

DEEPER STILL

Once many of the antibiofilm strategies have been used to over time weaken Lyme disease, there is often another layer that must still be addressed, which represents the deepest level. It is the level of healing damaged cellular tissue and potentially DNA damaged cells. Most chronic Lyme disease sufferers admittedly never reach this level of healing, because they don't know how. And maybe that's a good beginning. Once you have tried everything you know how, it's time to give up and let the body take over.

At the end of the chapter on Biofilms we discussed the complex process that takes place in chronic inflammation; how the body itself may play a larger role in its own damage than even the infected bacteria themselves. It may be worth rereading. Reversing this process is absolutely vital to going deeper. Unless the excessive fibrin/fibronectin which contains the source of the infection is slowly reduced over time, the bacteria can remain trapped within the epithelial extracellular matrix and intracellulary long after the systemic infection has subsided. Often deep seated resistant Lyme arthritis can represent this level, but also anywhere lesions have formed as a result of biofilm attachment which forced human cells to accommodate the infection just to survive, thus inducing DNA damage. In order to reach this deeper level of healing is it necessary to go way beyond even the reduction of biofilms. It is the level wherein we are required to reverse the activity that allowed the damage to take place in the first place. Let's briefly review.

During chronic infection, Borrelia Burdgorferi burrows deeply into specific tissues and ultimately attaches itself to cells by means of their fibronectin-binding proteins. This is a calculated maneuver. Since immune cells which would normally extract or engulf the bacteria have become down-regulated, or have developed myeloperoxidase deficiency, they are nearly paralyzed from removing the bacteria from this newly-formed microbe-cell bond. These human cells to which fibronectin-binding proteins become attached become damaged, yet are kept just enough alive in order to accommodate the bacteria which uses the cell as a means of protection. In turn, as a secondary means of self-preservation, the body itself sequesters or wards off the infected/damaged cells/tissues by layering the area with fibrin. However this also in turn actually becomes the perfect oasis for biofilm development. Fibrin matrix not only is intended to aid in the healing of injured cells, they can also act to seal-in these damaged/injured cell/germ complex accumulations. In time they can continue to proliferate while the body also continues to hold the infected cells in check. Thus, chronically injured or damaged tissue almost seems to spread, while the avascular fibrin deposits can continue to develop more and more over time. These accumulations represent the deepest level of infection that seem unaffected by antimicrobial medicines which simply cannot penetrate deeply enough to resolve the condition.

So what is the answer? And how can the body resolve this condition on its own, or at least begin to reverse it, when it is the body itself which is contributing to these formations? In other words, all of our efforts to resolve the condition, no matter what they involve, are an upstream battle, since no longer is the problem necessarily a microbe problem, but a condition the body itself is perpetuating. Therefore, unless the body itself can reverse its own efforts, this self-proliferation of its own disease will in fact remain unchanged.

Two almost universally overlooked therapeutic measures that can have a dramatic effect on Lyme, as well as other diseases, involve diet. We only briefly mentioned diet earlier. One significant aid to healing can be the elimination of the normal American diet. I became interested in diet when I read about a medical doctor that had used diet to completely reverse her Multiple Sclerosis. She called it the "hunter/gatherers" diet. Since MS has been associated with spirochete infections, this possible connection to Lyme disease told me that there is much more to diet than we have been told. Others have used what they call the *paleo* or cave man-diet which incorporates meats, but the reduction of grains and simple carbohydrates. I have used an even stricter diet such as one which incorporates large quantities of greens and vegetables, raw nuts, hemp protein, and healthy oils such as coconut, moringa, and olive oils, seaweeds and algae products such as chlorella and spirulina, while eliminating simple starches, sugars, and carbohydrates, particularly grains, and even most fruits and their juices. But as advantageous as these diets are, they are not likely to bring the level of healing that is necessary to actually reverse infection-damaged tissues and cells.

ENTER FASTING

Fasting has been used for as long as anyone can remember to accelerate the healing of certain illnesses, when all other medicinally-based methods alone have failed. It is often laughed at by those that don't truly understand the power of proper and correct fasting, and view it as some superstitious or religious practice that has no place in the arena of modern healing. However the benefits of fasting, as had been written about by some of the early physicians of the 20th century, were so dynamic and effective, that even to this day there does not exist a single medicine in the conventional medical arsenal that rivals the potential that fasting holds in many that have chronic and highly resistant diseases.

Today when one thinks of fasting, it is often associated with a short term, sometimes 2-4 day abstinence from solid food in order to give the body time to eliminate stored toxins and rest from the digestion process, for cleansing, or in an effort to lose excess weight. But even then these fasts are often supplemented with juices, or perhaps some fruit or milk, or whatever happens to be the current "in" fad. As beneficial as these may be, and to whatever degree they may be effective to fulfill what purpose the faster is trying to accomplish, these are not true fasts, and will not accomplish what a true fast can do. This will be explained forthcoming.

A true fast is the total abstinence from food which provides nourishment, with the exception of water, or also simply called a *water fast*. But the real key to an effective fast as it relates to the healing of chronic conditions, is the length of time the fast is done. Rarely does one ever hear of a fast that lasts more than a week. This is because the ancient practice of true fasting has become so foreign to those of us in the modern age of pharmaceutical medicines, it has almost become viewed as some pagan practice that has no relevance today, and certainly to the ignorant, has no scientific basis for which to considerate it a viable and legitimate healing practice. And so the idea of a longer extended fast truly does not compute in most peoples minds. After all, what's the point?

Long term water fasting does what no other form of fasting comes close to. But before we go into the science behind what happens in the body during an extended water fast, consider that this is not an uncommon "extremist" idea. Maybe the most famous fast that many people are familiar with was the 40 day fast of Jesus in the wilderness prior to embarking on his ministry.

During the ninth month of Ramadan, Muslims fast and abstain from water from dawn to sunset. Of course this form of fast is primarily done for spiritual reasons, and is actually not a true fast since they are permitted to a meal following sunset. Certainly fasting for spiritual reasons can sometimes form a stigma that prevents people from considering the physical benefits that fasting instills.

The idea of abstaining from food for an extended period of time for physical healing is in fact instinctive. It is quite common to observe that injured and diseased animals will naturally go into isolation and fast for even weeks at a time in order to heal by following their innate instincts. Upon healing their appetites return. Even in humans, we lose our desire for food during illness, or when the body is trying to heal from sickness or infection. It is simply instinctive. However nowadays, we have surrendered our body's natural instincts to heal over to the current conventional medical system which sees drugs as gods over the body's own innate wisdom to heal itself. But this system can never do what the body often can do for itself when fasting occurs.

Although fasting is in fact a quite natural process, it is counterintuitive to our "trained" scientific minds since the idea of being deprived of food is thought of as being an obstacle to health and healing. In fact, it is increasingly becoming understood that people live longer and healthier who eat less. In part, this is because even eating amounts of food whose caloric intake is considered to be "necessary" to maintain the persons body weight, can increase the metabolic processes necessary for the processing of that energy to age the body beyond its potential years. In other words, we don't need to eat as much as we have been told is necessary, and in fact will actually shorten our life span by doing so.

An interview with Dr. Michael Mosley in Mailonline revealed that some studies done in the US and Japan showed that people living in communities that typically have lower food intake, live longer. Rats fed a diet reduced by 40% lived up to 20% longer than rats eating a normal diet. That would be equivalent to a person living some 20 years longer.[1]

Dr. Rai Casey MD shares an often cited study that was done on earthworms.

> Experimental tests conducted in the 1930's at the Zoology Dept of the U. of Chicago showed that worms, when well-fed, grew old, but by fasting them they were made young again.

> In one experiment worms were fed as much as they usually eat, except one worm, which was isolated and alternatively fed and fasted. The isolated worm was alive and energetic after 19 generations of its relatives had lived out their normal lifespan.

> Prof. C.M. Childs said: "When worms are deprived of food, they do not die of starvation in a few days. They live for months on their own tissues. At such time they become smaller and may be reduced to a fraction of their original size. Then when fed after such a fasting, they show all the physiological traits of young

animals. But with continued feeding, they again go through the process of growth and aging (and die)."2

Obviously no one is insinuating that the longevity of humans will also translate into some multiple by fasting. But it does tell us that some phenomenon is taking place that is counterintuitive to what most associate with being "underfed". So that as interesting as studies like these are, fasting allows something to take place in the body that goes way beyond simply living longer. And understanding what that "something" is, will help us to see how fasting can aid the body in self healing that no other therapy can come close to.

The normal steps the body goes through during a fast are:

1. Converting foods in the gut to energy. Then once these are depleted,
2. Glycogen stored in the liver is released for plasma glucose conversion to be used universally throughout the body. Once these stores become depleted, the liver begins to-
3. Break down amino acids in a process called gluconeogenesis.
4. This is followed by actual catabolic (breakdown) of muscle tissue.
5. Finally, lipolysis, or the breaking down of adipose (fat tissue) for the conversion of energy.

When the body reaches the point that it begins burning its own fat reserves, this has the additional benefit of releasing stored toxins in these fat cells, which has been placing an additional toxic burden on the body. And when the body is continually forced to expend extra energy just to digest its own food, it can impede the ability of the immune system to work at its best to clear out toxins and wastes from the body. Lowering the digestion load is a huge advantage. You probably knew that already from your science class in school.

But something more happens in the body when we fast beyond the point of using excess energy reserves. The body goes into super charge mode enabling it to do what it cannot do when it is being forced to constantly be preoccupied with the task of utilizing energy just to digest food, impeding its ability to focus on optimal healing. There have been a number of studies which have demonstrated the benefits of fasting on immune modulating and increase of neutrophil activity. The reader is encouraged do his own research on the subject.

The reduction or elimination of solid foods as occurs during a juice fast does reduce the need for the body to exert energy just to make energy, and is a huge advantage over not fasting at all. But the drinking of juices or any other supplementation with food is not a true fast, and in fact may slow or impede the body from entering into a deeper form of healing that would only be in the beginning stages when doing these kinds of fasts.

Before moving on to explain the benefits of a true fast, it should be clarified that the use of this kind of fast that will be described is intended to be used for Level 6 healing. Particularly in the more acute infective levels of 1-5, fasting of this depth may have the affect of placing an excessive undo burden on the body's detox pathways by inducing such powerful herxes, that it may be overwhelming. The intention for employing a true and extended fast is to deal with the problems of Level 6 infection. What this means is that the Lyme sufferer will have already reached a level of healing wherein virtually all of the systemic planktonic infection has been eliminated, as well as has spent considerable time and effort reducing biofilm infection. The reason this is important will become evident. We are trying to first reduce the level of infection over time to such an extent prior to fasting, that once the fasting begins, the body can focus on healing rather than overwhelming the detox pathways and immune cells with the burden of ongoing infection that still has not been resolved from some of the other levels.

Is it possible to employ fasting during some of the earlier levels of infection? Would they be useful? Certainly they would. And periodic fasting to whatever extent can be tolerated by the Lyme sufferer would be advantageous. But what we are discussing here is an extended fast. And this kind of fast is intended to be used to focus deeply on a level of healing after other therapies have already been employed to take the Lyme patient as far as they are able. And what the body is about to embark on as one begins this kind of fast is in and of itself difficult and challenging for most people. To add to that significant herxes and the added burden that you will experience if you have not first eliminated as much of the biofilm-based infection as possible, may be too much for some people to maintain, and thus short circuit the entire fasting process. That is why we have reserved fasting for the final and deepest level of healing, which will allow the body to perform unfettered from the burden of yet unresolved excessive infection that other therapies are intended to deal with.

Some may disagree with this approach and are obviously free to begin fasting at the earlier levels of infection. What I have described here has three advantages: 1) It assumes that the infection has already been dramatically reduced to almost imperceptible levels, thus 2) will significantly reduce (and in most cases virtually eliminate) herx reactions once the fasting begins; which will in turn 3) dramatically increase the effectiveness of the fast to focus on healing rather than expending energy for battling excessive unresolved infection. As we begin to see exactly what happens in the body during an extended fast, and especially why we are using it to resolve deep-seated accumulations that have taken place as a result of chronic Lyme disease, this will make much more sense.

The purpose of fasting as it relates to Level 6 healing is to address chronically inflamed and DNA damaged cells and tissue, and to a large extent accumulated fibrin which may represent unresolved deeply imbedded infection which has been unaffected by all other forms of therapy. Chronically infected lesions, or what some doctors have termed "post-Lyme syndrome" or post Lyme arthritis, are often experienced by many sufferers which lingers long after the acute infection has subsided, and may not develop in all

Lyme patients. But to the extent they do, they represent a chronic source of inflammation, almost cyst-like in nature. As we describe the affects of a true extended fast, it will become clear that something is happening in the body that goes way beyond what occurs in short term fasts, or "fasts" which simply replace solid foods with other forms of energy such as juicing, fruit, milk fasts, etc. These are not true fasts, and may not go as deeply as a true extended water fast with regards to the physiological and chemical pathways of the body. Remember, this book about going deeper into healing.

Fasting has also been used by some Lyme patients in the past with some success; but virtually never, to my knowledge by anyone in the manner being described for the elimination of damaged and chronically infected cells that occur and hold on even after most of the systemic Lyme infection has been resolved. And so it would be difficult for anyone to prejudge what this kind of fasting can do since we are not speaking of using fasting as a general therapy against Lyme disease. This is very specific and targeted towards Level 6 healing—that level which represents the final, deepest and most resistant chronically Lyme-damaged tissue. Not only have few people attempted this form of healing, but the manner in which the fasting is employed, the length of time the fast takes place, and the severity and stage of the infection would all affect the degree to which healing would take place. So to use fasting in any other manner than will be described here as a means of healing Lyme disease would be a hit or miss proposition since the terms "Lyme disease", and "fast" can have very broad meanings.

I personally had attempted a watermelon fast for about a week during earlier levels of infection prior to my experience with antibiofilm substances, with no noticeable benefits whatsoever. I had heard the testimony of a woman that went on a watermelon fast for her Lyme disease, which subsequently went away with no further symptoms. However her's appeared to be early Lyme, not chronic, which would represent a much deeper and more resistant infection. And that form of Lyme would be affected in an entirely different manner than is represented in long-standing chronically damaged and entrenched tissues.

There are two uses of fasting as it relates to infections. The first is the level of the microbe, in which not only are germs deprived of readily available energy, but how fasting frees immune cells to become more active against pathogens. The second is how fasting acts upon the body itself in a process called *autodigestion*. This second level occurs in a long term extended fast, and is the level we will examine as it relates to reversing chronic illnesses.

In medical terminology, the words *autodigestion* and *autolysis* have several different meanings depending on the process you are describing. Often they refer to the body's own enzymes breaking down tissue, autodigestion, and can occur within the stomach for example following death. However our use of these terms with regards to fasting is defined as: the body itself, either by the use of endogenous enzymes (enzymes stored in the cells themselves), or any number of other processes such as phagocytosis, hydrolysis, catabolism, etc., as well as proteases and other enzymes which break down excesses in the body in the form of accumulations, cystic tissues, growths, tumors, injured or damaged tissues, aging cells, toxic excesses, lesions, scar tissue, etc. In this manner we are describing a process the body initiates during prolonged fasting in which the body begins to do some house cleaning by removing long-standing non-vital agglomerations or masses that up to this point have been tolerated.

According to an article written by Dr. Harold Goldhamer, Therapeutic Fasting, "Fasting allows the body an opportunity to generate an acute response in a chronic condition." [3] In order to affect long-term chronic conditions, a fast must reach a level that will address more entrenched resistance. This type of fasting goes beyond the commonly practiced juice or water fast usually done for several days for cleansing and detoxification. I learned that something happens in the body when a fast is extended for longer periods of time that would only be in its beginning stages if only performed for several days.

In the beginning days of a fast, the body is going to survive off of available fats in a process called *lipolysis*. But as the fast progresses, another process begins to accelerate called *autolysis*. In autolysis, cells essentially dissolve by their own enzymes. Autolysis occurs in dying, injured, or disease cells and tissues. This process can speed up dramatically during fasting. So in order to reach this level, sufficient energy stores must be depleted in order for the body to begin moving to autolyse diseased or damaged tissue. Otherwise, they will remain once the fast is ceased, and continue to plague to body in spite of all efforts.

A well researched article on fasting by Swayze Foster, <u>What the Body does during fasting</u>, explains the physiological benefits of fasting. He cites that fasting helps break down cholesterol deposits, initiates fibrinolysis (the break down of fibrin), phagocytosis is accelerated, diuresis (the excretion of salt and water from the kidneys), and autolysis is sped up. One source of nonessential material in the body is diseased tissue. "During the fast, the process of autolysis leads to the breakdown of this type of tissue which has hampered normal functioning." [4]

Dr. Herbert Shelton wrote an excellent article on the scientific benefits of fasting.

> *It is generally held by men with wide experience with the fast that abnormal tissues are broken down and eliminated more rapidly than normal tissue during periods of abstinence . . . More than a hundred years ago Sylvester Graham wrote: "It is a general law of the vital economy, that when, by any means, the general function of decomposition exceeds that of composition or nutrition, the decomposing absorbents always first lay hold of and remove those substances which are of least use to the economy; and hence, all morbid accumulations, such as wens, tumors, abscesses, etc., are rapidly diminished and often wholly removed under severe and protracted abstinence or fasting."—Science of Life, pp. 194-195.*[5]

"Fasting is a scientific method of ridding the system of diseased tissue, and morbid matter, and is invariably accompanied by beneficial results.".[6] "The essential tissues obtain their nourishment from the less essential." [7]

"The increase of erythrocytes, during the early part of the fast, he regarded as due to improved nutrition resulting from a cessation of overeating., by enzymic action, a process which has been termed *autolysis."[8]*

> Keep in mind that oftentimes it has been observed that shorter term fasts can also demonstrate remarkable healing for particular conditions. Although not common, I've read some doctor's reports of some types of tumors drying up after only a few days of fasting. Certain kinds of infections subside. However these are not necessarily due to the autolytic or autodigestion processes which become increasing more active as the fast progresses past several weeks. Rather, some of the healing taking place during a shorter term fast is often due to the deprivation of nourishment no longer feeding the infections, tumors, growths, etc. These will naturally subside on their own from being starved out. This is different from what happens in an extended fast where the body's own autolytic processes feed on these aggregations, rather than infectious growths dissolving on their own. What makes the extended fast so much more powerful is that both processes take place, rather than only one. And the autodigestion process is much more effective in the long term.

An important function of fasting is the increase in fibrinolytic activity. We previously discussed the accumulation of fibrin in biofilms and infected tissues. In prolonged fasting, the breaking down of fibrin accelerates. According to some studies, significant increase in fibrinolytic activity of the blood takes place after 36 hours of fasting, and lasts sometime after the fast.[9]

It is also known that although the percentage of neutrophils can be reduced in a prolonged fast, the phagocytic activity of neutrophils actually becomes greatly enhanced upon fasting. This is probably an additional mechanism induced by the body to aid in the elimination of toxic tissues, cellular debris, and pathogens which becomes part of the autodigestion process that takes place during fasting.

It was mentioned previously that there have been some researchers that have observed that DNA of Bb joins with human cells, which would represent a form of permanent damage to these cells. If in fact this is true, these diseased cells with DNA damage or modification may represent diseased epithelial and /or connective tissue cells which would be more susceptible to autolysis since the vitality of these cells has become greatly impaired. Certainly the deprivation of energy would have a detrimental effect on infectious bacteria like Bb. But the autolysis process experienced in fasting would go far beyond the level of the microbe, and induce the body's own autolytic mechanisms to force the digestion of diseased and low vitality tissues and cells. These activities can be illustrated to a much larger extent with the dissolution of tumors and cystic growths observed to take place upon extended fasts.

In an extended fast, the body begins to reduce and eliminate expendable stores or excesses, in an effort to rebalance the system as a whole. It can draw upon non-vital or damaged tissues which have become a chronic source of imbalance. In doing so the body has an opportunity for a sort of internal remodeling by converting non-essential stores and redirecting them for use as energy and/or their elimination. Non-essential growths which have been allowed to proliferate such as tumors, cysts, internal scarring, unhealed chronic wounds with their fibrin accumulation, etc, are now seen as unnecessary "parasites" that act as excessive burdens on the system.

One of the reasons why some "fasts" may not be as effective as they could be is because unless the body is deprived of energy at a level where autolysis is allowed the opportunity to draw upon these excess accumulations and tissue stores, it may not reach its intended level of healing. For instance short term 2-3 day fasts, or popular fasts which include juices, fruits, or any other method that supplements some food that provides sufficient energy to prevent or slow the autolysis initiative, would not be sufficient to allow healing to take place at these deeper levels.

Certainly short term juicing or fruit fasts may allow for the elimination of toxins, and perhaps even temporarily free the burden on immune cells which may allow them to function more effectively, thereby freeing the immune system as a whole to more aggressively eliminate pathogens. However deep seated chronic lesions, infectious tissues, or damaged cells which have become entrenched even at the cellular and DNA level, may require their autolysis, or removal by the body itself. This level of cleansing may only be possible with a true longer term fast that allows the autolysis mechanism to perform optimally.

Again, Dr. Shelton says,

> *The fasting body begins to grow smaller, and in order to maintain the integrity of its vital organs, it utilizes all the surplus material it has on hand. Growths, deposits, effusions, dropsical swellings, infiltrations, fat, etc., are absorbed and used to support these organs. With no digestive drudgery on hand, nature employs the long desired leisure for general house cleaning purposes. Accumulations of surplus tissues are overhauled and analyzed; the available component parts are turned over to the department of nutrition, while the refuse is thoroughly and permanently removed.* [10]

Another reason why an extended fast is more effective is that unhealthy cells and tissues do not process available energy as effectively as healthy cells. The body acts in a prioritized and orchestrated effort to maintain the integrity of vital tissues, and in order of their necessity or importance, will naturally seek to provide for their energy supplies. In a fast, damaged or diseased tissues, such as are known to occur in Level 6 infections, will not therefore be able to process sufficient energy to maintain them at the same level, since lower energy reserves will deplete their capabilities to remain active. Thus even if the autolysis process didn't exist at all, the lower energy provisions alone would significantly reduce their ability for self-proliferation, and inflammation-inducing capabilities. This alone would permit the body to heal at a deeper level.

What may be an icing on the cake with regards to benefits of fasting, and its potential to resolve chronic conditions such as is seen in Lyme disease, is that we now are aware of specific natural medicines which could be taken during a fast which not only would *not* provide energy to slow the autodigestion process, but would actually aid the body's efforts by providing targeted support. For example, the taking of fibrinolytic enzymes, niacinamide, berberine, EDTA, etc, will enhance the body's effort. In this manner, we are delivering an even greater potential for deeper healing than fasting alone.

But the kind of fast necessary to see these benefits have rarely been practiced by those suffering from chronic Lyme disease. Most simply are not aware of this possibility. And you certainly are not going to hear of this from the medical community which has long abandoned natural healing practices. In fact, I didn't become aware of the deeper potentials of extended fasting until a short time prior to publishing of this book. In the past I had tried the short term, and juice fasting, which did demonstrate some temporary reduction of symptoms and inflammation. But never the longer term fasts such as 3-6 weeks which are often necessary in order to experience the benefits mentioned in this section. However as this book was going to publication, I decided to delay it so that I may share with the reader my own experience with an extended fast.

I had shared earlier that with the use of the new approach to healing that has been shared in this book I had achieved the level of healing that I would estimate as perhaps 99% elimination of my Lyme condition. But even with that level, which is far beyond what many achieve who have developed long-entrenched chronic Lyme lesions and long-standing arthritic conditions, there remained yet some lower back trouble, as well as slight skin lesions, all of which represent areas of old injury, or deep accumulations of biofilms which had subsequently become reduced. These kinds of conditions we have learned in this book are prime targets for the chronic Lyme development.

> By the way, there may be some readers that have been fortunate enough not to have experienced some of these conditions described in this book, where localized chronically diseased tissues have formed as a result of their long-standing Lyme infection. However you may never seem to get completely well. In you, this may represent deeply entrenched infection, which may also find significant benefit from this form of fasting,

I wanted to see what effect longer term water fasting would have on these localized areas based upon what some of the research has been suggesting, as well as what many of the doctors had to say that have used fasting to eliminate and outright cure many highly resistant diseases in their patients. Since I had never performed a true extended water fast before, it was difficult in the beginning to know how it would affect me, and how long I felt I would be able to continue on it until I simply couldn't go any further. So I didn't have any particular goal in mind when I started. But I had aimed at 40 days.

Most that partake on a long-term fast testify that by around the third day it becomes very difficult. You are very weak and go through a lot of hunger pains. This is because by around the third day the body is beginning to make a major shift from living off its glycogen stores in the liver and any remaining food in the intestines, and begins converting muscle into energy, as well as shifting to fat stores. At the same time the stomach is reducing its size. These physiological changes can cause a lot of discomfort, and in some people can be enough to have them call it quits before they have barely begun because they assume this unpleasant feeling will endure throughout the entire fasting process. I too experienced this feeling, but had been prepared beforehand since I knew what to expect. My experience that followed this 3 day hurdle was similar to others that say following this time, the discomfort from these initial changes subside. You then begin to feel quite calm and clear headed. You feel relaxed and even serine. Fogginess in your thinking fades away, and you feel as though another part of you is being "reborn".

Perhaps this is the level that many seek that use fasting for spiritual purposes. Their body's are no longer being burdened by the digestion process which constantly draws blood away from the brain in order to digest food, and the excess metabolic processes the body is forced to manage while eating. Actually, the vital body systems require very little energy to perform, and are now free from their "enslavement" of being forced to constantly process food in order to more effectively focus on healing. In this manner, the body is quite literally being forced to shift from "maintentance" mode, to reversing, or a tearing down and removal process.

During the next several weeks I cannot say that I didn't involuntarily and spontaneously find myself dreaming of barbeque ribs and mashed potatoes smothered in gravy. But actually the experience was not nearly as discomforting as I imagined. In fact, as time moved on, I could sense some changes taking place, particularly in those very areas of chronic pain. They did begin to flare-up. But then would subside. As time proceeded I could feel myself experiencing healing like I've never experienced before. My skin began to look much younger as the body was moving deeper to eliminate toxins.

But I knew that the body was only in the beginning stages of removing deeper accumulations and diseased tissue which had long entrapped infected cells and microbes. By around 2 ½ weeks, I was experiencing clarity of thought and an ability to focus more effectively than at any time in my life. I seemed to be almost completely unimpaired by the normal grogginess or mental fatigue. They simply went away. Although admittedly I naturally felt somewhat weak from lack of food. The trade-off was well worth it.

By the end of the third week I was now experiencing definite healing, and knew something was happening. But I knew this was only the beginning stage. At this time, I was actually excited to find out how far I could go since I knew that healing can actually accelerate almost exponentially as the body is allowed to go deeper to perform the autolytic/housecleaning process. I was well intentioned to go all the way to 40 days.

However something unexpected happened, that I now see was part of the healing process. (Although this was my story, it will obviously be different in everyone.) I began to develop what I first thought was a cold at the time. As is my custom, I can usually stop a cold dead in its tracks by taking zinc gluconate lozenges. Within 2-3 days my cold is virtually gone. (Read the studies on zinc gluconate. You will find it to be the closest thing we have to an actual cure for the common cold.) However in this case it seemed to have no affect. But this wasn't new to me since I had periodically experienced this several times before.

Although I had never received an official diagnosis from a doctor, I have long suspected that I have had a mycoplasma co-infection along with my Lyme disease since I have additionally had symptoms 100% consistent with that illness even after all my systemic Lyme symptoms had disappeared (adding to the fact that mycoplasma has been found 70% of the time as a coinfection in Lyme disease.) Over the years I would periodically have a relapse into what seemed like a respiratory tract infection. At first this appears to be a cold, except it would last for sometimes 3-4 weeks, and I would experience a flare up of urinary tract inflammation, and low back pain, all of which are classic mycoplasma infection symptoms. Colds do not last for 3+ weeks, and they certainly don't relapse every few months with symptoms more consistent with mycoplasma.

The reason I tell you this is because this severe condition of upper respiratory infection caused me such suffering I felt I needed to go off of my fast just to recuperate. I was simply too weak to endure it any further. What I believe happened in hindsight was that due to the fast, the body may have finally reached a pocket of highly resistant and long-standing infection that had been released causing a relapse of symptoms (another reason I do not recommend this form of fast until one has first reduced the level of infection first by some of the other therapies). However, whether related, or just a pure coincidence that this happened during a prolonged fast, I was left with a reduced level of joint pain and quite noticeable reduction of skin lesion and inflammation.

After 4 days however, I resumed my fast. And after another week went by, although I was noticeably weaker, I was also noticing a dramatic reduction of pain. It was as if it was just "drying up".

Now I am not that naïve to believe that a mere 4 week fast would eliminate the degree of chronically inflamed tissue necessary to completely resolve the final vestiges of tissue damage and years of accumulations needed for complete healing. After all, I only lost about 15 lbs during that time. My 6' tall 185lb frame only went to 170 lbs. But this brief 4 week fast did in fact bring me to a deeper level of healing than I had ever experienced up to this point, and has suggested to me that I am on the right path. What this experience has prepared me for is a much longer term fast I plan to do very soon. I will report my progress to those interested. This experience also lent more evidence to me that in fact the remaining symptoms may not be Lyme disease at all, but rather are more consistent with mycoplasma, which in many cases can be even more resistant to treatment than Lyme disease. In any case, I am now especially confident that fasting is a very viable healing tool which may hold the key to perhaps completely reverse the last remaining vestiges of disease.

> For me personally, I have reached a level where any remaining "symptoms" are almost non-existent. I put "symptoms" in italics for this very reason. I now believe it is possible that even those with very deep long-standing chronic Lyme disease to reach a level of healing they never thought possible; and in some, to virtually and perhaps completely reverse the "disease" process to a point that it is no longer a "dis-ease". This book does not, and would not claim to hold the answer for every person to completely remove every last remaining vestige of damage they have experienced caused by this disease. After all, one can still see the scarring or damage left behind from measles, polio, chicken pox and other such illnesses which become cured, but then leave behind signs of their past inflictions. It is about giving to the sufferer the tools to *reverse* the disease to a level never before experienced, and certainly which conventional drug-based medicine denies is possible.

Particularly a prolonged fast over 3 weeks may require medical assistance from a health care professional trained in fasting to aid you and monitor you during this period. A lot happens, and a lot can happen if a fast is not done properly. It needs to be customized to fit the unique needs of each individual. Perhaps the most noticeable side effect from a extended water fast is the lowering of blood pressure, which can make you feel light-headed upon standing; another reason to take it slowly.

But keep in mind that fasting and starvation are not the same thing. In starvation, the body has gone passed the point of living off of its own energy reserves, to begin actually breaking down vital tissues.

The faster must not be allowed to prolong the fast to this point. The reader is encouraged to study fasting and understand the precautions and healing potentials prior to beginning. So although fasting itself is quite simple, monitoring your fast is important. But humans can go much longer without food than they think. It is important to reach the level in your fast where the autolysis process can begin removing damaged and diseased tissues in order to reverse the chronic conditions that have formed in the epithelial and other damaged cells throughout the body. The longer this process is allowed to work, the deeper the healing the body can perform.

The progression of the disease, and the length of time a person has had the disease will of course play a factor which determines the extent to which healing can take place. One of the dangers some practitioners of fasting have had in the past is that they became too aggressive in their desire to heal. Some "healers" in the past have not been prudent in their administration or management of fasting with regards to their patients. They pushed them to the point of endangering them beyond what the body was capable of performing within a given period of time. Fasting must be done as a healing tool to work with the body, not force it beyond its limits.

Remember that often in a fast, or when people lack or are deprived of food for long periods of time, they begin to suffer from malnutrition long before their energy reserves become depleted. The body requires vital nutrients to prevent malnutrition. Remember, we are speaking of therapeutic fasting, not suffering or starvation. Fasting without also being given the necessary nutrients such as vitamins and minerals during the fast, can in fact be disastrous. In the fast, our focus is to withhold energy so the body is induced to feed off of the non-vital accumulatons, not to rob it of essential nutrition. This is to be a time of healing, not dangerous deprivation.

Of course the primary objective with a long-term fast is to over time induce or intensify the body's autolytic or autodigestion capabilites by feeding off of non-vital growths and excesses. How one reaches that level however can vary. The ideal, fastest and most intensive would of course be to do one continuous fast for 4-6 weeks. But the prospect of such a dramatic fast on some people may be too much for some to even consider, let alone follow through to completion. This would be especially true for some who may already be carrying excess weight or energy reserves, as even a typical 40 or so day fast may not be sufficient for the body to begin sufficiently feeding off of non-vital deposits, damaged tissues, etc. Additionally, as we have said, the longer period fasts required to reach these deeper areas may cause some to begin experiencing malnutrition (of vital nutrients) before they actually deplete their energy reserves. And thus they may not be able to reach the level of their healing potentials.

So it may be more practical for some to do what I call a "step-down" fast wherein you take short breaks from your fast while continuing towards the target. For example if an individual weighed 190 lbs. and the potential weight to reach the optimal healing would be around 145 lbs, he/she may wish to take a day or two break from the fast following 2 weeks to resupply the body with light good nutrition. This may be some fruit, vegetables, quality protein such as fish for example. But avoid excess carbohydrates. Remember, you are only doing this to give the body a periodic break and resupply nutrients. This will have a positive psychological impact as well by giving yourself those intervals to look forward to, rather than seeing your fast as an "all or nothing" proposition, which may prevent some from beginning the fast in the first place, or stopping completely in the middle of the fast concluding that it is just too difficult. However this kind of fasting will inevitably take somewhat longer to do, and may not reach as deeply as a continuous fast. But for some the trade-off is worth it, and may be the only way others will be able to even consider the fast as a viable healing method. Remember the goal is to move in the direction of healing, not to see healing as a torturous journey.

But keep in mind that the final stage of the fast may be the most important of all, and may be the most difficult to discern when to actually end the fast for optimal healing. The deepest level of healing will likely take place the deeper the autolytic process is able to perform. It is for this reason that one should be encouraged to fast under the guidance of a healthcare practitioner who is familiar with fasting for healing purposes to help monitor your condition and advise when best to end the fast. This would be especially true during the final stage of fasting. Again, the reader is highly encouraged to research the topic of fasting further in order to fully understand the benefits and cautions. The following are excellent sources to begin:

Fasting and Eating for Health: A Medical Doctor's Program for Conquering Disease by Joel Fuhrman and Neal D. Barnard 1995

The Miracle of Fasting: Proven Throughout History for Physical, Mental, & Spiritual Rejuvenation by Patricia Bragg and Paul C. Bragg 2004

Fasting Can Save Your Life by Herbert M. Shelton and Ronald G. Cridland 1981

The Miracle Results of Fasting: Discover the Amazing Benefits in Your Spirit, Soul and Body by Dave Williams 2005

Of course using fasting as a tool to help reverse the effects of chronic Lyme will be new to most practitioners. So your studies should be tempered with that intent in mind.

Rest

The process of fasting for healing certain conditions involves more than just the elimination of food. This kind of fasting also requires significant rest. The healing processes can be especially impeded if the body is not receiving adequate rest. Physical exertion diverts energy away from this process. It robs the body from using this time to its maximum and effective benefit. Therefore, when considering this kind of fast, it needs to be done as part of an overall program which allows for the body to rest while the fasting is done. If the fast is not done properly, not given sufficient time, or the proper rest is not allowed, the desired benefits may not be experienced, and one may conclude this method is not effective. And since we don't know the degree of resistance or how any person will respond to this form of therapy, there is no way to know what level of healing you may achieve unless a full extended fast done properly is performed. And in fact it may be necessary to perform several fasts before the desire level of healing is achieved.

It is hoped that this short primer on therapeutic fasting can be a new beginning and new hope for the chronic Lyme sufferer. The one caveat with regards to fasting that admittedly may be slower to heal is that often hardened accumulations of excessive mineral deposits can be slower to reverse than soft tissue. However once you have begun the process, you are well on the road to reversing the disease process to achieve a level of healing you may have never thought possible. The following are a few supplements that may aid the body during a fast, and may be a consideration.

- EDTA (Essential Daily Defense by Longevity Plus)
- Serrapeptase, Nattokinase (Neprinol AFD by Arthur Andrew Medical)
- Berberine (Glycosolve or GlycoX 500)
- Humic Acid/Monolaurin (Humic-Monolaurin Complex by AllergyResearchGroup)
- Ecklonia cava extract (Seanol)
- Non-GMO lecithin granules

CONCLUSION

Level 6 healing of Lyme disease is often a level most resistant to therapy for the chronic sufferer. However as we have said previously, diseases such as Lyme may require the use of every weapon in our arsenal. And with this new understanding of fasting, an even deeper level of healing is now possible. In fact, with this understanding that fasting holds the potential for reversing and even healing chronic conditions, some may want to consider using fasting after some of the other methods have been used. As early as the 1920's a Dr. J.H. Tilden MD was using fasting in his practice to cure a myriad of diseases.[11] Among these were relapsing fever and syphilis, today both of which are known to be sourced from spirochete infections. Therefore this therapy holds strong potential for Lyme sufferers at all levels, and particularly when used in conjunction with many of the therapies offered in this book.

In many people, the deepest level of Lyme disease infection is localized DNA damaged cells and tissue. These can linger for far longer even after most of the biofilm-based infection has been resolved. There is a limit to what any particular or combinations of medicines can do before the body must take over on its own. And the length of time it can take the body to heal these deeper conditions when given the right support will vary with each individual. We know that these conditions are possible to heal. For myself, I no longer consider myself to have Lyme disease. It is simply gone. And I am also no longer afraid of it returning. I suppose that one of the consequences of the many years I have personally suffered is the empowerment I now feel over this disease. Never again will I be its victim. I used every tool provided by the Creator to conquer the enemy and have regained the land. Yet to so many who still bow down to the god of government interference which remains a part of the American medical system, they may never know the heights and depths of healing that are possible when entering into the rediscovered paradigm provided to us in nature by the Creator.

Words such as "autolysis" and "autodigestion" are almost exclusively understood today as impractical academic terms to the modern medical community. But the power that is unleashed by the body itself during a prolonged fast often accomplishes what no medical doctor can do with even the most sophisticated medicines that conventional medicine can muster. That is because the innate wisdom and super-intelligence possessed by the body itself is far superior to even the wisest of men. It seems that sometimes the most difficult task of man is to simply get out of the way so the body can heal itself. And perhaps modern science is just now beginning to understand advice from ancient wisdom—"this kind goes out only by prayer and fasting".

Good healing.

ENDNOTES

1. *Want to live longer? Ditch the diet, cancel your gym session - just eat less.* By Liz Thomas Article in Mailonline July 31, 2012 http://www.dailymail.

co.uk/health/article-2181370/Want-live-longer-Ditch-diet-cancel-gym-session--just-eat-less.html Retrieved Feb. 3, 2013

2. Dr. Rai Casey MD sharing her experience with fasting. http://www.notmilk.com/hs/casey.html Retrieved Feb. 3, 2013

3. *Therapeutic Fasting: An Introduction to the Benefits of a Professionally Supervised Fast.* Alan Goldhamer D.C. Article on TrueNorth Health Center website http://www.healthpromoting.com/learning-center/articles/therapeutic-fasting Retrieved Feb. 3, 2013

4. *Introduction to fasting: What The Body Does When You Fast* by Swayze Foster Article from Raw Food Explained.com website http://www.rawfoodexplained.com/introduction-to-fasting/what-the-body-does-when-you-fast.html Retrieved Feb. 3, 2013

5. Shelton, Herbert N.D. *The Science and Fine Art of Fasting* Natl Health Assoc (January 1994) Chapter 5: Autolysis Printed online at http://www.soilandhealth.org/02/0201hyglibcat/020127shelton.iii/020127.ch5.htm Retrieved Feb. 3, 2013

6. Ibid. Chapter 6 *Fasting is not starving.* http://www.soilandhealth.org/02/0201hyglibcat/020127shelton.iii/020127.ch6.htm

7. Ibid, Chapter 7 *Chemical and Organic Changes During Fasting* http://www.soilandhealth.org/02/0201hyglibcat/020127shelton.iii/020127.ch7.htm

8. Ibid.

9. *Effect of fasting on fibrinolysis and blood coagulation.* Miettinen M. Amer J Cardiol 1962;10:532-534 and *Fasting and non-fasting fibrinolytic activity.* Menon, IS. Lab Prac 1967;16:469-470.

10. Shelton, Herbert N.D. *The Science and Fine Art of Fasting* Natl Health Assoc (January 1994) Dr. Herbert Shelton, Fasting Chapter 10. http://www.soilandhealth.org/02/0201hyglibcat/020127shelton.iii/020127.ch10.htm

11. Tilden, John H. *Impaired Health: Its Cause And Cure Vol 2* Health Research, Mokelumne Hill. California Year 1921 http://chestofbooks.com/health/natural-cure/J-H-Tilden/Impaired-Health-Its-Cause-and-Cure-Vol2/ Retrieved Feb. 19, 2013